Tibial Plateau Fractures

Tibial Plateau Fractures

MASON HOHL, MD
Clinical Professor
Department of Orthopaedic Surgery
UCLA School of Medicine
Los Angeles, California

W.B. SAUNDERS COMPANY
A Division of Harcourt Brace & Company
Philadelphia London Toronto Montreal Sydney Tokyo

W.B. SAUNDERS COMPANY
A Division of Harcourt Brace & Company

The Curtis Center
Independence Square West
Philadelphia, Pennsylvania 19106

Library of Congress Cataloging-in-Publication Data

Hohl, Mason
Tibial plateau fractures / Mason Hohl.—1st ed.

p. cm.

Includes bibliographical references and index.

ISBN 0–7216–7015–6

1. Tibia—Fractures. I. Title.

[DNLM: 1. Tibial Fractures. WE 870 H719t 1997]

RD560.H64 1997 617.1′58—dc20

DNLM/DLC 96–9599

TIBIAL PLATEAU FRACTURES ISBN 0–7216–7015–6

Printed in the United States of America.

Last digit is the print number: 9 8 7 6 5 4 3 2 1

To the memory of my beloved wife, Blanche

Preface

This monograph sets forth my approach to the art and science of tibial plateau fractures based on 45 years of experience with the uncertainties, imponderables, and vagaries of these challenging joint injuries. The main purpose of the monograph is to provide fracture surgeons with a concise guide to effective treatment of tibial plateau fractures. Another purpose is to provide in-depth information derived from the study of more than 1533 plateau fractures and the collected wisdom of the more than 1100 authors who have contributed to the literature. The reference list contains as many references as I was able to obtain. Many are annotated in order to assist future researchers in deciding which might warrant their attention. The demographic and statistical information contained in this volume is derived from a large series of plateau fractures collected over many years.

If use of this volume aids the fracture surgeon in improving the care of patients, or if it helps motivate him or her to do clinical or laboratory research on plateau fractures, my task will have been completely worthwhile.

The original stimulus to study plateau fractures came in January 1950 when, as a junior resident, I was looking for a challenging research project. After rounds at Los Angeles County General Hospital with three orthopaedic surgeons, I listened to a discussion of discouraging results so often obtained after treatment of tibial plateau fractures. Nonoperative treatment resulted in deformed but often functional knees, while operative treatment frequently resulted in knee stiffness. This stimulated me to review cases from the hospital and present the results of plateau fracture treatment to the Western Orthopedic Association in 1952 and 1954 and to the American Academy of Orthopaedic Surgeons in 1955. Ever since then this subject has remained my primary research, publication, and teaching interest.

During the early years I was influenced by many astute and skillful surgeons including Paul E. McMaster, Alonzo Neufeld, Samuel Matthews, and J. Vernon Luck. In 1950, Doctor Luck was developing and testing his concepts of "arthrofibrosis." When he learned of my interest in plateau fractures, he designed a research project using primates left over from poliomyelitis viral research. In these controlled experiments, defects were created in the articular cartilage and cortex of both knees to study the effect of immobilization and mobilization on articular healing. The study results definitively established that small full-thickness defects through cartilage and bone heal with a "hyaline-like" cartilage if the knee is allowed to move actively. However, if the knee is immobilized for two months, fibrous pannus envelops the defect, scarring to the fat pad and synovial membrane in the healing process. This study provided a scientific basis for moving joints with articular fractures early.[459]

A major change in data handling occurred with the installation of the first mainframe computer at UCLA Medical Center in the 1960's. Fracture records were put on punch cards for data storage and processing so that complex data analyses became possible. Evolving technology allowed a minicomputer and finally a microcomputer to do much superior analyses with the aid of Revelation software and a Revelation programmer, Blaise Wrenn. Doctor Fred Dorey of the

UCLA Division of Orthopaedic Surgery aided in statistical matters. I am very grateful to them both.

These efforts over so many years were supported by my wife, Blanche, who helped me to tabulate statistics for presentations and articles by spreading case records around the den almost every night. For years of patience and understanding, she has earned her rest.

My daughter Judy spent endless hours reading and editing the manuscript and my son William, orthopedic surgeon and physician, gave valued criticism as well as encouragement. My thanks to both of them. Lewis Reines, President of W.B. Saunders Company, gave me the courage to finish.

MASON HOHL

Contents

CHAPTER 1

Historical Perspectives

In early civilization, treatment of fractures was guided by those who set themselves up as healers. Some were good observers and passed their wisdom on to later generations. The management of fractures thus began. When it became possible to visualize the position of fractures by x-ray, major changes in treatment took place and led to internal fixation and later to rigid fixation of anatomically reduced fractures.

Fractures that involved joints were more easily diagnosed by x-ray, but the methods of treatment employed early in the 20th century largely ignored joint physiology. The scientific basis for treating joint fractures developed much later as the result of clinical observations and later laboratory investigations that defined the healing processes that took place when fractures involved articular surfaces. The principles of treatment of joint fractures that evolved included accurate reduction of articular surfaces with early movement of the joint.

Expectations of outcome after treatment of a fracture have also changed radically over the years as our ability to achieve reduction and fixation has improved. Today, the goal of treatment is to restore strong, stable, well-aligned, and fully moveable extremities; in other words, to restore normally functioning joints. This, of course, proves impossible in the case of most joint fractures but, nonetheless, remains the goal.

This chapter contains a brief overview of many important developments in the diagnosis and treatment of tibial plateau fractures. These developments provide the current scientific basis for treating these fractures.

HISTORY

Tibial plateau fractures have proved to be fascinating therapeutic challenges during nearly 2 centuries of written experience. More than 1100 articles, theses, and books have documented the trials and tribulations of treating these capricious joint fractures. Most developments that have led to our current state of knowledge about articular fractures of the proximal tibia are mentioned in this chapter. There remain many gaps in our knowledge; however, through the diligence and curiosity of future investigators, fracture treatment will doubtless be improved. These future contributors need to be aware of where we have been and how we have arrived at our current state of knowledge.

Early Text Description

Textbooks on fractures written early in the 19th century referred to instability about the knee without a clear description of plateau fracture until Sir Astley Cooper,[195] in his 1825 treatise on fractures, clearly described the fracture as follows:

> *The head of the tibia is sometimes obliquely broken; and if it be fractured into the knee joint the treatment which it*

requires is similar to that which is necessary in the oblique fracture of the condyle of the os femoris; that is, first: The straight position of the limb, because the femur preserves the proper adaptation of the fractured tibia by forming a splint to its upper portion, and keeping the articular surfaces in apposition. Secondly: A roller to press one part of the broken surface against the other. Thirdly: A splint of pasteboard to assist in the preservation of that pressure. And fourthly: Early passive motion to prevent ankylosis.

Cooper's description was accurate despite the lack of x-rays, and his recommendation of early motion remains valid today.

Classification

In 1845, fractures involving the knee joint were separated from nonarticular fractures of the proximal tibia by Bonnet,[101] but an accurate description of a fracture began with the first detailed autopsy by Walther in 1852.[1098] Heydenreich,[439] in a classic 1877 thesis, provided a classification of fractures involving the knee joint based on autopsy specimens from patients who died as the result of injury. At that time such categorization had little practical value since the diagnosis was entirely clinical as determined by the site of leg instability and crepitation. After 1900, when x-rays became commonplace, the diagnosis of fracture and its classification were simplified.

Plateau fractures were described by Barr[51] as either undisplaced or displaced, moderately or severely. The concept of displacement was considered to be important as recently as 1979 by Apley[29] and by many others before. In 1932, Goodwyn considered both displacement and knee stability to be important. Cubbins and associates[219] used the terms minor or major and also described compression and split fracture types. Over the years many have described crush (compression or impression) and split (wedge or cleavage) types. Palmer (1951) used the terms split, compression, and T or Y.[811] Hohl and Luck[459] in 1956 described undisplaced and four types of displaced plateau fractures: (1) local compression, (2) split compression, (3) total condylar depression, and (4) split (see Chapter 3). The AO group simplified the categorization of these fractures to minimally displaced, split, impression, split compression, and bicondylar. MacDonald[651] suggested the use of stability as a treatment criterion in 1961, an idea further developed and used by Rasmussen[873] in his important follow-up study of fractures treated only on the basis of knee instability. Moore observed certain proximal tibial articular fractures that defied standard classification and had poorer results with an increased incidence of vascular and ligament injuries.[723] In 1981, Moore published the concept of fracture-dislocation of the knee with five types in addition to five standard plateau fracture types. Muller and associates published a comprehensive and complex alpha-numeric classification system that encompasses almost every proximal tibial fracture pattern that occurs.[757] In 1993, Tscherne and Lobenhoffer[1058] suggested that some plateau fractures, fracture-dislocations, and comminuted fractures have associated soft tissue injuries that they graded from 0 to 3, depending on their severity.

As future classifications evolve, it is important that these be beneficial to surgeons and researchers who deal with fractures and who attempt to make meaningful comparisons of alternative treatment methods that are sufficiently detailed to include almost every fracture configuration encountered and simple enough to be readily recalled. The particular descriptive terms are less important than are their adoption and universal use.

Closed Treatment

In 1852, Thamhayn provided the first case report describing treatment of plateau fractures. Using leeches and traction, he restored the patient to active life.[1038] Duplay and Merot (1876) performed a knee examination under anesthesia, noting fracture instability, after which they performed closed reduction.[280] Cases reported in about 1860 were treated by massage, splint, cast, or extension (traction) until the knee again stabilized by fracture healing. Wagner wrote of the benefits of using traction in an 1887 case report.[1093]

After the x-ray came into use, treatment objectives became more defined. One of the goals was restoration of joint surfaces. Accomplishment of such reduction by closed means required considerable ingenuity, and the result was that an impressive variety of closed treatment methods were described. Forrester[343] used a C clamp to help reduce and impact plateau fractures and a hinged cast for knee motion. In 1941, a cast with anterior and posterior hinges to control valgus-varus alignment was used successfully by Dobelle.[267] In 1952, Badgley and O'Connor[39] developed a traction apparatus that maintained valgus knee alignment while encouraging knee movement. Fairbank (1954) made a plea for the use of traction treatment and early knee motion.[318] In 1956, Apley reported very successful traction management of plateau fractures.[28] Turner advocated traction treatment based on favorable experience.[1061]

Ilfeld and Hohl (1959) described a method of fracture reduction using heavy traction and compression for displaced and comminuted plateau fractures.[482] Traction of 60 to 70 lb on a fracture table reduced many such fractures quite well. Additional closed manipulation was carried out as needed, and the fracture strongly impacted using a C clamp or Bohler clamp. Reduction was maintained by a traction apparatus that allowed knee movement during fracture healing. Chaix also described the benefits of traction mobilization in the treatment of plateau fractures.[165, 166]

In 1952, Fyshe used the Stader splint as an external fixator.[359] Anderson and Loughlen (1954) did a closed reduction on a fracture table using pins above and below the knee incorporated in a cast to ensure healing in proper alignment.[19] Mooney described cast bracing for plateau fractures.[720, 721] Sarmiento and associates (1977) noted gradual displacement of the medial plateau during closed treatment of bicondylar fractures with an intact fibula.[940] The fibula provided support against distal displacement of the lateral plateau but not the medial plateau. Percutaneous fixation after closed reduction, which has been used for several decades, has recently been championed by Yuan-Zhang and associates[1149] and Duwelius and Connelly.[289]

Open Reduction

Fassbender was given credit by Riedl for performing the first open reduction of a plateau fracture in 1901.[324] Riedl did the second open reduction (1907) in a split-compression type of fracture that he had been unable to reduce by closed manipulation.[892] After opening the fracture, he noted that the depressed articular fragment was holding the fracture apart. He disimpacted and elevated the depressed fragment, after which the split fragment sprang back into position. In 1909, Meerwein reported that Wilms used two nails to hold reduction of a plateau fracture, which was perhaps the first internal fixation of such a fracture.[696] Open reduction using wire or plate was mentioned by Blake (1913), who also noted that missed diagnoses of plateau fracture was leading to liability actions.[87]

Dehelly (1927) used grafts under surgically elevated plateaus after open reduction.[240] Over the years cortical grafts, iliac grafts, and various processed bone and bone substitutes have been used to support depressed joint fracture surfaces.[127, 181, 273, 492, 691, 819, 890] Cotton and Berg described "fender fractures" in

1929 and was an early advocate of open reduction.[204] After a few years, however, he also became discouraged and almost abandoned surgical treatment. The general frustration with open methods of treatment came from problems of fracture exposure and reduction, internal fixation, complications, and postoperative care, all of which contributed to a high incidence of permanently stiff knees.

During the 1930s and 1940s, conservative treatment was believed by most to produce the best functional results. A few surgeons continued to develop materials and techniques for fracture fixation. Webb developed a bolt for condylar compression.[1104] In 1939, Lichtenauer described the use of a wire loop to fix the tibial condyles.[627] The Y incision for visualization of both tibial condyles was described by Schmidt.[958]

In 1952, Jacobs reported the successful use of the patella to substitute for an articular surface after severely depressed fractures.[494, 495] Five years later, Lee described the use of the iliac crest for the same purpose.[601] In 1963, buttress plates were developed by the AO group.

The Swiss A.S.I.F. group deserves great credit for developing exposures, techniques of reduction, internal fixation devices, and postoperative care regimens.[756] Those following these techniques faithfully were compelled to re-evaluate the traditional expectations of results. Instead of aiming for a well-aligned knee that was nearly normal, it rapidly became the goal to restore a normal knee. The use of rigid fracture fixation, restoring articular anatomy, permitted earlier knee motion so that near-normal function began to be possible after open reduction in some plateau fractures. Kuss used plates and screws successfully.[576] In 1968, Schauwecker and Weller described the inframeniscal approach to the tibial plateau.[953] Both Ruedi[913] and Muggler and associates[752] emphasized the need for rigid fixation and early motion of the knee. Olerud developed a comprehensive approach to both condyles in which the tibial tubercle was osteotomized.[792] Tubercle osteotomy and later fixation were improved by Fernandez in 1988.[327]

Beginning slowly in the 1950s and increasing in momentum through the 1960s and 1970s, a wave of enthusiasm for open reduction overtook many fracture surgeons. Published results of rigid fixation showed that those experienced in the use of side plates and cancellous screws and who trusted these devices sufficiently to encourage immediate or early motion of the knee were getting improved results as measured by most criteria. Less experienced surgeons who treated these fractures were noted to have more technical problems in achieving reduction and fixation, and their results were not as good.[950] Although closed treatment methods are used successfully by some surgeons, most surgeons are currently treating more than half of tibial plateau fractures by operative methods.

External Fixation

Percutaneous pins were used to stabilize fractures following closed reduction, and the next step was to develop devices to couple pins together to stabilize fractures.[19] Stader developed one of the early devices. The later devices developed for long bones had problems in maintaining control of articular fragments until small wire half-ring devices were used after closed reduction.[85, 663, 760, 971, 1063] Use of these systems in comminuted fractures is leading to better results because of fewer complications than open reduction and plating techniques.[1063]

Arthroscopic Methods

Reiner (1982) discussed the potential of using the arthroscope for diagnosis after joint fractures.[880] Caspari and associates,[155] Jennings,[604] and Lemon[610] reported good results using arthroscopy as a guide to fracture reduction and percutaneous grafting and fixation. Parisien reported some success in lysis of intra-articular adhesions following knee joint fracture.[814]

Experimental Studies

In 1879, using cadaver knees, Segond experimentally produced tibial plateau fractures as well as ligament injuries.[978] The Segond fracture, a capsular avulsion fracture from the anterolateral upper tibia, was first described by him. Bistolfi (1931) clearly described the mechanism of production of plateau fractures in a classic biomechanical study.[82] In 1929, Hulten, after stressing cadaver knees, concluded that either a plateau fracture or a ligament injury resulted, but not both.[472] An intact collateral ligament was deemed necessary to produce a bony compression fracture. Despite this observation, small numbers of ligament injuries associated with plateau fractures began to be reported.[146, 344, 411, 548]

Haldeman created defects in rabbit joint cartilage and noted that the cartilage lesions did not heal unless the subchondral bone was also injured.[418] Hohl and Luck (1956), using primates, noted that immobilization of knees with a full-thickness cartilage defect into subchondral bone promoted the development of intra-articular adhesions, whereas cage ambulation and free movement produced a smooth, hyaline-like cartilage articular surface.[459] Stumpfegger[1025] found adhesions covering the articular surface and meniscus at an open procedure long after fracture and believed that these were the after-effects of articular fracture. Mitchell and Shepard created fractures in rabbit knees and assessed articular healing after rigid or nonrigid fixation.[713] Kennedy and Bailey, in 1968, using sophisticated laboratory machines with cadaver knees, produced knee fractures that matched some of those seen clinically.[538] Akeson and associates (1984) investigated the weakening and disorganizing effect of immobilization on knee ligaments and provided another argument for more functional management of tibial plateau fractures, possibly even when these fractures were associated with ligament injuries.[9]

Soft Tissue Injuries

Segond, using cadaver knees, either produced fractures or ligament injuries in 1879.[978] Richet, in an autopsy in 1880, discovered a medial plateau fracture associated with rupture of the lateral collateral ligament.[889] Martin (1960) investigated plateau fractures and the diagnosis of ligament injuries in cadaver studies.[679] On the basis of Hulten's work on cadaver knees, it was long believed that plateau fractures and ligament injuries could not coexist.[472] In 1929, Cubbins and associates noted that the meniscus could block fracture reduction.[220] Fowler[345] (1911) described a plateau fracture with knee dislocation, while Jones and Smith[515] (1913) made the point that ligament laxity gives late disability following plateau fractures. Forster and associates (1961) examined consecutive patients with tibial plateau fractures by valgus and varus stress x-rays and noted that 20% had ligament injuries combined with plateau fractures.[344] This study stimulated interest in and awareness of combined ligament and bony injuries. In 1972, Wilppula and Bakalim noted late knee instability due to ligament injury.[1122] Moore and associates found little knee instability in a long-term follow-up of plateau fractures.[727] Hohl and Hopp[457] and Delamarter and associates compared the operative repair of torn ligaments with no repair and concluded that operative repair produced better knee stability.[244]

Diagnosis

Fagerburg used tomography to improve the radiologic diagnosis of plateau fractures and to document fracture displacement and depression with greater accuracy.[316] Moore and Harvey noted that an anteroposterior knee x-ray, taken with 10 degrees of caudal angulation to match the posterior slope of the plateaus ("plateau view"), allowed a more accurate assessment of the depth of depression than a standard anteroposterior view.[725] Computed tomogram technology dramatically increased available imaging information, especially in more comminuted and displaced fractures.[263, 864, 865, 1100] Magnetic resonance imaging (MRI) was noted to reveal fractures that were not evident even with multiple x-ray views.[71, 711] Jensen and associates showed on late follow-up MRI studies that soft tissue fills plateau defects.[508]

Early Knee Movement

In 1825 Cooper recommended early passive movement to prevent ankylosis.[195] Fripp believed that early movement of the knee was important for a good result, regardless of the method of treatment used.[355] Luck developed the concept of traumatic arthrofibrosis to describe fibrous adhesions that developed almost routinely after joint fracture.[646] He believed that this scar tissue was responsible for the often slow and incomplete recovery of motion after joint fractures. Hohl and Luck (1956) reported on the healing of defects made in articular cartilage and cortex of primate knees.[459] If the knee was not allowed to move, a dense core of adhesions developed from the subchondral bone and spread to all the articular structures. If the knee was not immobilized, the defect healed smoothly with fibrocartilage with few adhesions. This experimental study demonstrated conclusively the beneficial effect of knee movement during the early healing of joint articular defects. Apley demonstrated good clinical results using traction while encouraging knee movement.[28] In 1980, Salter and associates described the concept of continuous passive motion (CPM) that has led to the use of CPM machines in the postoperative care of some plateau fractures.[928]

Result Assessment

Much of the confusion about the results of tibial plateau fracture treatment derives from the often inadequate definitions of the case material analyzed and subjective categorization of the quality of result obtained. Too often, dissimilar fractures and displacements with closed or open treatment are compared. It would be refreshing to study only local compression fractures without other fractures or ligament injuries in the same extremity in which the measurable articular depression was between 10 and 12 mm. Those fractures treated by closed means, traction, or cast could then be compared meaningfully with the results of various methods of open reduction. The follow-up evaluation, in terms of varus-valgus deformity, instability, range of movement, knee extension, and the late development of arthritic changes, would then be extremely meaningful. The subjective responses of the patient in terms of pain and ability to use the knee compared with normal need to be factored into the total picture. Furthermore, since many of the objective findings are time related, there needs to be a minimum of 1 year follow-up time.

One of the oldest orthopedic result grading systems used separate anatomic and functional results. Often there was little or no correlation between them. Many other systems, simple and complex, have been used by one or more authors without any system being universally as acceptable as is the Harris Hip Rating, which is a composite and logical system for comparing results. Some acceptable system of this type must be used by future authors. The AO Group is currently promoting a unique system of documentation and reporting of results.[816] Use of such a system would provide readers with a more concise perspective on the quality of results.

In 1970, with these concerns in mind, the author devised, and has since used, a 100-point rating system to assess the results of treatment of tibial plateau fractures.[449] The subjective rating totals 30 points, with pain rated from 0 to 20

Table 1–1. POINT RATING SCALE (100-Point Maximum)

	POINTS
SYMPTOMATIC (Maximum of 30 points)	
Pain (maximum of 20 points)	
None	20
Barometric	18
After hard use	16
Limits use	14
Painful walking	10
Limits walking	5
Rest pain	0
Activity (maximum of 5 points)	
Unlimited	5
Minimal limitation	4
Limited sports	3
Limited walking	2
Cane needed	0
Patient assessment (5 points)	
Normal knee	5
Near normal	4
Good	3
Fair	2
Poor	1
FUNCTIONAL (Maximum of 45 points)	
Knee motion (maximum of 30 points)	
More than 135 degrees	30
120–134 degrees	26
105–119 degrees	23
90–104 degrees	20
75–90 degrees	15
60–74 degrees	10
Less than 60 degrees	0
Lack of extension (10 points)	
Full extension	10
Lacks 1–5 degrees	5
Lacks 6–10 degrees	2
Lacks more than 10	0
Crepitus (5 points)	
No crepitus	5
Fine crepitus	4
Coarse crepitus	3
Constant crepitus	1
Locking	0
ANATOMIC (Maximum 25 points)	
Deformity (10 points)	
No deformity	10
5 degrees	8
10 degrees	5
15 degrees	2
20 or more degrees	0
Instability (10 points)	
No Instability	10
5 degrees	8
10 degrees	5
15 degrees	2
20 or more degrees	0
Arthritis (5 points)	
No arthritic changes	5
Minimal changes	4
Moderate changes	2
Severe changes	0

points, activity level rated from 0 to 5 points, and the patient's assessment rated from 0 to 5 points. Arbitrarily in this rating, knee movement is rated from 0 to 30 points; full knee extension is rated from 0 to 10 points; and lack of crepitus is rated from 0 to 5 points. These 45 points relate to knee function. The anatomic rating considers knee alignment and stability of 0 to 10 points each and absence of arthritic change by x-ray as 0 to 5 points. The practical value of such a rating is that any specific fracture type or treatment can be evaluated with a single composite numeric result. It would not be possible to have a good result with knee fusion or with any major anatomic or functional impairment. Excellent results are between 91 and 100 points. These results are essentially for normal knees for practical purposes with no significant pain or functional impairment. Results between 81 and 90 points are good results that satisfy the majority of patients and restore them to activity. These patients often lack complete knee extension or full flexion, and their knees may be slightly malaligned or unstable and mildly painful at times. As a rule, the activity level of such patients is mildly impaired. Fair results are rated between 71 and 80 points, where the patient and the physician recognize that the knee is fairly functional but has limited use (Table 1–1).

There will be references in this volume to point rating results for various groups of fracture types and displacements. Use of point ratings puts results in a simple numeric format for purposes of easy comparison between methods of treatment. A sharper focus on one aspect of the result can be obtained by using only the anatomic, functional, or subjective ratings. Also elements of the point rating, such as pain, range of movement, stability, or arthritis, can be compared.

THE FUTURE

It is never easy to predict future developments, but it appears that increasing availability of excellent techniques and devices for fracture fixation and rising patient expectations to obtain a normal knee after often catastrophic injury are leading to a greater dependence on open treatment methods. Economic forces dictate fewer hospital days and also favor the use of surgery rather than traction.

History, hopefully, will never let us forget the efforts and learning curves of so many investigators who have brought the art and science of treating plateau fractures to its current status. Nevertheless, there is much yet to be contributed in the basic and clinical science of managing patients with tibial plateau fractures.

CHAPTER 2

Diagnosis of Plateau Fractures

The extent of soft tissue and bone injury must be accurately ascertained in order to formulate an optimal treatment program for each tibial plateau fracture.[458, 1058] To obtain this information, a thorough physical examination and imaging study of the injured knee are required. The ultimate selection of treatment takes into account the type and the extent of soft tissue and bone damage, the future needs of the patient, and the risks, benefits, and known results of the various therapeutic options.

PHYSICAL EXAMINATION

The patient with a tibial plateau fracture often presents in an emergency room after having sustained a knee injury from a motor vehicle accident or other cause (Table 2–1).

The knee is inspected for skin condition, swelling, and deformity. Abrasions and open wounds are carefully evaluated, because their presence affects the timing and the type of definitive treatment that can be employed. The knee is often diffusely swollen and tender. Areas of tenderness are usually adjacent to the fracture or overlying the site of ligament injury. Knee alignment is compared with the uninjured knee. Valgus deformity is observed most frequently, but varus deformity, recurvatum, or procurvatum can occur depending on the fracture configuration.

Table 2–1. MECHANISM OF INJURY IN 1406 TIBIAL PLATEAU FRACTURES

	FRACTURE TYPES							
Mechanism of Injury	**MD**	**LC**	**SC**	**TO**	**SP**	**RIM**	**BIC**	**Total**
Automobile-pedestrian	142	172	100	79	8	44	53	598
Automobile versus automobile	41	40	19	22	7	8	33	170
Slip and fall	28	55	39	25	5	1	15	168
Fall from a height	33	68	44	35	9	3	32	224
Motorcycle	26	21	27	16	8	6	27	131
Athletics	9	14	10	4	1	3	4	45
Automobile versus bicycle	3	1	3	0	1	0	2	10
Direct blow	1	5	4	2	0	0	2	14
Miscellaneous	15	14	6	3	2	1	5	46
Totals	298	390	252	186	41	66	173	1406

MD = Minimally displaced; LC = Local compression; SC = Split compression; TO = Total depression; SP = Split fracture; RIM = Rim fracture; BIC = Bicondylar fracture.

Arterial circulation to the lower leg and foot must be evaluated at an early stage by palpation of arterial pulses about the ankle and foot. If arterial compromise is suspected, arteriography is performed immediately and appropriate management is instituted.[801] Compartment syndrome is uncommon but occurs sufficiently often that it must be considered, especially in more comminuted fractures.[23, 393] Thus, the anterior, peroneal, and posterior compartments of the leg should be examined for unusual tension. If there is increased leg pain or tension, compartment pressures should be measured. An increasing or high compartment pressure mandates that a fasciotomy be carried out promptly.

Peroneal nerve function should be tested and documented prior to treatment by noting the ability of the patient to feel sensation on the dorsum of the foot and to extend the foot and toes.[68, 764, 1058]

The knee should be palpated for areas of tenderness along joint lines, condyles, and ligament attachment sites (Fig. 2–1). In lateral plateau fractures, for instance, it is important to know whether there is tenderness over any portion of the medial collateral ligament that could indicate injury.[457]

Knee stability should be assessed in every injured knee, except those with a bicondylar fracture or with tibial or femoral fractures. It is often possible soon after fracture to test stability by applying valgus and varus stresses to the knee without using sedation or anesthesia.[68, 344, 458, 873, 911] Apprehensive patients or those in much pain can be adequately stress tested after a hemarthrosis is aspirated and some lidocaine is left in the joint. The stability of the uninjured knee should first be tested to provide a standard by which to judge the stability of the injured knee.[457, 724, 727] The technique is to apply valgus and then varus forces slowly, first in extension and subsequently in a few degrees of flexion, noting the angular deviation and endpoint, compared with the normal knee (see Fig. 2–2*A*, *B*). Since instability may persist unless it is corrected, this test provides a useful way to predict the need for operative reduction.[873]

Cineradiographic studies made by the author during stress testing frequently demonstrated additional fracture displacement, with the fragments springing back into the pre-stress position upon removal of the deforming force.[458] No harm to the knee is known to have resulted from stress testing and would be unlikely to occur when the magnitude of these applied forces is compared with the forces that originally caused the plateau fracture.

Documentation of valgus and varus stress testing by x-ray recreates the mechanism of injury and indicates graphically whether the collateral ligament is intact.[344] Abnormal widening of the cartilage space is diagnostic of collateral ligament rupture[679] (Fig. 2–3).

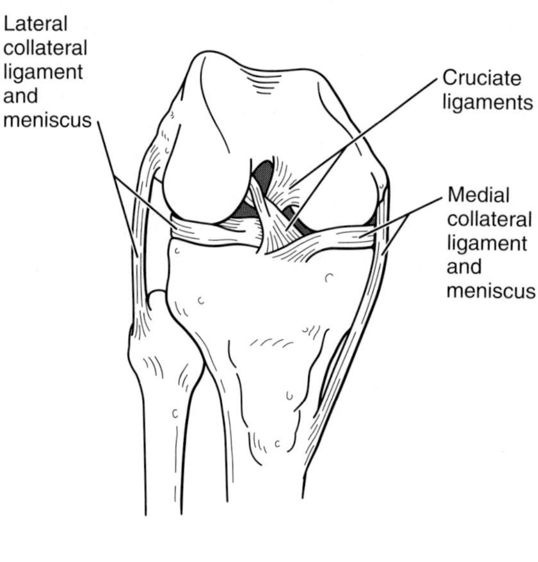

Figure 2–1. Drawing of an outline of a knee with collateral ligaments shown.

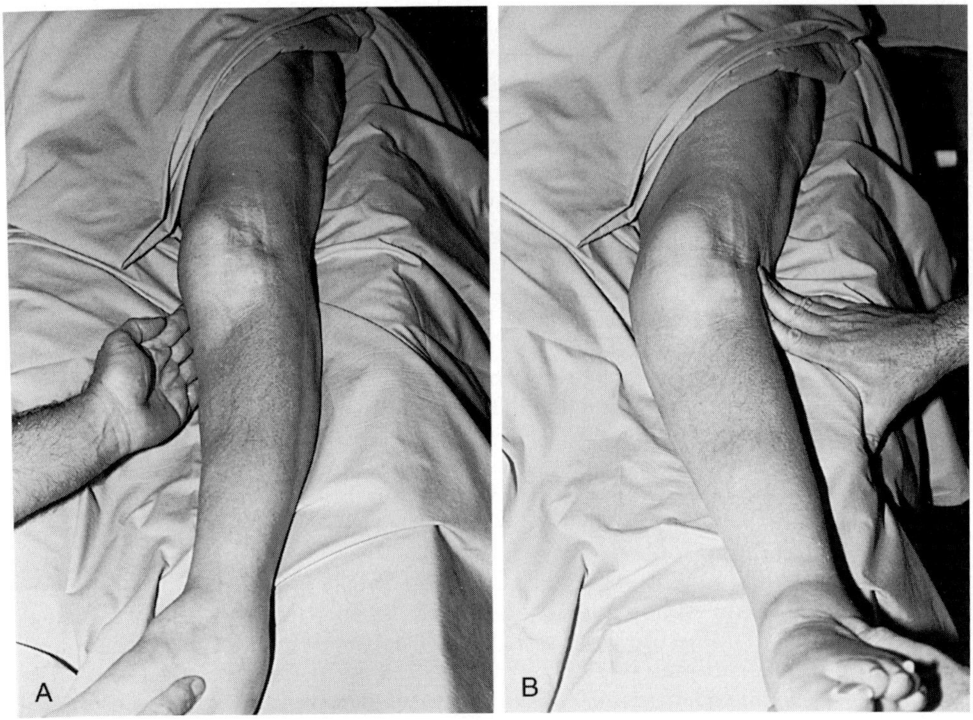

Figure 2–2. *A*, Left knee with a lateral tibial plateau depressed fracture. Note the knee swelling. *B*, Valgus stress testing in a lateral plateau fracture. Note the valgus deformity compared with *A*.

IMAGING TECHNIQUES

X-ray evaluation provides information about the type of fracture, the degree of displacement, and the quality of bone. In many plateau fractures, anteroposterior and lateral views provide insufficient information for determination of an optimal treatment plan.[185, 533, 778, 805, 846, 1100] Additional x-ray views need to be considered. Oblique projections give information about the location of fracture

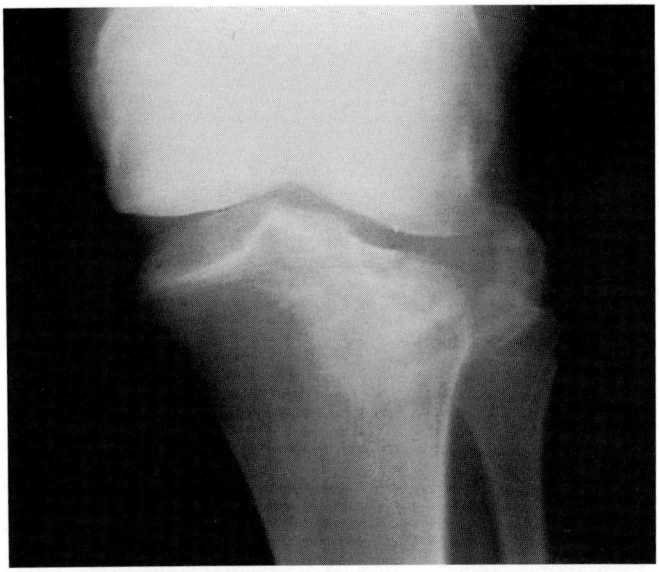

Figure 2–3. Stress x-ray of a local compression plateau fracture. Note the medial joint space widening.

lines and depressed areas. The amount of plateau depression and displacement is important to determine, although the exact number of millimeters of depression does not necessarily provide an indication for or against operative treatment. The plateau view of Moore,[725] taken with a caudal tube angulation of 10 degrees to match the normal posterior slope of the plateau, gives more accurate measurements than does a standard anteroposterior view (Fig. 2–4).

Today, however, most surgeons prefer tomograms or computed tomograms for compression-type fractures or those in which the degree and the direction of displacement are unclear.[263, 302, 316, 431, 770, 844, 864, 957, 1100] With these studies accurate measurement of depression and displacement can be made.

Anteroposterior and lateral tomograms provide sharp images of depressed articular fragments.[302, 316] Unfortunately, such studies are becoming less available, and computed tomography (CT) scans seem to be taking their place.[263, 864]

Computerized axial tomography is capable of providing an image of the proximal tibia in several reconstructed planes.[151, 263, 864] These images graphically demonstrate fracture lines and the direction and degree of fragment displacement (Fig. 2–5). CT scans are valuable in any displaced plateau fracture but are most useful in bicondylar fractures and should be used as a preoperative planning tool.

Magnetic resonance imaging (MRI) is not useful in the same way that the CT scan is; however, it demonstrates fracture lines or bone bruises and is helpful in making the diagnosis of a fracture when fracture lines are not evident in conventional x-rays.[71, 711] Suspected local compression fractures and minimally displaced fractures often show up clearly in MRI studies (Fig. 2–6). Although exact fracture displacement is not so clearly evident in these studies, cruciate, collateral, and meniscal injuries accompanying plateau fractures are well visualized.[2]

Collateral ligament injuries may often be diagnosed or at least strongly suspected by findings present in conventional x-rays.[242, 244, 457] The initial anteroposterior view may suggest or show cartilage space widening (Fig. 2–7), avulsion

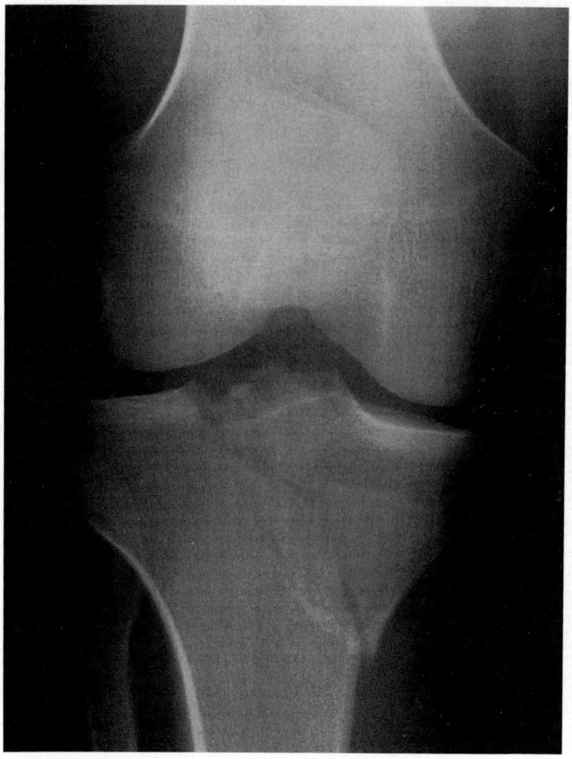

Figure 2–4. Total depression fracture of the medial condyle. Each plateau is clearly seen without superimposition of the anterior and posterior articular margins.

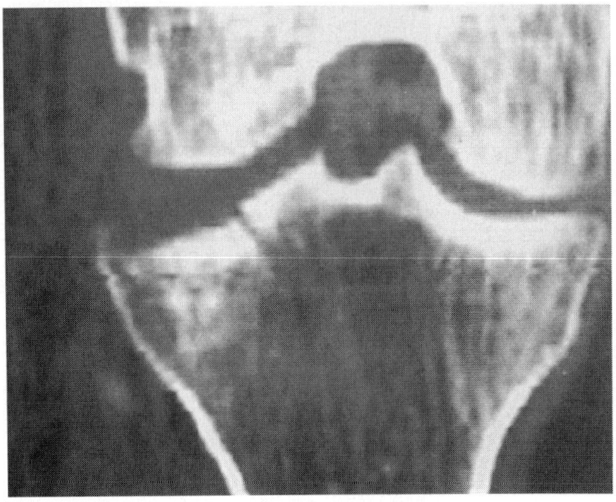

Figure 2–5. Computed tomography scan of a local compression fracture from an anteroposterior view.

of tibial spines, or a plateau rim avulsion, any one of which is sufficient to diagnose a coexisting injury to knee ligaments.[244, 457] Such findings were noted in 15% of proximal tibial articular fractures in the author's series and suggested the correct diagnosis in 77% of all confirmed ligament injuries.[244] The actual amount of knee instability is documented by stress x-rays (see Fig. 2–3).[68, 244, 344]

ARTHROGRAPHY

Arthrography is rarely used with the freshly fractured knee. As noted previously, however, fracture depressions can be visualized using arthrography and, occasionally, torn menisci diagnosed.[18, 715] Today, arthroscopic visualization of the knee has superceded arthrography.

ARTHROSCOPIC EXAMINATION

Advocates of the use of diagnostic arthroscopy before definitive treatment of plateau fractures argue that the status of intra-articular structures can best be evaluated by this means, and fragments of bone and cartilage that are free in the joint can be removed.[1072] The author advocates arthroscopy for intra-articular diagnosis in selected plateau fractures. These fractures include those in which

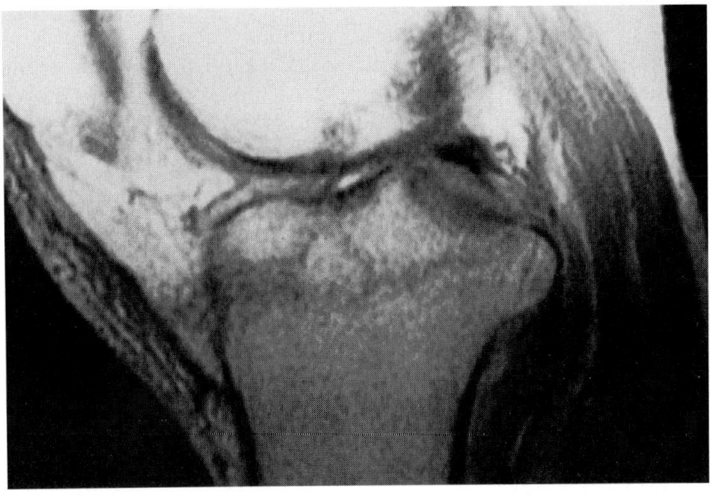

Figure 2–6. Lateral magnetic resonance image of a minimally displaced fracture that is barely visible by x-ray.

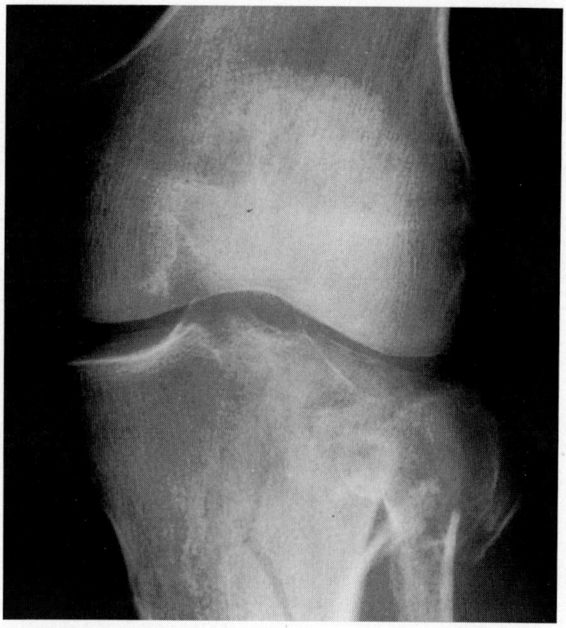

Figure 2–7. Anteroposterior x-ray of a split compression fracture. Note the suggestion of medial cartilage space widening.

there are loose fragments or a suspected torn meniscus, or those in which the fracture may be reduced and fixed percutaneously or treated by arthroscopic-assisted reduction.[68, 155, 346, 404, 423, 456, 466–468, 491, 492, 504, 835, 880, 881]

If an arthroscopic examination is to be done, a midline patellar tendon or a parapatellar port on the side opposite the fracture is created to avoid the necessity of subsequently performing open reduction in the area of this portal. As a rule, both compartments can be adequately visualized from one portal. Hemarthrosis and clots are washed from the knee, allowing an assessment to be made of the state of both menisci, cruciate ligaments, and articular surfaces. It is important to perform the examination expeditiously to avoid an accumulation of irrigation fluid in the tissues if subsequent open reduction is to follow.

In the next few years the role of arthroscopy in the diagnosis and treatment of plateau fractures will become more clearly defined, but to date arthroscopy has proved helpful in the management of many patients.[346, 404, 423, 468]

SUMMARY

The diagnosis of tibial plateau fractures requires a physical examination for soft tissue problems and imaging studies to determine the exact nature and extent of damage to articular surfaces and to the proximal tibia. Only following such a complete evaluation can the optimal treatment be planned to provide the best opportunity for recovery from the injury.

CHAPTER 3

Classification of Proximal Tibial Articular Fractures

At least 50 morphologically different fracture patterns involve the proximal tibial articular surface. Although surgeons have used a variety of methods to group these fractures, the ideal classification has not yet evolved.[77, 112, 179, 219, 228, 278, 363, 448, 458, 459, 464, 465, 471, 475, 757, 811, 947, 950, 965, 1000, 1058] A classification should be simple enough for clinical application and at the same time sufficiently detailed for investigators to accurately communicate their experience in the treatment of a particular fracture configuration.[986] The more sophisticated treatment becomes, the more important it is to utilize such a classification. If all those who publish their treatment results would use a uniform classification, rapid progress in the development of optimal treatment protocols could be anticipated. The author's classification, described in this chapter, and the older AO classification with the Schatzker modification have been used successfully for many years and have aided communication among investigators.[448, 458, 459, 756, 950] The newer AO alphanumeric classification system is being used increasingly but thus far has proved somewhat too detailed for most to apply.[757] The author believes that in the next few years a universally usable system will evolve.[986]

One reason for a classification is to simplify selection of the best treatment method for a particular fracture. Another reason is to allow clinical investigators to make meaningful comparisons of results obtained in the treatment of similar fracture patterns. These two reasons justify the adoption of some universally acceptable classification. To put classifications into perspective, it is important to briefly review how they developed.

Background

Fractures involving the knee joint were distinguished from nonarticular fractures of the proximal tibia by Bonnet in 1845.[101] Accurate morphologic description of plateau fractures began with the first detailed autopsy by Walther in 1852.[1098] Heydenreich,[439] in his classic 1877 thesis, provided a classification of fractures involving the knee joint based on autopsy specimens from patients who had died from their injuries. His categorization had little practical value in those early times since diagnosis was entirely clinical as determined by the site of leg instability and crepitation. After 1900, when x-rays became common, accurate diagnosis and such fracture classification were applicable.

Plateau fractures were described by Barr in 1940 as either undisplaced or displaced, moderately or severely.[51] The concept of displacement was considered important as recently as 1979 by Apley[29] and by many others before him. In 1932, Goodwyn considered both displacement and knee stability important.[385] Cubbins and associates used the terms minor and major and also described compression and split-fracture types.[219] Over the years many authors have described crush (compression or impression) and split (wedge or cleavage) types.[112]

Palmer (1951) used the terms split, compression, and T or Y.[811] In 1956, Hohl and Luck,[459] on the basis of 700 fractures, described undisplaced fractures and four types of displaced plateau fractures: compression (local and split), total and split (Fig. 3–1). The AO group[756] simplified the categorization of these fractures into minimally displaced, split, impression, split-compression, and bicondylar. Schatzker added subcondylar fractures to the AO classification.[947] MacDonald[651] suggested the use of stability as a treatment criterion in 1961, an idea further developed and used by Rasmussen[873] in his important follow-up study of fractures wherein treatment was based solely on the presence or absence of knee instability. Moore observed certain proximal tibial articular fractures that defied standard classification and had poorer results because of a high incidence of vascular and ligament injuries.[723] In 1981, he described the concept of fracture-dislocation of the knee with five types in addition to standard plateau fractures. In 1993 Tscherne and Lobenhoffer separated fractures into plateau, fracture-dislocation, and comminuted.[1058]

Current Classifications

In recently used classifications, fractures involve either one or both condyles and are either minimally displaced or displaced. Some have used the terms minor or major to denote degree of fracture displacement.[724] Several fracture types were produced experimentally by Kennedy and Bailey in a laboratory study (1968), but they were unable to produce all of the configurations observed clinically.[538] They showed that the application of abduction force produced split, total, and rim fractures. Axially applied forces caused compression or impression fractures. Combinations of axial loading and valgus forces produced split-compression fractures. Explosively applied axial forces often produced bicondylar fractures.

Moore[723] used Hohl's 1967 classification (Fig. 3–2) until, in 1981, he developed the concept of fracture-dislocation of the knee to classify approximately 10% of fractures that he observed were associated with a higher incidence of soft tissue injuries (nerve, vascular, or ligament) than had been noted in other plateau fractures. He retained minimally displaced, local and split-compression, total and bicondylar fractures as plateau fractures and placed split, entire plateau, rim avulsion, rim compression, and four-part fractures into his fracture-dislocation types (Fig. 3–3).

Schatzker[947] modified the AO classification by adding subcondylar fracture as a separate type (Fig. 3–4). The AO group perceived the need for a comprehensive classification of all fractures and produced an alphanumeric system that

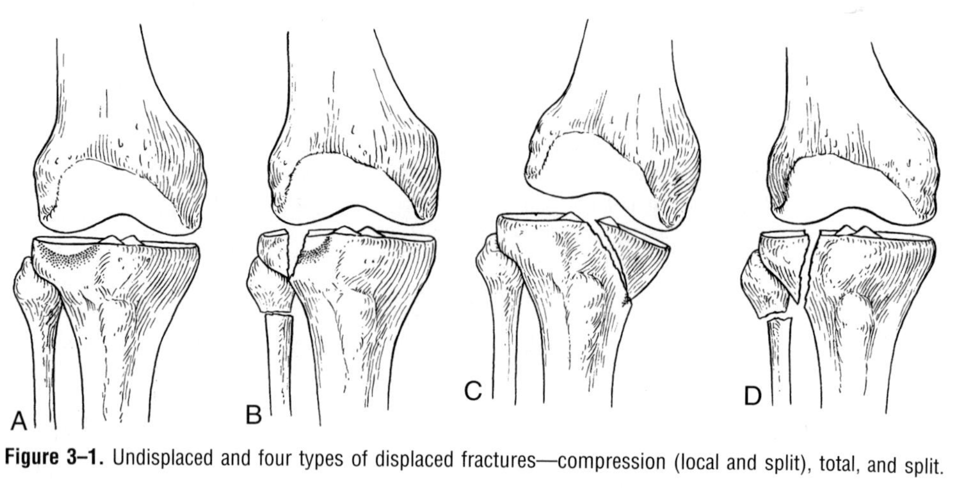

Figure 3–1. Undisplaced and four types of displaced fractures—compression (local and split), total, and split.

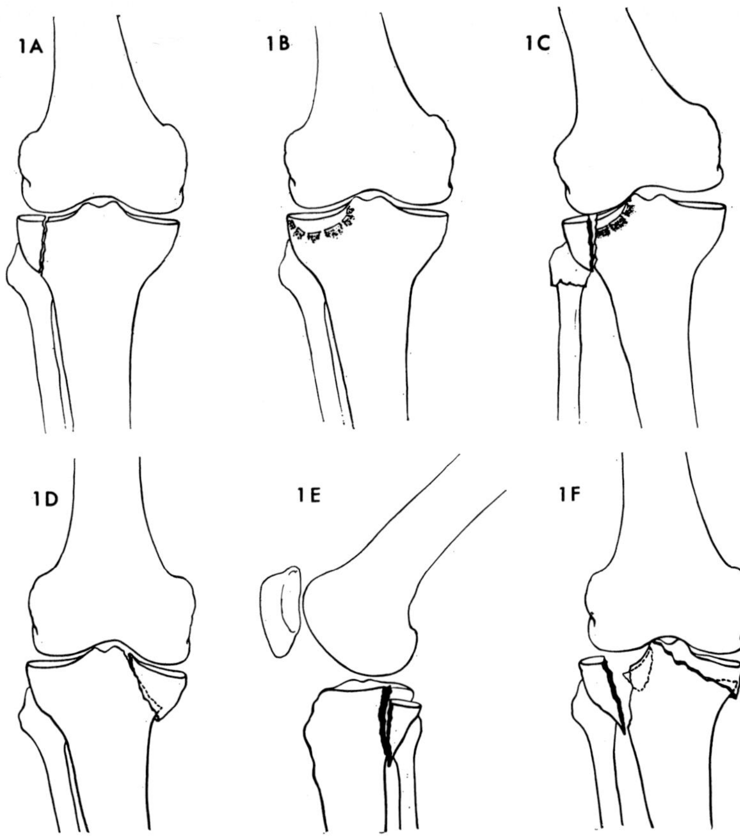

Figure 3–2. Hohl's 1967 plateau fracture classification. (From J. Bone Joint Surg., 49A: 1456, 1967.)

includes the bone, the region of the bone, the severity of the fracture, and its morphology.[757] Although at first difficult to understand and to apply, it has the advantage of accommodating most observed proximal tibial articular fractures (Fig. 3–5).

Today, the most commonly used classifications are the AO, the Schatzker modification, the Hohl and Luck (1956), and the Hohl (1967).

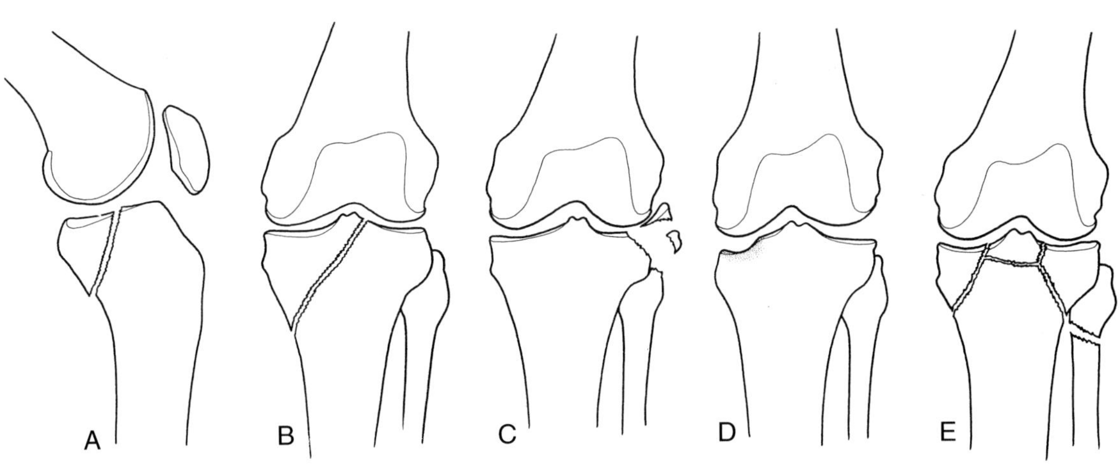

Figure 3–3. Moore's 1981 classification of fracture-dislocations of the knee. *A*, Split fracture; *B*, Entire plateau fracture; *C*, Rim avulsion; *D*, Rim compression; *E*, Four-part fracture. (From Fractures of the tibial plateaus. *In* Evarts, C. M. (Ed.): Surgery of the Musculoskeletal System. New York, Churchill Livingstone, 1990.

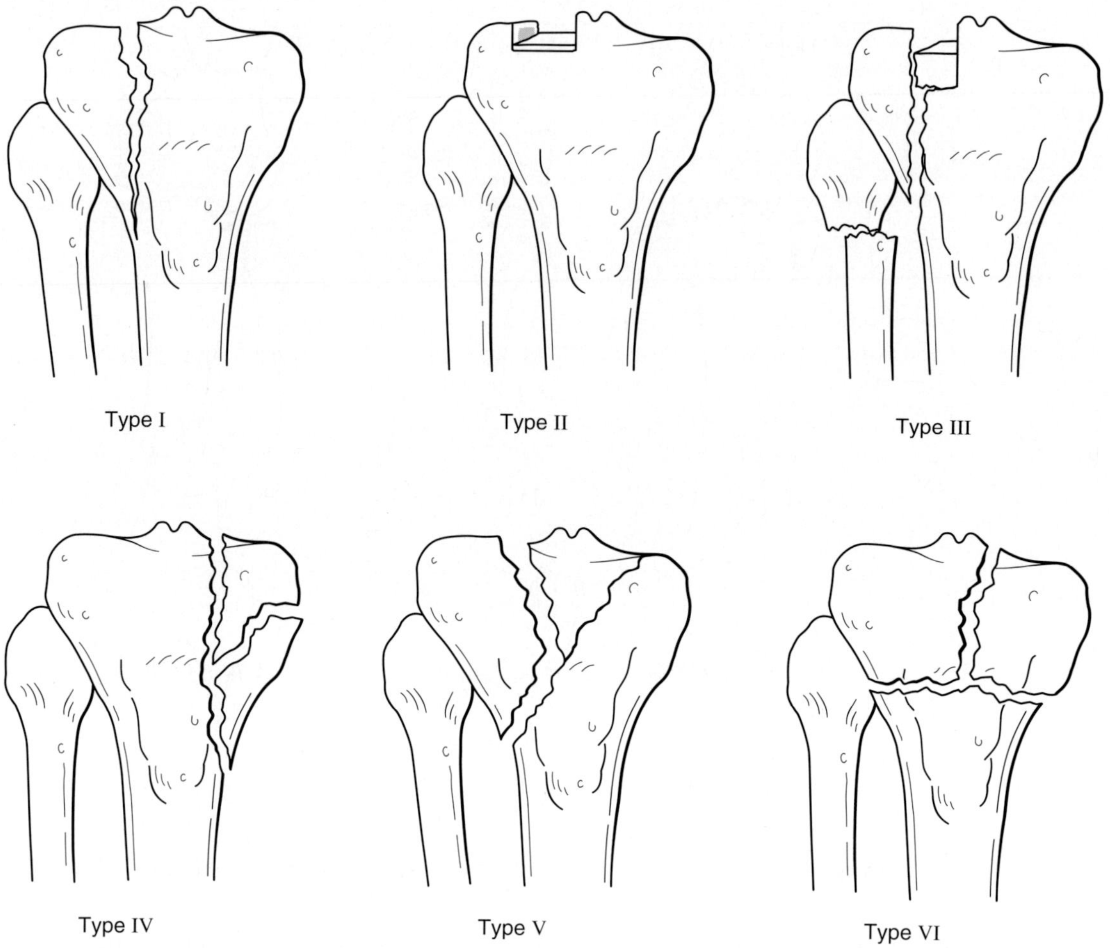

Figure 3–4. Schatzker's classification. (From Tile, M., and Schatzker, J.: The Rationale of Operative Fracture Treatment: Fractures of the Tibial Plateau. New York, Springer-Verlag, 1996, pp. 280–285.)

Author's Classification

The favorable clinical results observed after treatment of minimally displaced fractures (regardless of fracture configuration) indicated the desirability of making these a separate type.[77, 459] A minimally displaced fracture, as defined by the author, has less than 4 mm of displacement or depression as measured on x-rays or imaging studies. Displaced fractures, those with 4 mm or more displacement, are separated into six types by their morphologic characteristics (Fig. 3–6).

MINIMALLY DISPLACED FRACTURES

The concept of minimal displacement takes into account the known thickness of articular cartilage, 4 mm on the lateral plateau and 2 to 3 mm on the medial.[695, 728] The healing process in articular cartilage has seemed clinically to accommodate displacement within these ranges. Twenty-two percent of the author's series of 1533 proximal tibial articular fractures are minimally displaced.

DISPLACED FRACTURES

Fractures with depression or displacement of 4 mm or more comprise 78% of tibial plateau fractures in the author's series. These fractures are subdivided into the following six distinct types.

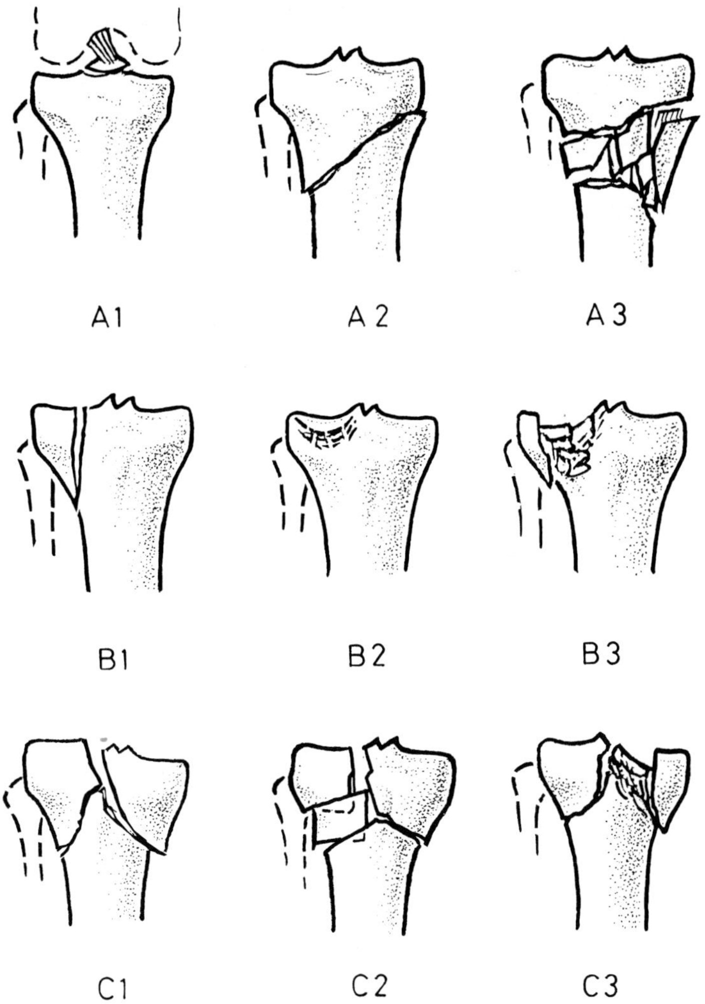

Figure 3–5. AO group's numerical classification. (From Mueller, M., et al: Classification of Fractures. Berlin, Springer-Verlag, 1990, p. 15.)

Local Compression

Local compression fractures are impression or compression fractures in which a part of the weight-bearing articular cortex and subchondral bone, usually of the lateral tibial plateau, is fractured and depressed by valgus and compression forces applied through the femoral condyle. The anteroposterior location of the depressed articular surface varies depending on the knee flexion angle at the moment of injury. Local compression fractures account for more than one third of displaced fractures.

A small vertical split fracture of the plateau margin may cause confusion as to whether the fracture should be classified as a local or a split compression fracture. If the fragment does not have sufficient articular surface (usually less than 1 cm width) to support the femoral condyle, the fracture is classified as a local compression fracture.

Split Compression

A split compression fracture occurs with valgus and compression forces. The impact of the femoral condyle initially splits off an articular fragment, and

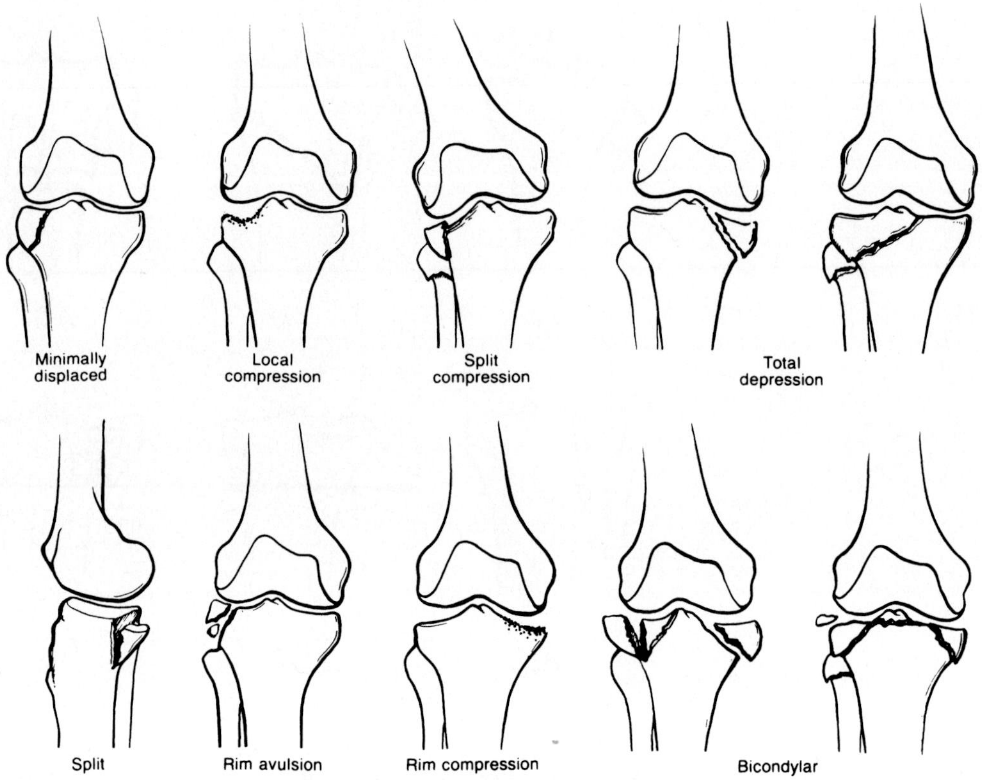

Figure 3–6. Hohl's 1991 classification. (From Tibial plateau fractures. *In* Rockwood, C. A., Green, D. A., and Bucholz, R. W. (Eds.): Fractures. Philadelphia, J. B. Lippincott, 1991.)

the continuing force pushes some of the remaining articular surface into the proximal tibia.[538] The split fragment usually has 1 cm or more articular surface that, when reduced and fixed to the proximal tibia, maintains knee alignment regardless of whether the depressed area of articular surface has been reduced. Split compression fractures comprise 23% of displaced fractures.

Total Depression

A total depression fracture is an oblique fracture extending through the upper tibia from or near the tibial spines to the cortex on the same or the opposite tibial condyle. Moore[723] divided these fractures into total or entire condyle fractures depending on whether the fragment includes the tibial spines. I recombined them, however, because both variations were observed to behave similarly in treatment and results. These fractures involve either medial or lateral condyle and constitute 17% of displaced fractures. Note that the fractured condyle is depressed as a whole, so there is little articular damage.

Split

A split fracture usually involves the medial condyle with a major articular fragment split from its posterior aspect in the *coronal* plane. Less commonly, the anterior portion of either condyle is involved. The fracture is identified in an anteroposterior x-ray view by the characteristic double-horizon appearance of the fractured plateau (Fig. 3–7). A lateral view demonstrates the size and distal displacement of the fracture fragment. This type of fracture should not be confused with the split or wedge fracture mentioned in other classifications,

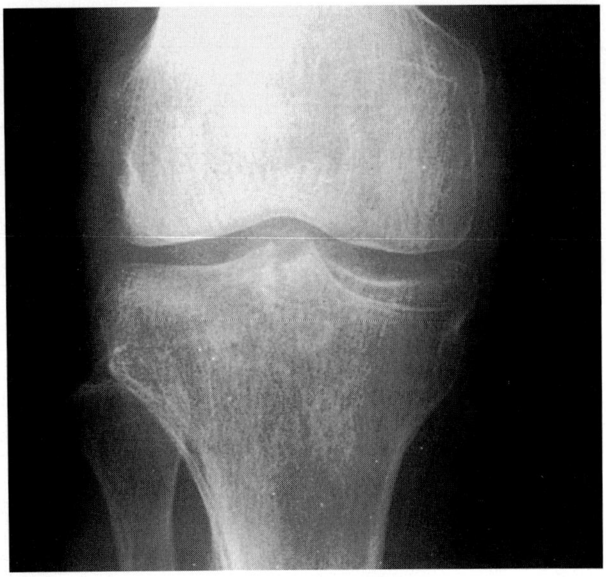

Figure 3–7. Anteroposterior split fracture. Note the double horizon appearance of the medial plateau.

which is a *sagittal* plane fracture of either plateau.[110, 937] Although only 3% of displaced plateau fractures are in this category, their uniqueness and management difficulties set them apart.

Rim Fracture–Dislocations

Rim avulsion and rim compression fracture–dislocations are characterized by either an avulsion or compression fracture of the margin of the tibial plateau. Six percent of displaced plateau fractures are rim fractures. Rim avulsion fractures displace proximally because of capsular attachments to the fragment. The collateral ligament on the side of the avulsion is also stretched or torn. Valgus or varus stress x-rays of the knee reproduce the mechanism of injury and demonstrate widening of the cartilage space on the side of the avulsion and may temporarily further displace the avulsed fragment. Rim compression fractures are caused by impact of the femoral condyle on the margin of the plateau. Such an injury cannot occur until the contralateral collateral ligament has been torn or stretched (Fig. 3–8). Rim compression fractures are associated occasionally with a rim avulsion fracture of the opposite condyle.

Bicondylar Fracture

Bicondylar fractures involve both tibial plateaus, often with comminution, and in a wide variety of fracture configurations. Fifteen percent of displaced fractures are bicondylar fractures.

Schatzker added another group of bicondylar fractures with a coexisting subcondylar fracture.[949] The author has chosen to consider subcondylar fractures as fractures associated with the plateau fracture, like the tibial shaft, patellar, or femoral fractures (see Chapter 14).

SUMMARY

Most tibial plateau fractures seen clinically are similar to one of the fracture types described earlier. It is important for the fracture surgeon to recognize the x-ray appearance of each type in order to consider the particular treatment

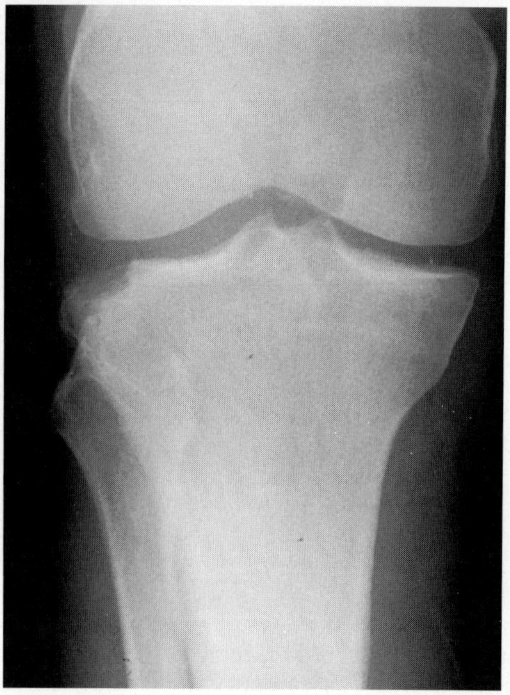

Figure 3–8. Rim compression fracture of the lateral plateau.

options for that fracture type and select the best treatment for the patient. Those who analyze their results should make every effort to classify their fractures in such a manner that others can properly and accurately use the data for comparison purposes.

CHAPTER 4

Soft Tissue Injuries and Plateau Fractures

Fractures of the tibial plateau are frequently accompanied by injuries to vascular structures, nerves, skin, menisci, and ligaments. Bennett and Browner found that more than half of 30 plateau fractures studied prospectively had soft tissue injuries.[68] If left untreated, such injuries often cause permanent impairment of leg function even with a fracture healed in anatomic position. Early diagnosis and treatment of both bony and soft tissue injuries should increase the number of good and excellent results.

VASCULAR INJURIES

Two serious vascular injuries seen after plateau fracture are popliteal artery laceration and compartment syndrome. Both injuries occur more frequently after bicondylar fractures or plateau fractures with coexisting subcondylar fractures.[728, 801] There were 14 arterial injuries and eight compartment syndromes in the author's series.

Arterial Injuries

The possibility of arterial injury should always be considered, especially in comminuted and displaced fractures.[728] Even if foot pulses are initially normal, arterial obstruction can still occur within the first few days of injury. Thus circulatory status should be monitored carefully for several days after an injury. If there is any doubt about the adequacy of circulation, arteriography and vascular consultation should be obtained without delay (Fig. 4–1). An arterial occlusion after a tibial plateau fracture may be partial or complete and is frequently located near the trifurcation of the popliteal artery.

Occlusion of the popliteal artery is a surgical emergency, and circulation must be re-established prior to definitive treatment of the plateau fracture. It is advisable to accomplish arterial repair and fracture fixation during the same procedure since a return to surgery a second time may for one reason or the other become impossible or may be inadvisable. Rigid fracture fixation should be used whenever possible. Prophylactic calf fasciotomies to prevent compartment syndrome should be considered after arterial injury.

Arterial repair is not always successful in restoring complete circulation, and amputation is a possibility. Careful monitoring of pulses and venous return is important during the first few weeks after repair.

Compartment Syndrome

Compartment syndrome produces a different type of pain than does a tibial plateau fracture. The character of the pain is a persistent, deep boring ache and

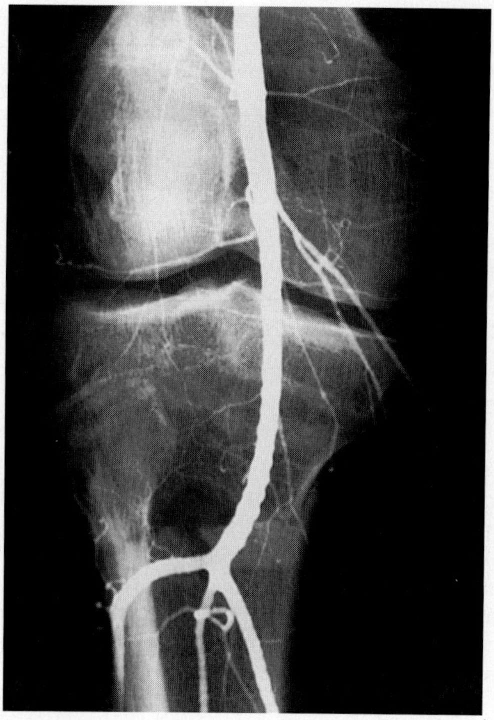

Figure 4–1. Tibial plateau fracture with a normal arteriogram.

numb feeling in the leg and foot that tends to increase slowly after injury and occurs without limb movement. Immobilization of the limb controls pain at the fracture site but does not control pain from compartment pressure. The pain, usually located distal to the area of fracture, is most frequently over or within the anterior compartment of the leg. As hours pass, the pain stabilizes and hypesthesia in the leg and foot becomes more pronounced. Ultimately, muscle necrosis takes place in the affected compartments and then no treatment is effective.

If compartment syndrome is suspected, all circular bandages should be removed and the leg should be examined. If compartment syndrome is impending, the affected compartments will be tender to touch and feel tight. Symptoms and findings that suggest increased compartment pressure indicate the need to measure compartment pressures. Accurate measurements can be made by using one of the catheter techniques. If the pressures measured are within normal range, they should be rechecked after a few hours to ascertain the trend. Clinical findings involving increasing pressures or high pressures mean that a fasciotomy should be performed without delay to relieve the compartment syndrome.[23, 393] The finding of pink contractile muscle at fasciotomy is a good prognostic sign, but pale nonreactive muscle is already partially or completely necrotic. The results of an early fasciotomy are generally good, but over the hours of delayed diagnosis and treatment results rapidly deteriorate.

LIGAMENT INJURIES

Ligament injuries occur in 10 to 33% of proximal tibial articular fractures[2, 68, 242, 243, 344, 457, 553, 556, 879, 903, 1010, 1058, 1122] (Table 4–1).

The incidence of ligament injuries in rim compression and rim avulsion fracture types theoretically should approach 100%, because lengthening or tearing of capsular and collateral ligaments is required for these fractures to occur.

Many ligament injuries occur as avulsions of bony ligament attachments,

Table 4–1. FRACTURE TYPES AND LIGAMENT INJURIES IN THE AUTHOR'S SERIES

	FRACTURE TYPES (N = 1500)							
LIGAMENT STATUS	**MD**	**LC**	**SC**	**TO**	**SP**	**RIM**	**BIC**	**Total**
Ligament injury	29	51	52	59	13	39	25	268
Percent injury	7%	12%	19%	30%	28%	54%	14%	18%

MD = Minimally displaced; LC = Local compression; SC = Split compression; TO = Total depression; SP = Split fracture; RIM = Rim fracture; BIC = Bicondylar fracture.

with or without a fleck of bone pulling off with the ligament.[411] A ligament injury frequently seen in patients older than 50 years of age is avulsion of the medial collateral ligament from the femoral condyle in lateral plateau fractures (Fig. 4–2). Avulsions of the ligament from the femur heal well with immobilization. At times, some ossification occurs in the region of the avulsion from the medial femoral condyle.[70, 727] Unfortunately, without visualizing the site of ligament injury at surgery, its nature cannot usually be determined. Magnetic resonance imaging (MRI), however, may demonstrate the site of injury.[2]

Patients younger than 40 years of age have bone-ligament attachments that are stronger than the ligament itself, and tears occur more often within ligament substance. When healing of an intraligament tear takes place, it does so by ingrowth of scar tissue. Without surgical repair, such healing may take place with enough lengthening to result in late knee instability. Isolated medial collateral ligament injuries have been shown to heal well with nonoperative treatment.[486, 922, 933] I believe, however, that in the presence of a tibial plateau fracture, collateral ligament injuries should be identified and repaired, along with the bony injury, to ensure the best opportunity for later knee stability.[243, 553, 1058, 1122]

Traditional after-treatment of torn collateral ligaments, whether surgically repaired or not, is immobilization for several weeks. More recently protective

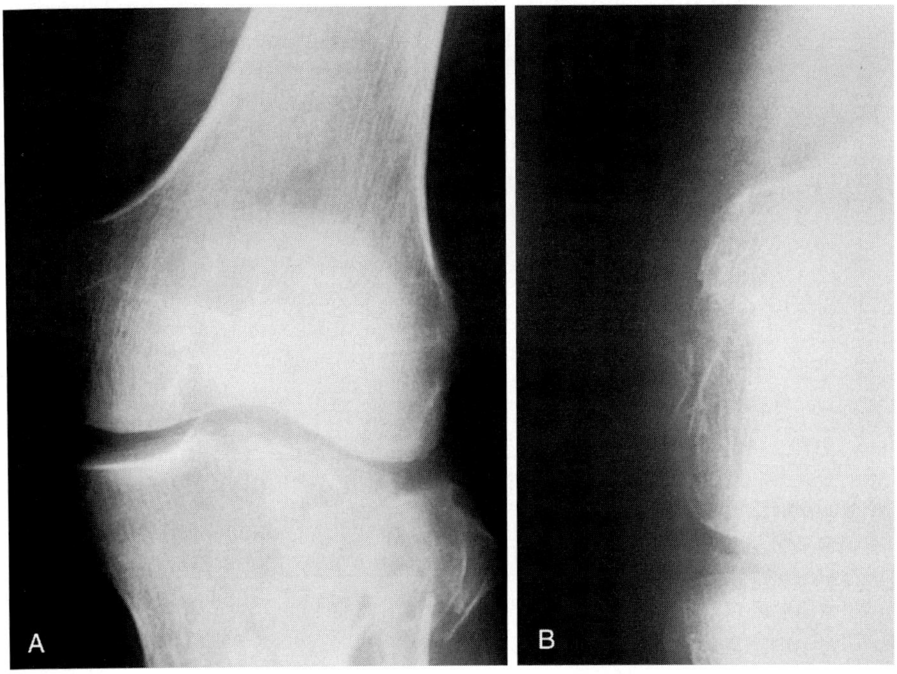

Figure 4–2. Split compression fracture of the lateral plateau. *A*, Note the slight medial cartilage space widening. *B*, A close-up view of an avulsed medial femoral fragment from the medial collateral ligament attachment.

braces have been used instead of rigid casts.[879, 933] I have used cast braces for a long time, and more recently I have used fracture braces for postoperative treatment of patients with repaired ligament injuries with no loss of knee stability. There is evidence that protected movement of collagenous tissues enhances strength and function.[9, 1137, 1138] The cause of late knee instability is usually related to uncorrected depression in the tibial plateau; however, unrepaired collateral ligament injuries can also be a factor. Results in the author's series indicate that knees with repaired collateral ligaments were more stable than were knees left with unrepaired ligament tears[243, 553] (Table 4–2).

Diagnosis

Fracture surgeons should be aware of the possibility of collateral or cruciate ligament injury in tibial plateau fractures. As the injured knee is examined, palpation along the course of ligaments may elicit tenderness. Tender areas, usually on the side of the knee opposite the fracture, may indicate the site of collateral ligament injury. Varus and valgus knee stability is tested with the knee in extension and also in a few degrees of flexion. Stress testing can often be done in the emergency room, but many surgeons perform stress testing under anesthesia in surgery prior to reduction and fracture fixation. If instability of 5 to 10 degrees or more is found, it is due either to fracture displacement, collateral ligament injury, or a combination of both. Initial x-rays may show widening of cartilage space or avulsed bone at ligament attachments, providing a significant clue to the presence of injury to the ligament (Fig. 4–3). The exact cause of knee instability is easily determined by stress x-rays. These x-rays may show only further fracture displacement, but in the presence of collateral ligament injury they will show cartilage space widening in the opposite compartment to the fracture.[68, 344, 448, 679] Stress x-rays that show only 2 or 3 mm of opening of the tested compartment probably indicate an intact or mildly stretched ligament. If there is an opening of 5 to 20 mm, the collateral ligament is severely torn (Fig. 4–4).[448]

Cruciate ligament injuries occur in some plateau fractures, especially the split type, and are frequently associated with collateral ligament injury as well.[2, 243, 1106, 1122] Either of the cruciate ligaments may be torn through its substance or may avulse from femoral or tibial attachments with bone. Bennett and Browner found 10% anterior cruciate tears in their prospective study.[68] At arthrotomy or arthroscopy, the cruciate ligaments can be directly assessed. An arthroscopic knee examination allows a much more complete internal knee inspection than is possible with an arthrotomy. Injuries to the cruciate ligaments will, therefore, be documented more frequently in the future.[1072]

Technique of Repair

Ligament repair logically should follow fracture fixation to help secure normal ligament length. A midline approach can be used for both fracture fixation and ligament repair; otherwise, two incisions are used, one on each side

Table 4–2. RESULTS WITH AND WITHOUT COLLATERAL LIGAMENT REPAIR

STATUS OF TORN LIGAMENT	NO. OF PATIENTS	NO. OF POINTS	AVERAGE INSTABILITY
Collateral ligament repair (All had ORIF of the fracture)	19	80	4.5 Degrees
Torn collateral—no repair (13 of 20 had ORIF of the fracture)	20	73	7.8 Degrees

ORIF, Open reduction and internal fixation.

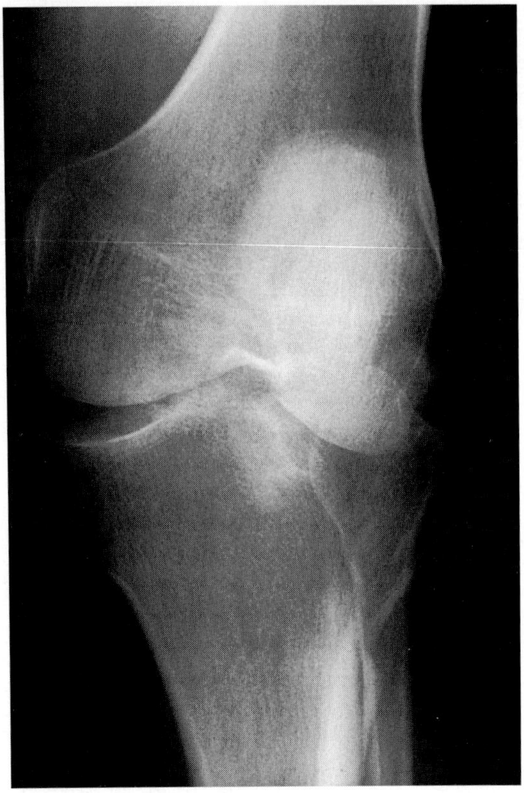

Figure 4–3. Lateral tibial plateau fracture with widening of the medial cartilage space.

of the knee. For avulsions from the femoral condyle, a short incision and suture to bone or stapling is all that is required to restore knee stability (Fig. 4–5). For insubstance tears, a layer-by-layer exposure and repair produces the best stability.

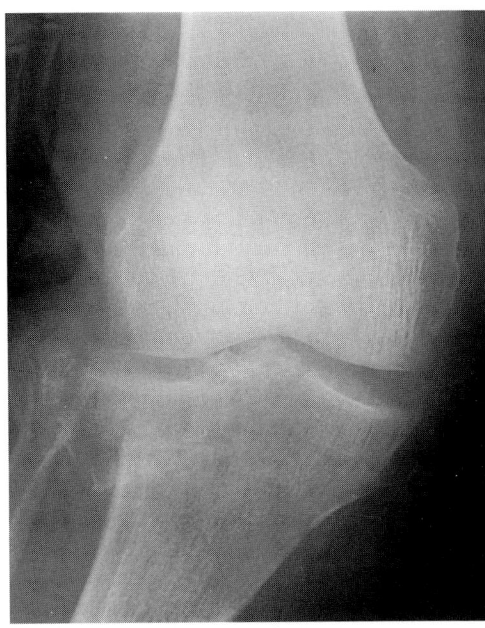

Figure 4–4. Stress x-ray with medial cartilage space widening.

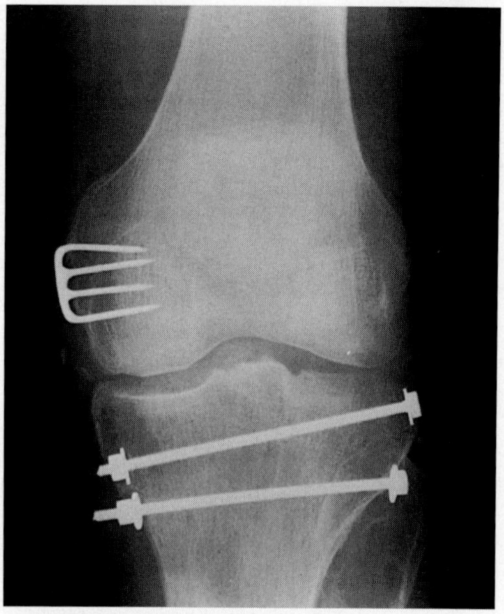

Figure 4–5. Staple fixation of the medial collateral ligament avulsed from the femoral condyle.

Post-ligament Repair Management

Protection of repaired ligaments is advised for at least 5 or 6 weeks. A long leg cast has been used for many years to protect both the plateau fracture and repaired ligament. Unfortunately, this type and duration of immobilization led to the formation of dense intra-articular adhesions that made rehabilitation of the knee slow and often incomplete. Recent trends, yet unproven scientifically, employ cast-bracing or fracture-bracing to allow knee movement, which is limited initially and then gradually increased as much as possible. To date, earlier movement with such protection has not adversely affected late knee stability in the author's series. Research by Akeson and colleagues supports minimizing immobilization after ligament repair.[1137, 1138] I employ immediate knee movement with the protection of a fracture-brace.

MENISCAL INJURIES

All mechanisms of injury that produce tibial plateau fractures, of necessity, place great stress upon the meniscus and thus may loosen its peripheral attachments or tear its substance.[1096] The more severe the fracture displacement, the more likely is meniscal injury. At times, especially in split compression fractures, the meniscus displaces into the fracture defect. The incidence of meniscal injury at arthrotomy for fracture reduction has been reported to be between 10 and 86%.[68, 274, 556, 899, 1058] Some reports deal almost exclusively with the meniscus in the fractured compartment, since the other meniscus was not observed. When arthroscopic inspection of both compartments was done, the observed incidence of meniscal pathology rose to 50% or more.[1072] Abdollahi and associates, using MRI, found that 74% of plateau fractures had meniscal pathology.[2] In the author's series there were only 16% diagnosed meniscal injuries (Table 4–3).

In the early years of open treatment of tibial plateau fractures, it was routine to remove the meniscus in order to visualize fracture reduction. In 1951, Palmer advocated preserving the meniscus, as have many others since then.[811] Because the meniscus has such important functions in knee stability and weight-bearing and its presence seems to help guide healing pannus and scar tissue after plateau fracture, it should not be removed for fracture visualization.[280, 811, 1096] Removal of the meniscus is only indicated in cases of irreparable damage. Peripheral tears

Table 4–3. MENISCAL INJURIES AND FRACTURES TYPES

Fracture Type	MD	LC	SC	TO	SP	RIM	BIC	Total
Meniscal Tear (%)	1%	14%	33%	12%	18%	17%	21%	16%

MD = Minimally displaced; LC = Local compression; SC = Split compression; TO = Total depression; SP = Split fracture; RIM = Rim fracture; BIC = Bicondylar fracture.

are readily repaired and these repairs, or the resuture necessitated by the inframeniscal surgical approach, rarely produce late meniscal derangement.[161] In the author's series of 189 open meniscal repairs after surgical or traumatic detachment, there are no known internal derangements requiring additional meniscal surgery.

Late meniscal complications are rare after plateau fractures, probably because of the pannus that tends to stabilize the meniscus after fracture.[454]

Diagnosis

The diagnosis of meniscal injury is usually made at surgery or arthroscopic examination.[68, 556, 899, 1058, 1072] Arthrography has not proved to be helpful in fresh fractures.[772] MRI has demonstrated many meniscal injuries and may prove to be a useful preoperative tool in many patients.[2]

Management

The meniscus should be preserved except when it has been damaged irreparably.[811] Complete radial tears provide an indication for removal. Minor trimming or peripheral suturing will salvage most torn or displaced menisci. Slowly absorbable sutures attaching the periphery of the meniscus to the coronary ligaments restore the normal anatomy.[1125] I believe that resutured menisci should be managed in the same way as the fracture, whether by immediate motion, cast-brace, or plaster cast.

PERONEAL NERVE INJURIES

Because of its anatomic location and course, the peroneal nerve is damaged occasionally by the trauma that produces a tibial plateau fracture. Severe angular distortions of the knee at the moment of injury may elongate the peroneal nerve sufficiently to produce stretch injury. Also, direct trauma to the nerve can occur as the result of a lateral blow against the fibular head and neck. Rarely stretch injury from surgical retraction or damage from direct pressure against the neck of the fibula in traction or in a cast may produce nerve injury.[68, 762, 1058]

Diagnosis

The initial evaluation of an injured extremity should always include an assessment of sensory and motor nerve function. It is a simple matter to record the ability of the patient to contract the anterior tibial muscle and to dorsiextend the great toe against resistance and to test for sensory abnormality. The presence of splints or bandages should not prevent this examination from taking place. If the peroneal nerve is damaged, there will be an area of hypesthesia over the dorsum of the foot that extends to the area between the great and second toes. It is important to ascertain whether the peroneal nerve or the sciatic nerve has been damaged. Motor and sensory examination of the entire limb may be required to make this determination. Electromyograms (EMGs) are helpful in both the diagnosis and prognosis but are useless in the first 2 to 3 weeks after injury. Serial EMGs offer an objective assessment of reinnervation and are helpful in determining the need for later exploration of the peroneal nerve.

Treatment

Treatment of peroneal nerve injury is usually conservative and includes serial observations of nerve function clinically and by EMG. Indications of nerve recovery, although frequently noted within 6 weeks of injury, may require as much as 3 months. If an EMG shows that reinnervation is occurring, more patience is needed. If by 3 months there has been no clinical or EMG sign of recovery, surgical exploration of the nerve should be considered. The timing of exploration depends on the status of fracture healing. It is best to have the fracture healed and movement restored before exploring the peroneal nerve.[762, 1058] The findings at late exploration in five patients by the author varied a great deal from neuroma of the nerve to scarring. In this limited experience with peroneal palsies, significant recovery of nerve function has not resulted from exploration. An ankle-foot orthosis to lessen footdrop makes walking safer and more comfortable.

OPEN FRACTURE

Open fracture of the proximal tibia and knee joint is often a difficult and serious problem, depending on the extent of the fracture, the skin wound, and contamination. The types of open wounds as classified by Gustilo and Anderson vary from grade 1 punctures from within to massive grade 3 injuries with nerve and vascular involvement. Tscherne and Lobenhoffer proposed a classification of soft tissue injury about the knee from grades 0 to 3, depending on their severity.[1058] The trauma that produces an open fracture often causes serious or even critical injuries elsewhere. The priorities, after preserving life and limb, are to prevent infection in the contaminated wound by débridement and stabilization of the fracture.

Treatment

In general, parenteral antibiotics should be administered in the emergency room. Débridement under anesthesia in surgery should be accomplished as soon as possible to prevent the spread of contamination to uninvolved tissues. The decision whether to close a wound depends on its location, size, and degree of contamination. If the wound is from within and not grossly contaminated, wound closure is indicated. Any greater degree of contamination suggests leaving the wound open initially and redébriding every few days with a delayed primary or secondary procedure at a later date. If such a course is elected, bony stabilization must be accomplished. Traction has long been the standard method of stabilization, because limb alignment is maintained and access for wound care is possible. The introduction of metallic fixation in an open wound is always a calculated risk but is justified in some plateau fractures. It should be used in its simplest form, which does not require additional tissue dissection and does not take up much space within the wound, which might create additional tension on closing sutures. Percutaneous screws, pins, or wires that are inserted from uninvolved areas of skin can stabilize some fractures with minimal risk. Small pin external fixators, including the Ilizarov apparatus, have been used about the knee with success (Fig. 4–6). The fixator may span the knee with pins into the distal femur to maintain alignment or, depending on the fracture, just in the tibial fracture area to stabilize a subcondylar or upper tibial shaft fracture.[86, 126, 214, 238, 359, 641, 663, 729, 760, 971, 1063] As previously noted, the first priority is elimination of wound contamination. Once this has been accomplished, limited

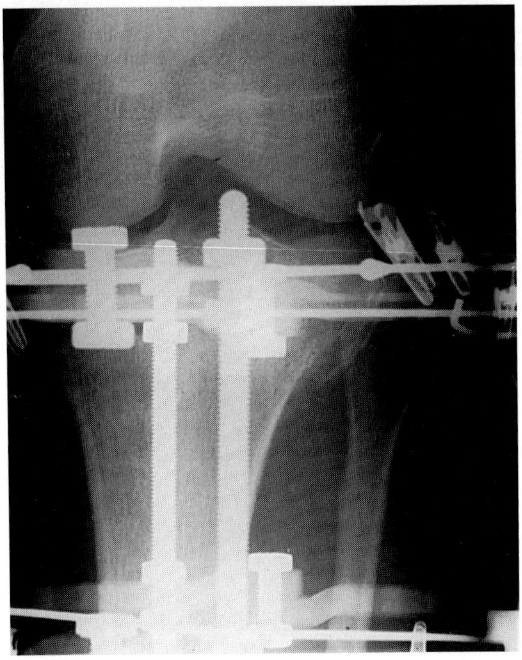

Figure 4–6. External fixator applied to stabilize a plateau fracture with an associated subcondylar fracture.

open reduction may be possible at 2 to 3 weeks, or fracture treatment may be continued in traction or external fixation.

Prognosis

The prognosis after open fracture involving the tibial plateau region is frequently for permanent disability, including limitation of knee motion. The author's series included 35 open fractures with three quarters having ipsilateral fracture as well. The 1 year rating was 76 points. Nine patients had wound infection, but only one patient developed osteomyelitis. There were nine good results and 14 poor results among these open fractures.

SUMMARY

Soft tissue knee injuries should be anticipated and, therefore, looked for routinely in proximal tibial articular fractures. Such injuries can have a devastating effect on the ultimate outcome of knee function and must be managed appropriately to minimize their permanent effects.

CHAPTER 5

Treatment Techniques

The number and diversity of treatments that have been used in the management of tibial plateau fractures is a tribute to the ingenuity of surgeons who were stimulated by dissatisfaction with earlier methods. Although many treatment techniques have passed into history, some have been improved, and new ones have been developed.

The principles of treatment evolved slowly as the reaction of joints to injury was discovered and as the benefits of accurate articular reduction were noted in both clinical and experimental studies. These observations resulted in the premise that joint fractures should be moved early to minimize the development of intra-articular adhesions and that anatomic reduction of articular fractures favors good results. Clinical observers had long been aware that satisfactory functional results were routinely obtained after traction treatment and that unsatisfactory functional results often followed knee immobilization or operative treatment.

In general, the best treatment is the simplest and least risky that gives promise of accurate articular surface reduction, restoration of leg alignment, and knee stability, while permitting early rehabilitation.

In this chapter, currently used treatment methods are considered in relation to indications, advantages, disadvantages, and complications that may result from their use.

CLOSED MANAGEMENT TECHNIQUES

Closed management of plateau fractures has always been popular because it is relatively simple, with minimal risk to the patient, and gives favorable results in fractures with lesser articular displacements (Table 5–1). However, uncorrected articular offsets or displacements cause significant degradation of long-term results.[123, 634, 635] Before 1973, 77% of tibial plateau fractures in the author's series were treated closed. Since 1973, closed treatment was used in only 31% (Table 5–2). More recent treatment methods in the several types of fractures are shown in Table 5–3.

Table 5–1. INITIAL FRACTURE DISPLACEMENTS AND POINT RATING (TREATED CLOSED OR OPEN)

FRACTURE DISPLACEMENT	CLOSED TREATMENT Point Rating	OPEN TREATMENT Point Rating
0–3 mm	85 (N = 65)	85 (N = 7)
4–7 mm	79 (N = 80)	83 (N = 20)
8–11 mm	75 (N = 75)	81 (N = 94)
12–15 mm	68 (N = 17)	69 (N = 55)
>15 mm	70 (N = 19)	75 (N = 28)

Table 5–2. CLOSED AND OPEN TREATMENT OVER THE YEARS (AUTHOR'S SERIES)

TREATMENT (%)	MD	LC	SC	TO	SP	RIM	BIC	TOTAL (%)
Closed before 1973	99.6	86	62	83	75	88	80	77
Closed 1973–1994	84	26	9	31	10	39	30	31
Open before 1973	0.4	14	38	17	25	12	20	23
Open 1973–1994	16	74	91	69	90	61	70	69

MD = Minimally displaced; LC = local compression; SC = split compression; TO = total depression; SP = split fracture; RIM = rim fracture; BIC = bicondylar fracture.

Functional Management

Tibial plateau fractures with small displacements and little tendency to redisplace are treated appropriately by functional methods of early knee movement and muscle strengthening, perhaps using a brace or soft dressing, until fracture healing is evident by x-ray. The main concern in utilizing this treatment is the potential for loss of fracture position.

Some minimally displaced fractures do well without external support; however, others have a tendency to displace further. Fractures that are especially susceptible to displacement are oblique fractures involving the medial condyle or plateau fractures with an associated subcondylar fracture. Whenever functional management is used, x-rays should be taken every few days until evidence of bony healing is present and to ensure that reduction is maintained. Significant loss of reduction demands a change of treatment, which might include open reduction and internal fixation.

Some displaced fractures may also be treated successfully by functional methods with follow-up x-ray evaluation to detect further fracture depression

Table 5–3. TREATMENT USED BETWEEN 1973 AND 1994 (N = 529)

	FRACTURE TYPES							
% TREATMENT CLOSED	MD	LC	SC	TO	SP	RIM	BIC	Total (%)
Functional	4	1	1	1	1	1	1	2
Fracture-brace	3	1	0	2	0	1	2	2
Cast-brace	12	11	3	6	0	3	4	7
Plaster cast	34	11	3	8	1	4	7	13
Traction	7	6	3	3	0	1	8	5
Closed reduction	1	3	0	4	0	0	4	2
Closed 31% Total	61	33	10	24	2	10	26	31
	FRACTURE TYPES							
% TREATMENT OPEN	MD	LC	SC	TO	SP	RIM	BIC	Total (%)
Open reduction (ORIF)	5	25	50	20	6	7	28	27
ORIF and cast	4	44	50	27	8	8	27	32
ORIF—traction	2	2	3	0	0	0	2	2
Arthroscopic reduction	1	23	4	1	1	1	2	6
Closed and percutaneous	0	0	0	2	0	0	1	<1
External fixator	0	1	1	3	3	0	1	2
Open 69% Total	12	95	108	53	18	16	61	69

MD = Minimally displaced; LC = local compression; SC = split compression; TO = total depression; SP = split fracture; RIM = rim fracture; BIC = bicondylar fracture.

or displacement. An example is a local compression fracture, depressed 5 to 8 mm, in an older patient whose needs for knee stability and alignment are not as important as is the maintenance of function. One must, however, accept the inevitable malalignment and instability that accompany the residual articular depression resulting from such treatment.

Cast Immobilization

Plaster casts have long been used in the management of plateau fractures because of convenience and ease of use. Another reason has been the general belief that casts "immobilize" a fracture until it is healed. Krackow and Vetter observed that a long-leg cast, even molded about the thigh, permits limited valgus-varus and flexion-extension movement.[564] Such movement is sufficient to promote loss of fracture reduction in a tibial plateau fracture.[35, 564] In experimental and clinical studies, Sarmiento and associates demonstrated that certain fracture configurations, especially those that involve the medial tibial plateau with an intact fibula, tend to depress in casts.[940]

Another disadvantage of more than a few weeks of cast immobilization is the complex joint reaction termed "arthrofibrosis" by Luck.[646] In this uncommon condition, fibrous pannus envelopes the interior of a joint and limits movement, often permanently. Apley described "plaster disease," which is a more frequently noted condition that also develops from immobilization.[29] This syndrome includes stiffness in the joint as well as reactive demineralization of the distal femur and proximal tibia. Many months of difficult rehabilitation are required to obtain maximum function once either arthrofibrosis or plaster disease has set in.

Plaster casts are certainly useful for short periods to protect knees against additional injury in patients who are not trustworthy or compliant. Long-leg casts should extend from high on the thigh down to (and including) the foot, holding the knee in the extended position. This position helps to prevent the development of flexion contracture. A knee immobilized in flexion often requires many weeks or months of therapy just to regain normal extension.[454] I have observed that after prolonged physical therapy, stiff knees regain flexion more readily than extension.

Hinged Casts and Braces

The role of bracing, either fracture- or cast-bracing, in plateau fracture management is becoming more clearly defined.[122, 224, 237, 243, 289, 720, 721] Fractures with a tendency to redisplace are less likely to lose position in a modern brace than in a cast because of the shape of the thigh cuff and the ability to stress the brace against expected displacement. Recent orthotic developments have made fracture-bracing as effective as cast-bracing. Either of these bracing methods can be used in certain unstable fractures or when it is necessary to maintain continuing varus or valgus stress to prevent fracture redisplacement. Nonetheless, even with these techniques, some fractures do displace in a cast-brace or a fracture-brace, making it important to observe fracture position by x-rays during the healing period.[940] The expense of these braces makes it important to use them appropriately and not to use them when more cost-effective methods will suffice.[243]

The technique of cast-brace application is well known, but a few points deserve mention. The fracture surgeon should hold the limb to minimize pain and to protect fracture position. The lower leg cast part of the brace is applied first, followed by the thigh portion over a plastic quadrilateral socket.[122] Once these casts are in place, the hinges are loosely affixed using an alignment jig and hose clamps. The proper location for hinges is then determined by gently flexing and extending the knee and by correcting their location as necessary. For surgically elevated and grafted local compression fractures or others with one weak or unstable condyle, the cast-brace should be stressed in a direction opposite to the fractured condyle to help prevent fracture redisplacement. The surgeon stresses the leg with the knee extended. For lateral plateau fractures, varus stress is used; for medial plateau fractures, valgus stress is applied. While the stress is being exerted, the hose clamps are tightened to maintain this position. The hinges are then permanently affixed with fiberglass or plaster. An x-ray taken in a cast-brace that is properly stressed opposite the fracture should show some widening of the cartilage space. Weight-bearing cineradiographic studies made by the author of knees in a stressed cast-brace demonstrated continued lateral cartilage space widening despite weight-bearing. This does not indicate that weight-bearing is a good idea or that such cartilage space widening can be maintained in every patient for the 8 weeks necessary to fracture healing.[721] Cast- or fracture-braces have been successful in maintaining reduction in many patients.

Local compression fractures that have been reduced and grafted by open or arthroscopic techniques need postoperative protection. In such patients braces require more patient compliance and physician attention than do cast-braces and need frequent adjustment and tightening as thigh atrophy takes place. Bicondylar fractures, especially those with an intact fibula, have a tendency to displace into a varus position. This tendency is reduced but not eliminated by the use of bracing.[940]

A yet unproven, and therefore controversial, use of bracing is to protect collateral or cruciate ligament repairs after fixation of a plateau fracture. In a brace the ligament repair is protected against major stresses, and the knee is allowed movement within a predetermined range.

In a series of 141 cast-braces used after plateau fracture, it was evident that some were used in cases in which lesser support would certainly have been sufficient.[243] In stable minimally displaced fractures, except for the total depression subtype, soft dressing, postoperative splint, or plaster cast is adequate treatment. A cast-brace would be helpful, especially in a noncompliant patient. The same reasoning applies after rigid internal fixation of plateau fractures. In these cases, a removable support or soft dressing is usually sufficient in compliant patients. The drawbacks of braces are their cost, weight, bulk, and an often 90-degree limitation of knee motion.

Traction

Traction is a useful and reliable method of plateau fracture management that permits knee movement while helping to correct and maintain fracture position (Fig. 5–1). Many fractured knees, treated in traditional traction, were noted to have lost normal valgus knee alignment when compared with the uninjured knees.[728] Improved traction methods, such as Badgley and O'Connor's method and Moore and associates' modification, help maintain the normal valgus orientation of the knee.[39, 728] The disadvantage of traction is the expense of hospital confinement for 3 to 6 weeks until the fracture becomes sufficiently stable for a brace or other form of support to be used. Thus, despite the good functional results reported after traction treatment, most fracture centers today rely increasingly on operative methods.

Traction is an option when open reduction is contraindicated. Some contraindications for surgery are extraordinary risk because of systemic condition, loss of skin or infection in the area of the knee, or a fracture so comminuted or osteopenic that in the judgement of the surgeon open reduction could not result in rigid fixation or reasonable restoration of articular surfaces.

Traction can be applied temporarily through the skin or for long periods through a skeletal tibial pin. Skin traction is useful for a few days in patients confined to bed for other injuries, but skeletal traction should be used when

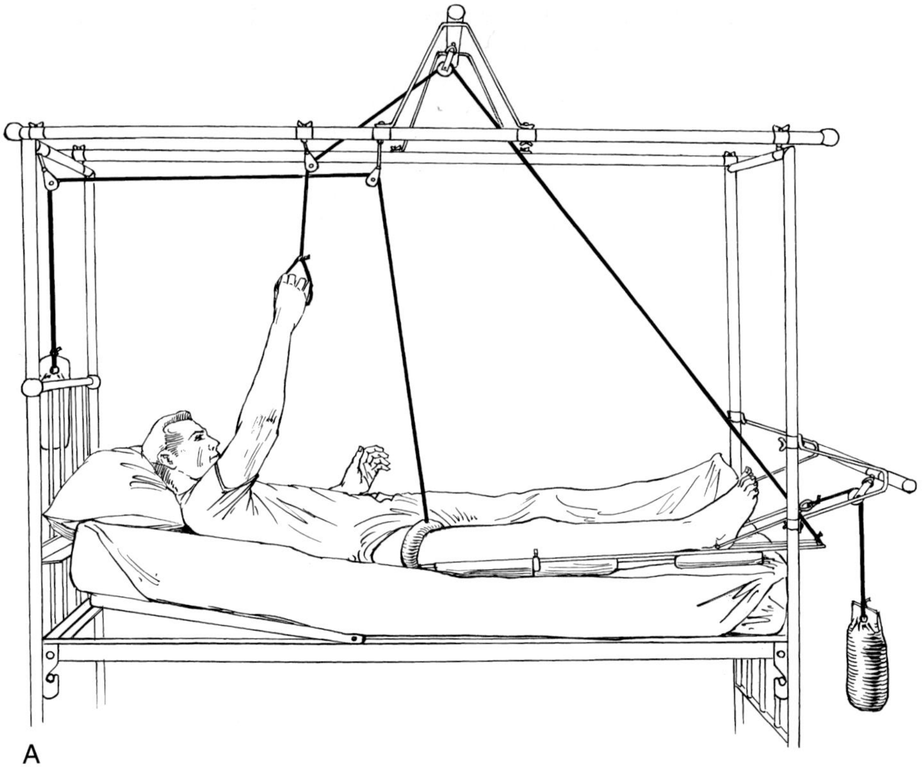

A

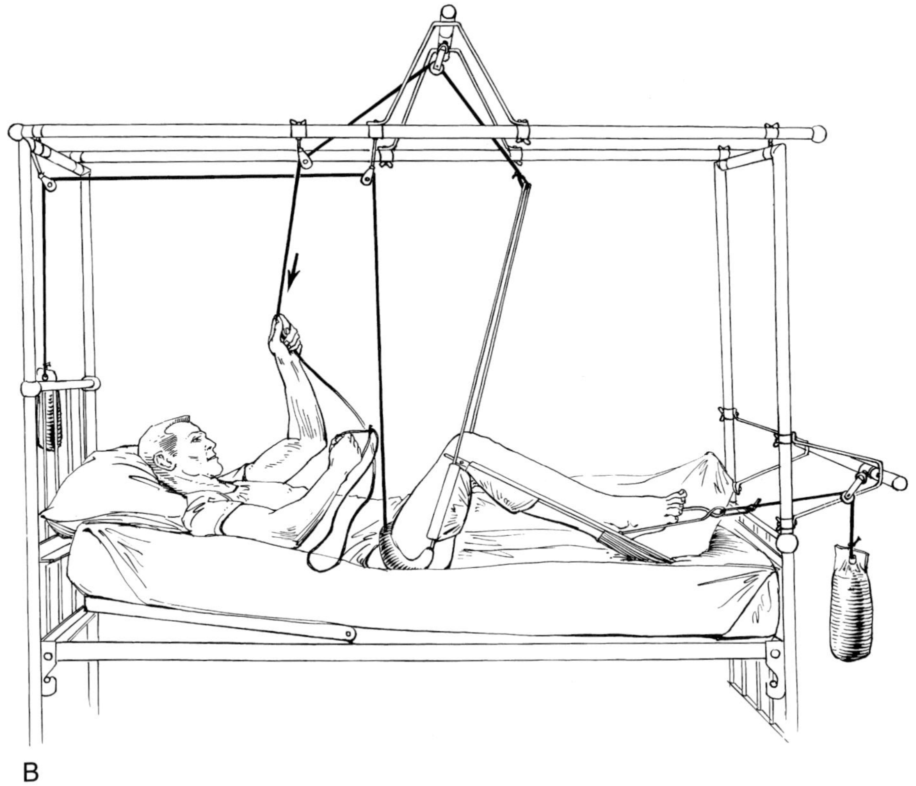

B

Figure 5–1. *A* and *B*, Traction setup that allows passive knee motion. (From Hohl, M.: Tibial plateau fractures. An instructional course lecture. J. Bone Joint Surg., 49A:1460, 1967.)

traction is to be the definitive treatment. The traction pin is best placed in the distal tibia but has been used in the mid-tibia and in the calcaneus.[28] Apley's traction method permits 90 degrees of knee motion. Ilfeld and Hohl's exercise method and others using splints and pulleys also promote good knee motion in traction (Fig. 5–1).[482] The major advantage of the use of traction is the ability to keep the knee moving while reduction and alignment are maintained. French fracture surgeons have called this the traction-mobilization method.[165, 278]

Whenever traction is used, the resting position should leave the knee fully extended in order to minimize the likelihood of later knee flexion contracture. Various rope and pulley combinations can be utilized to begin passive knee movement while maintaining traction. As the fracture begins to heal, traction weight is gradually decreased for more active knee movement and muscle strengthening.

Disadvantages of skeletal traction may include less than anatomic fracture reduction, loss of normal knee valgus alignment, pin tract infection, and expense of lengthy hospitalization. Advantages are the ability to move the knee early while maintaining reduction and alignment without the risk of wound infection. After traction treatment, patients uniformly show good function of the knee with a minimum of intra-articular adhesions and deformity.[28, 29, 165, 278, 989, 1058]

Closed Reduction

For a century closed manipulative reduction under anesthesia has been used in the attempt to restore articular alignment. Its current use is reserved for patients in whom open reduction is contraindicated or to obtain reduction prior to the insertion of percutaneous fixation devices.[275, 289]

The problem with this method is not so much the difficulty of obtaining adequate reduction but of maintaining reduction once it has been achieved. Plaster casts are very unlikely to maintain fracture reduction after closed manipulation. Skeletal traction seems to be the only reliable closed method for preventing redisplacement, but it must be continued for about 4 weeks before a brace or cast-brace can be safely applied.[482] Percutaneous pinning and external fixation techniques are semiopen methods to maintain reduction obtained by closed means and are now being used more frequently.[85, 100, 540, 562]

Ilfeld and Hohl described a method of closed reduction under anesthesia with the patient on a fracture table.[482] In this technique the knee is first aspirated of hemarthrosis, then a traction pin is placed through the distal tibia or os calcis and 60 lb of traction are applied. An x-ray or image intensifier is used to assess the adequacy of reduction. If one condyle remains below normal articular level, it may often be reduced by pounding it proximally with a padded mallet. Once the condyles are at normal level, lateral compression using a Böhler or C clamp is used to impact the fracture. In order to maintain reduction, the patient is transferred to bed with 20 lb of skeletal traction, and passive and later active knee exercises are instituted until early fracture union occurs. Traction is maintained with decreasing weights for between 3 and 6 weeks, after which a cast-brace may be used if further support of the fracture is necessary.

Closed Reduction and Percutaneous Fixation

After successful closed reduction utilizing traction and angular forces, screws or pins may be inserted percutaneously to maintain reduction. This technique is especially helpful for fractures with larger fragments and is gaining popularity because of the availability of cannulated screw systems.

Once reduction is obtained, guide pins are inserted percutaneously to hold major fragments to the opposite intact condyle. Cannulated screws are a convenient way to use the technique. After measurement of the necessary length, the screws with washers are inserted over the guide wires and then tightened. The guide wires are removed, and the fracture is carefully assessed for stability. Several screws may be required to accomplish fixation and stability. Even then, bracing or cast immobilization is advisable.[361, 424, 540, 562, 663] Follow-up care includes serial x-ray examinations, and the examiner must look for any loss of fracture position. Until the fracture is consolidated, it is advisable to continue external support.

Another method involves the use of small wires placed through the reduced proximal tibial fracture and fixed to a half-ring that is in turn supported by an external fixator into the mid-tibial region.[85, 126, 214, 641, 663, 760, 971, 1063] This technique is useful even for open fractures. Fracture reduction can also be accomplished by pressure exerted through olive wires and normal knee alignment maintained. Perhaps its best use is with larger fragment plateau bicondylar fractures that have an associated subcondylar or proximal tibial shaft fracture.

The advantage of these techniques is the avoidance of many of the complications of open reduction with the ability often to provide near-anatomic reduction and early knee motion. The results of this method are now becoming available; it may be superior to open reduction in some patients.[90, 100, 275, 289, 424, 540, 562]

OPEN REDUCTION

A surge of enthusiasm for open reduction developed in the 1960s based on the recognition that new internal fixation devices combined with techniques of reduction did have the ability to fix fractures rigidly and accurately. This meant that external support, such as a cast, would be needed for only a short time if at all.[910] Rigid fracture fixation has allowed earlier knee movement after open reduction and consequently, improved functional results.[950] Of the author's 529 plateau fractures treated since 1970, 69% have had open or arthroscopic reduction.

Open reduction should have defined objectives based on the particular type of fracture being treated. For instance, in local compression fractures, the depressed articular surface needs to be elevated and supported by grafts aided possibly by wires or screws under the condyle. In split-compression, total depression, and split fracture types, rigid fixation using screws or plates should be obtained in a high percentage. Rigid fixation should always be the goal so that early knee movement can be instituted. In bicondylar fractures, anatomic reduction and rigid fixation cannot always be achieved, and limited internal fixation, external fixation, or closed treatment methods provide useful alternatives.

Tibial plateau fractures that were less than rigidly fixed were shown to have poorer results than those in which rigid fixation was achieved.[950] Stiff and deformed knees may be the result of a poorly fixed fracture, a worse result than might have been achieved by closed treatment.

There are many potential problems associated with the open reduction of plateau fractures. The obvious concern with any open procedure is the ever-present risk of wound healing problems, including deep wound infection reported in 2 to 38% of patients in the literature.[608, 1091] Open procedures are often technically demanding and difficult, leaving the surgeon feeling frustrated and unsatisfied as to fracture reduction and fixation. Schatzker pointed out that only 26 of 41 internal fixations resulted in rigid fixation.[950] The results in fractures that were rigidly fixed were superior to the others.

Loss of fracture reduction occurred in almost 20% of plateau fractures in the author's series regardless whether closed or open treatment had been used. This is attributable to several factors, including the nature of the fracture and the effectiveness of external support or internal fixation devices. Despite the very best technique in bicondylar fractures or fractures through osteoporotic bone, some loss of reduction will inevitably occur (Table 5–4).

A disadvantage of internal fixation is the frequent need to remove fixation

Table 5–4. LOSS OF REDUCTION AFTER METHODS USED IN OPEN REDUCTION AND INTERNAL FIXATION

	REDISPLACEMENT					
INTERNAL FIXATION	**None**	**1–2 mm**	**3–4 mm**	**5–6 mm**	**≥ 7 mm**	**Total**
Screw	26	3	3	1	0	33
Screws	64	11	7	3	2	87
Tibial bolt	34	2	6	2	3	47
Tibial bolts	32	4	7	3	0	46
Wires or pins	13	2	4	1	0	20
Bone graft only	11	3	3	3	1	21
Plate and bolt	12	2	3	1	0	18
Buttress plate	71	5	8	3	2	89
Medial and lateral plates	11	0	1	0	0	12

devices that cause deep tissue irritation. In general, it is best to delay removal of metal for several months after x-ray evidence of healing has been noted. For a few weeks after removal of screws in the upper tibial shaft, there is some weakening of the torsional strength of the bone. The patient must therefore be careful when using the limb until strength is restored.

Arthroscopic Methods

The role of arthroscopy in the management of plateau fractures is still being defined.[346, 404, 423] A brief arthroscopic inspection of the knee compartments for soft tissue and articular injury has proved to be helpful in assessing intra-articular damage and convenient for débridement of loose fragments of cartilage and bone.

Certain fractures may be reduced and fixed under arthroscopic control. Local compression fractures, especially those with only a few depressed fragments, may be elevated through a tibial flare window and grafted while the intra-articular reduction is confirmed through an arthroscope and image intensifier. The dead space under the elevated articular surface is bone grafted. A screw or pin inserted percutaneously under the elevated fragment may help to maintain reduction. Following arthroscopically assisted reduction, a fracture- or cast-brace is used to unweight the elevated condyle.

Split compression fractures may also be reduced under arthroscopic control and the split fragment fixed with two or three cannulated screws inserted percutaneously. Many total depression fractures may also be viewed arthroscopically and fixed percutaneously by screws or a buttress plate after closed reduction. Reduction should also be checked by an image intensifier or x-ray to ensure articular restoration.

The advantage of arthroscopic methods lies in the minimal additional insult to soft tissues about the knee, low morbidity, and rapid restoration of motion and strength.

INDICATIONS FOR CLOSED MANAGEMENT OR OPEN REDUCTION

Now that various forms of available treatment methods have been described, it is important to consider general indications for their use. A more detailed discussion of indications is found in chapters on individual fracture types.

Indications for Closed Management

Most fractures can be treated by one of the closed methods, but this may not represent ideal management for a particular fracture. When traction and early mobilization are used, the functional result is likely to be good. When skin condition is not ideal or the patient's general health is not good, closed treatment may be the best option. When skin condition is not ideal, it is better to use closed methods to avoid wound problems and osteomyelitis.

In general, undisplaced and minimally displaced fractures do very well when treated by closed methods, ranging from knee braces to a cast or traction. Any fractured knee that is unstable to clinical examination should benefit from an open procedure that restores bony or ligamentous stability.

Some types of displaced fractures, by the nature of their bony configuration (total and some bicondylar fractures), lend themselves to closed reduction techniques. These methods are often more demanding and difficult to accomplish than open techniques but are fraught with fewer serious complications.

Indications for Closed Reduction and Percutaneous Fixation

Percutaneous fixation is a method applicable to some fractures that can be reduced by closed manipulation or by arthroscopically assisted reduction. Such fixation is not always rigid and may not adequately resist the muscle forces that tend to cause fracture redisplacement. To prevent this complication continued traction or brace protection may be required until the fracture heals.

The percutaneous technique requires anesthesia and closed manipulation and often a fracture table. After the fracture is reduced, a guide pin is inserted across the fracture under imaging intensifier control. A cannulated drill and tap are then used, and finally the screw with a washer is inserted over the guide pin. Two or three screws may be required to ensure stability. A fracture- or cast-brace is used to minimize stresses on the knee to lessen the likelihood of loss of reduction.

Indications for Open Reduction

As a general rule, unstable fractures are benefited by open reduction and internal fixation. Some stable fractures with a propensity to redisplace slowly should also be considered for internal fixation. Undisplaced fractures with associated subcondylar, tibial spine, or other ipsilateral fractures that are treated by the open method should also be internally fixed.

There is no magic number of millimeters of depression or displacement that provides an indication for open reduction. Instead, analysis of the particular fracture, its stability, displacement, and configuration provides information from which the method of treatment is selected.

Ninety percent of split-compression fractures were treated surgically in the author's series during the last 20 years. Local compression fractures are operated on because of deformity or knee instability noted by stress testing. However, the anteroposterior location of the depressed area and its depth must be considered. Total and entire fracture types do best with internal fixation, thus avoiding the uncertainty that goes with closed methods. Bicondylar fractures are a special challenge to reconstruct and require an experienced surgeon, proper operating conditions, and appropriate internal fixation materials.

Open fracture in the proximal tibial region demands thorough débridement to minimize the possibility of wound infection. Wounds seen early and débrided may permit simple internal fixation to be used to fix major fragments about the knee joint. Grossly contaminated wounds preclude primary internal fixation if at all possible. Instead, an external fixator provides one option for fracture control in the presence of serious soft tissue injuries with comminuted and unstable fractures or fracture-dislocations. Another option is traction, which is useful in almost every patient. Late bony and soft tissue reconstructive procedures can be performed after skin cover has been obtained.

Indications for Arthroscopic Reduction

The ideal fractures for arthroscopic-assisted reduction are the local compression and split fractures. Total depression and split compression fractures may also be treated by those experienced in this method. Bicondylar fractures have been generally considered to be too complex for its use. Uhl and associates reported on limited percutaneous fixation with arthroscopic visualization of reduction in bicondylar fractures;[1063] thus, there may be some role for arthroscopic débridement and inspection in almost any plateau fracture.

SUMMARY

Many methods of treatment are possible for any tibial plateau fracture. The challenge is to select and implement the best method for a particular fracture configuration, while taking into account the patient's future requirements and the skill and experience of the surgeon. When all of these factors come together, the chances for a superior result are very good. There are no magic formulas that point to the best treatment, but a good and useful general guide is the stability of the injured knee. The stable knee most likely will do well regardless of treatment method selected. The unstable knee, on the other hand, will most likely obtain the best result by internal fixation.

CHAPTER 6

Surgical Approaches and Techniques

In the last 20 years open reduction has been used increasingly in the treatment of tibial plateau fractures because of greater safety and predictability of results. Improved preoperative diagnosis and better surgical approaches and internal fixation systems have made rigid fixation possible in many displaced plateau fractures. Rigid fixation, in turn, has allowed early knee movement, bringing ever closer the goal of restoring a knee with a tibial plateau fracture to normal.

Three surgical approaches for open reduction of lateral, medial, or bicondylar fractures are described. The use of these approaches allows as much exposure of the articular surface and tibial shaft as is required to reduce a fracture and apply plates and screws to the tibial condyle and shaft. Such surgical wounds tend to heal readily and predictably. Because many knees with plateau fractures will eventually develop traumatic arthritis, whenever possible skin incisions that are not likely to interfere with later knee replacement should be planned. Other approaches with their advantages and disadvantages are discussed briefly.

Regional or general anesthesia is recommended. After anesthesia has been induced, the uninjured as well as the injured knee should be examined for collateral and cruciate ligament stability. Stress testing by applying varus and valgus force with the knee in extension and in 20 degrees of flexion allow assessment of collateral ligament stability. Instability, caused either by fracture movement or ligament tearing, can be graphically displayed on stress x-rays if desired.

A pneumatic tourniquet is inflated to an appropriate pressure with the knee flexed 90 degrees. This gives adequate freedom of knee movement and allows optimal visualization of the joint without the limiting effect of the tourniquet on the quadriceps mechanism.

APPROACH TO THE LATERAL TIBIAL PLATEAU

I prefer a curvilinear skin incision beginning over the lateral femoral condyle and crossing the joint line at the lateral border of the patellar tendon.[455] Some surgeons, however, prefer to use a lateral parapatellar approach. The disadvantage of such an approach is that it is often more difficult to expose the posterior aspect of the joint than the approach to be described. The advantage of the parapatellar approach is that it could later be incorporated in a midline skin incision to accommodate late knee replacement.

The landmarks are the patella, the lateral tibiofemoral joint line, the tibial tubercle, and the fibular head (Fig. 6–1). The skin incision begins laterally over the femoral condyle distal to the origin of the lateral collateral ligament and passes across the joint line anterodistally near the patellar tendon. At the lateral edge of the patellar tendon the incision curves distally down the tibial shaft, 5

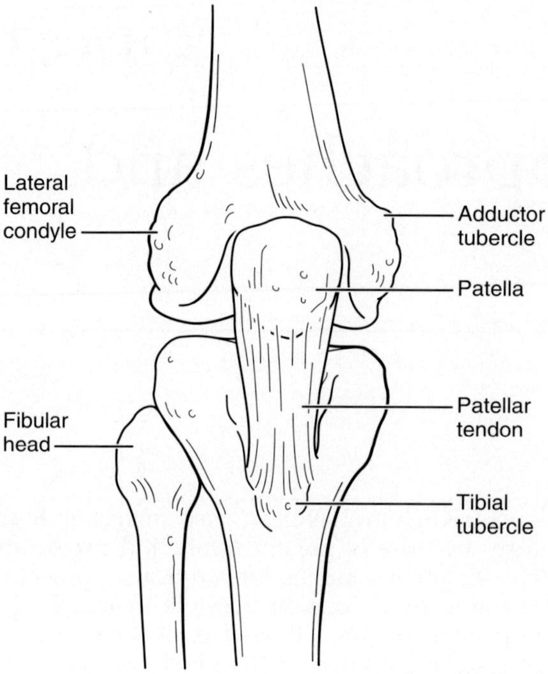

Figure 6–1. A drawing of landmarks on the upper tibia.

or 6 cm (Fig. 6–2). The skin incision may be readily extended down the tibial shaft if a long plate is required or a cortical graft needs to be harvested.

The subcutaneous tissue is divided in the line of the skin incision. The fascia lata is identified as a discrete band attaching to Gerdy's tubercle. Although I use osteotomy of Gerdy's tubercle rarely, it is used by many surgeons to facilitate wider visualization of the tibial articular margin from anterior to posterior. If osteotomized, it must be reattached by screw after fracture reduction.

I prefer to flex the knee 80 degrees or more to move the iliotibial band posteriorly. The joint line, which is usually near the proximal edge of the now nearly horizontal iliotibial, is located using a needle. The joint is entered by

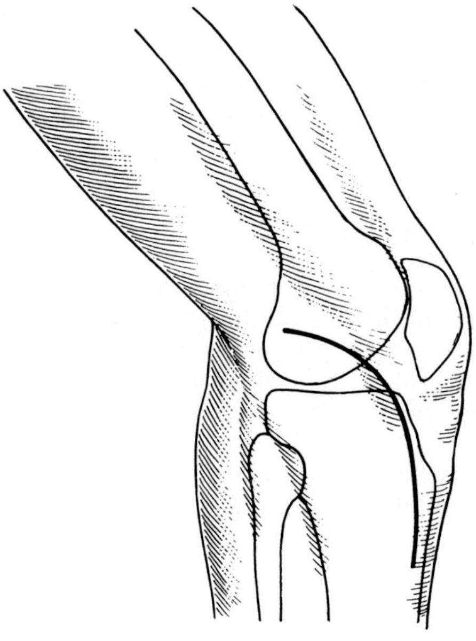

Figure 6–2. A drawing of a lateral skin incision. (From Laurin, C. A., Riley, L. H., and Roy-Camille, R. (Eds.): Atlas of Orthopedic Surgery, Vol. 3. Paris, Masson, 1992, p. 353.)

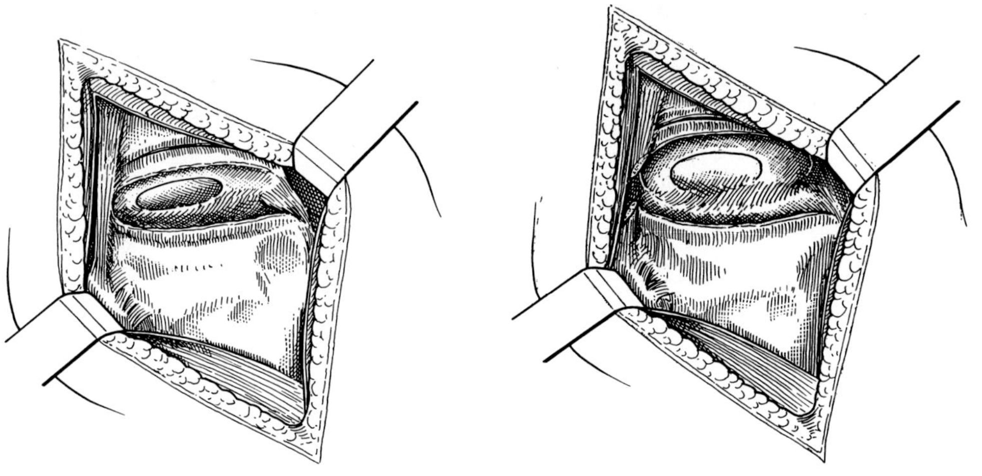

Figure 6–3. Lateral approach with capsular retraction, meniscotibial incision, and varus stress. The meniscus remains with the lateral femoral condyle, permitting visualization of the tibial plateau. (From Laurin, C. A., Riley, L. H., Roy-Camille, R. (Eds.): Atlas of Orthopedic Surgery, Vol. 3. Paris, Masson, 1992, p. 353.)

incising the capsule and meniscotibial ligament from anterior to posterior.[161] Varus stress on the knee permits visualization of the lateral tibial articular surface as the meniscus remains with the femoral condyle (Fig. 6–3). If more exposure of the plateau, especially posterior, is required, the lateral collateral ligament is divided obliquely and is later resutured. Division of the lateral collateral ligament is rarely necessary, however.

If the lateral flare of the tibia is to be windowed or used for fracture fixation, it is exposed by elevating the anterior tibial muscle from the flare of the tibia. A combination of sharp dissection and periosteal elevation is used. Care must be taken not to injure the anterior tibial artery as it passes into the anterior compartment just distal to the proximal tibiofibular joint (Fig. 6–4).

A femoral distractor may be used to maintain distraction of the lateral compartment, making fracture reduction easier and more certain. The distractor pins are placed anterolaterally in the femur and well distal to the surgical site in the tibia. After the distractor has been tensioned, the joint space is maintained open. This facilitates any windowing, reduction, grafting, or fixation.

I advise preservation of the meniscus whenever possible.[161, 1096, 1125] Peripheral

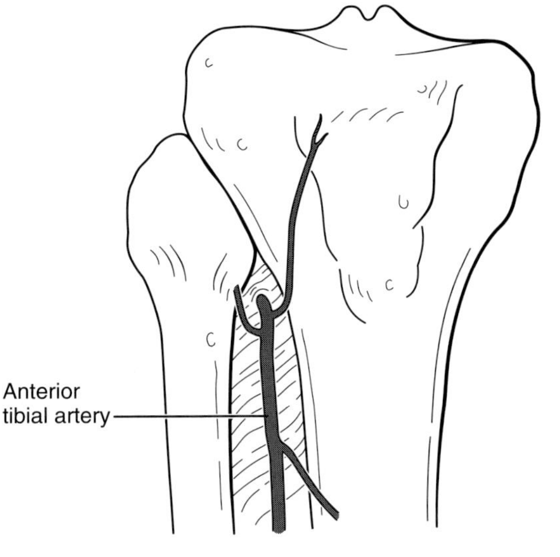

Figure 6–4. The anterior tibial artery arises in the popliteal space and passes just distal to the proximal tibiofibular joint.

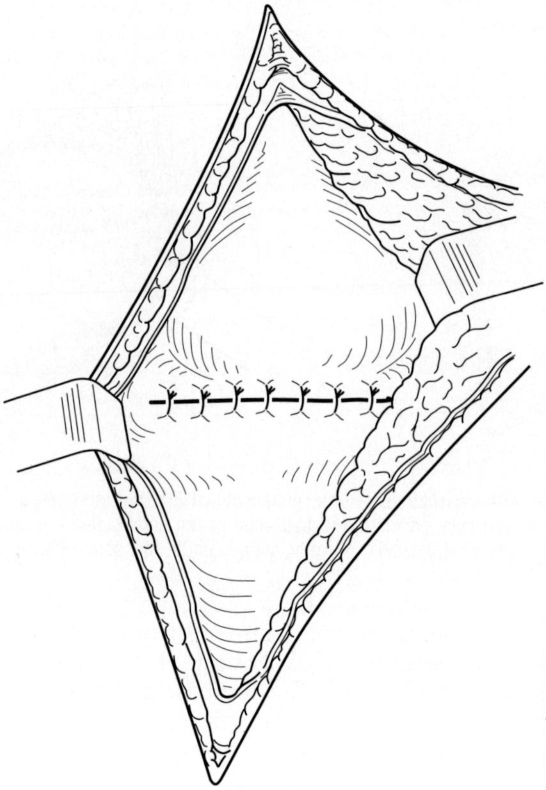

Figure 6–5. Technique of meniscal repair after inframeniscal detachment. Interrupted sutures join the meniscus to the inframeniscal ligament. (From Laurin, C. A., Riley, L. H., Roy-Camille, R. (Eds.): Atlas of Orthopedic Surgery, Vol. 3. Paris, Masson, 1992, p. 377.)

detachments or torn menisci are repaired using slowly absorbable sutures. Several sutures hold the meniscus in position until healing has occurred (Fig. 6–5). Because of the value of the meniscus in guiding pannus after fracture and its function in weight-bearing, it should never be removed for visualization of the fracture.[317, 1096] Only severe meniscal injury justifies removal.

The joint capsule is closed in the same line as it was opened and Gerdy's tubercle, if osteotomized with the fascia lata, reattached strongly by screw and washer. If the lateral collateral ligament was divided, it is repaired strongly using suture. I close the anterior compartment fascia loosely to avoid problems associated with increasing anterior compartment pressure from postoperative swelling. If there is a subcondylar fracture or a proximal tibial shaft fracture, it is advisable to release the anterior compartment fascia for a few inches below the knee. Prior to skin closure, I test the sutures by flexing the knee to a right angle. Skin clips or interrupted sutures are used for skin closure. Suction drainage of the knee decreases postoperative pain and swelling.

APPROACH TO THE MEDIAL TIBIAL PLATEAU

The landmarks are the patella, medial femoral condyle, tibial tubercle, and tibiofemoral joint line (see Fig. 6–1). The types of fracture involving the medial tibial plateau differ from those involving the lateral plateau. For instance, the total depression fracture of the medial plateau does not usually require arthrotomy but simply exposure of the medial upper tibia for accurate fracture reduction and internal fixation. The skin incision in these cases need not be the entire medial utility approach but only the more distal portion of it, exposing just the tibial flare.

Inspection of the interior of the knee can be done arthroscopically or by arthrotomy. The trend today is to cleanse and inspect the knee arthroscopically.

If arthrotomy is performed, a skin incision is made beginning over the medial femoral condyle near the adductor tubercle and extended obliquely anterodistally toward the patellar tendon and distally along the subcutaneous surface of the upper tibia (Fig. 6–6). The knee joint is entered through a vertical parapatellar capsular incision centered on the joint line. To expose the tibial articular surface, the meniscotibial ligament is incised just distal to the meniscus. This is best accomplished with the knee in at least 90 degrees of flexion to shift the superficial tibial collateral ligament posteriorly. Valgus stress on the knee and retraction will then permit visualization of the medial tibial plateau and the medial meniscus.

If the posterior aspect of the medial plateau needs to be exposed, a vertical skin incision is made along the posterior border of the medial collateral ligament. The attachments of the semimembranosus along the upper tibial margin are released, leaving sufficient soft tissue for later resuture. A vertical incision through the capsule posterior to the medial collateral ligament is made, and the meniscotibial ligament is incised for articular exposure. This allows a limited but sufficient view to accurately reduce a coronal split fracture of the posterior margin of the medial plateau. Another approach to the coronal fracture from the posterior aspect of the medial plateau is a popliteal incision in which the medial head of the gastrocnemius is partially divided to expose the fracture. Screws or even a buttress plate can then be readily inserted.[233]

Median parapatellar approaches have been used for generous arthrotomy; these are especially useful when cruciate ligament repair or replantation of an avulsed intercondylar eminence is required. Medial meniscectomy should be avoided, except when the meniscus is severely damaged.

Closure begins with suture of the meniscal margin to the coronary ligament. Then further closure is effected layer by layer. The capsule is closed and if part of the semimembranosus has been released, it should be repaired strongly to preserve posteromedial knee stability. The skin is closed with metallic clips that permit movement with security of the wound.

APPROACH TO BOTH TIBIAL PLATEAUS

Simultaneous visualization of both tibial plateaus for internal fixation is difficult. Over the years a number of approaches have been used, including separate medial and lateral approaches, the "Y," and the midline.[327, 416, 487, 792, 934, 958] Since the majority of patients with displaced bicondylar fractures develop later traumatic arthritis, and some of these knees will eventually require joint replacement, the recent trend has been to use a midline approach. Although this approach provides excellent access to the femoral condyles and tibial plateaus simultaneously, reduction of certain fractures, such as coronal plane fractures, requires the knee to be extended to permit their reduction and fixation. In these unusual fractures, two incisions rather than one may be advisable. The midline

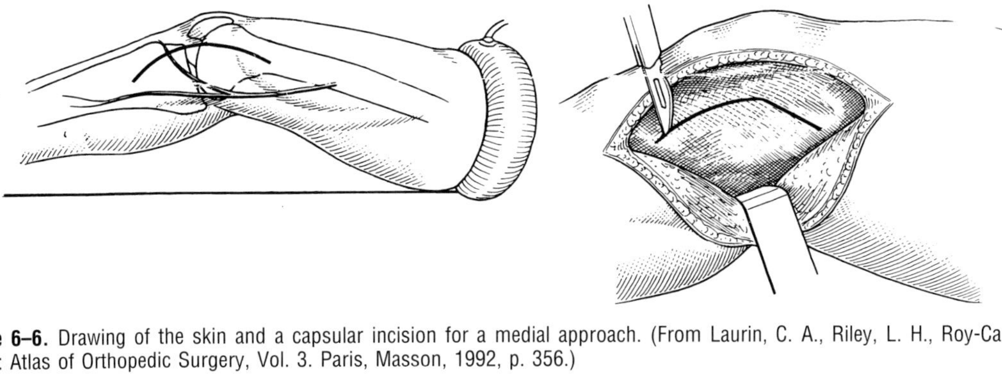

Figure 6–6. Drawing of the skin and a capsular incision for a medial approach. (From Laurin, C. A., Riley, L. H., Roy-Camille, R. (Eds.): Atlas of Orthopedic Surgery, Vol. 3. Paris, Masson, 1992, p. 356.)

approach gives access to both plateaus, the intercondylar notch area and the cruciate ligaments. As in all extensive approaches there is concern about stripping of soft tissues from fracture fragments and the proximal tibia because of the possibility of bony devitalization and wound infection.

Technique

The midline approach begins with a long vertical skin incision from above the suprapatellar pouch, curving slightly either medial or lateral to the patella and then distally just lateral or medial to the tibial tubercle (Fig. 6–7). The amount of distal exposure depends on whether a plate will need to be used. The skin, subcutaneous tissues, and knee joint capsule are incised. This allows limited visualization of both compartments after the patella has been everted and the knee is flexed. For fractures requiring simple internal fixation, the lateral compartment may be entered in the inframeniscal interval, and the flare of the tibia can be exposed as for a lateral plateau exposure. The medial plateau can be similarly exposed.[455]

For simultaneous and complete exposure of both plateaus and the intercondylar notch, it is necessary to reflect the extensor mechanism proximally.[327, 455, 487, 792] There is a risk involved if the proximal tibia is comminuted in the region of the tibial tubercle. If the tibial tubercle is to be osteotomized, it should be outlined by drill holes, and a substantial boneblock should be removed with the patellar tendon insertion as suggested by Fernandez.[327] Predrilling of the tubercle fragment and the tibial bed should be accomplished before the fragment is loosened (Fig. 6–8). The tubercle is raised from its bed, separating the patellar tendon from the capsule around the tendon margins to the inferior patellar pole. The infrapatellar fat pad is maintained with the reflected tendon and patella. This permits complete exposure of the intercondylar area from in front. The menisci are mobilized in the inframeniscal interval. If the menisci are both divided near their anterior attachment, they can be reflected with the femoral condyles. This approach gives excellent simultaneous exposure of the entire proximal tibial surface. One or two femoral distractors, with pins above and below the knee, maintain distraction and permit easier handling and more accurate reduction of articular fragments.

Closure of the midline approach is performed in the reverse order of the

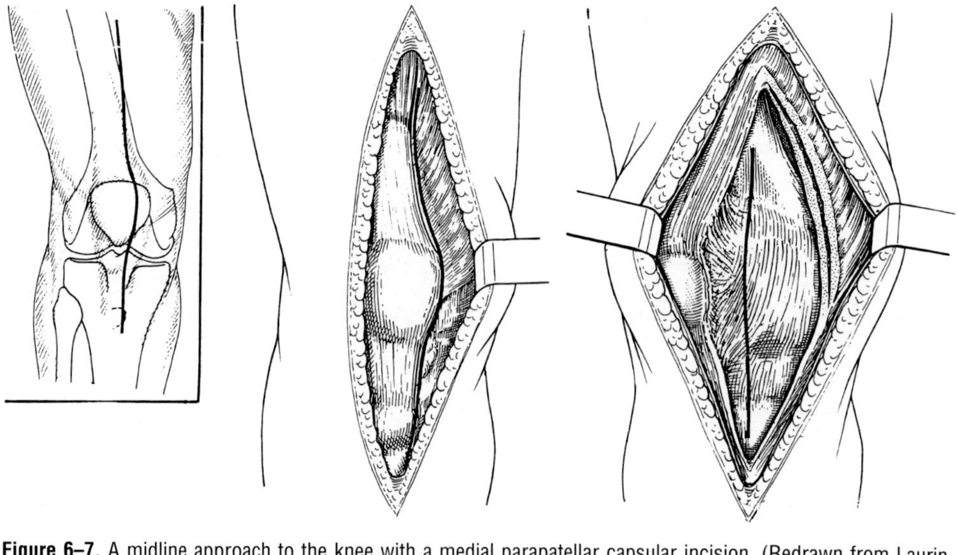

Figure 6–7. A midline approach to the knee with a medial parapatellar capsular incision. (Redrawn from Laurin, C. A., Riley, L. H., Roy-Camille, R. (Eds.): Atlas of Orthopedic Surgery, Vol. 3. Paris, Masson, 1992, p. 354.)

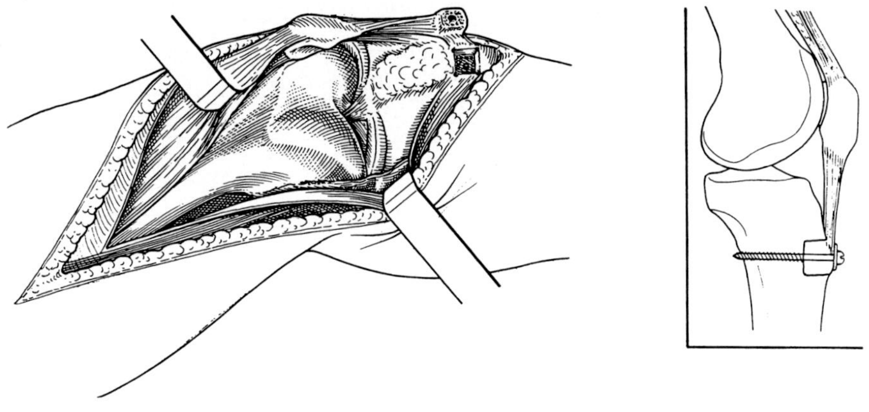

Figure 6–8. Osteotomy of the tibial tubercle. Note the drill hole in the tubercle for later reattachment. (Redrawn from Laurin, C. A., Riley, L. H., Roy-Camille, R. (Eds.): Atlas of Orthopedic Surgery, Vol. 3. Paris, Masson, 1992, p. 352.)

approach. The meniscal incisions are closed by interrupted sutures, and the meniscotibial ligaments are resutured. The tubercle is positioned in its original bed and secured by one or more screws that must engage the posterior tibial cortex. Suction drainage should be used. The synovia and capsule are then sutured in the parapatellar areas to the patellar tendon. Finally, the subcutaneous tissue and the skin are closed by skin clips so that continuous passive motion can be used early. After any of the extensive approaches has been used, wound healing becomes the first priority; the second priority is movement. The skin should be inspected frequently, and knee movement should be discontinued temporarily if skin problems develop.

An alternative to osteotomy of the tibial tubercle is division of the patellar tendon, reflecting the patella and infrapatellar fat pad proximalward. If the patellar tendon is divided, it will require resuture and probably further protection either by cast immobilization or preferably by a separate loop of wire from the patella to the tibial tubercle to prevent stretching or disruption of the repair. Thus, early motion of the knee may not be possible after patellar tendon repair, and the result might be a very stiff knee. Division of the patellar tendon should not be done unless other methods cannot be used.

The "Y" approach has been used for many years to visualize both tibial condyles.[958] The high incidence of wound slough and deep infection after its use has led many surgeons to use other approaches. Most surgeons now use either the midline approach or separate medial and lateral approaches.

SUMMARY

Preoperative planning of the surgical approach to treat a particular plateau fracture is crucial to the ease and success of the procedure. It is difficult to accurately reduce articular fragments if they cannot be seen. It is even more difficult to apply plates and insert screws through an inadequate approach. Prolonged firm retraction of skin edges is one cause of wound problems; therefore I advocate the use of generous approaches.

CHAPTER 7

Undisplaced and Minimally Displaced Fractures

Between 20 and 25% of proximal tibial articular fractures are undisplaced or displaced less than 4 mm. These are referred to as minimally displaced fractures even though they may resemble one of the other fracture types (Fig. 7–1). They occur in all age groups and involve one or both tibial plateaus. Seventy-five percent of minimally displaced fractures in the author's series involved one plateau, and 25% involved both (Table 7–1).

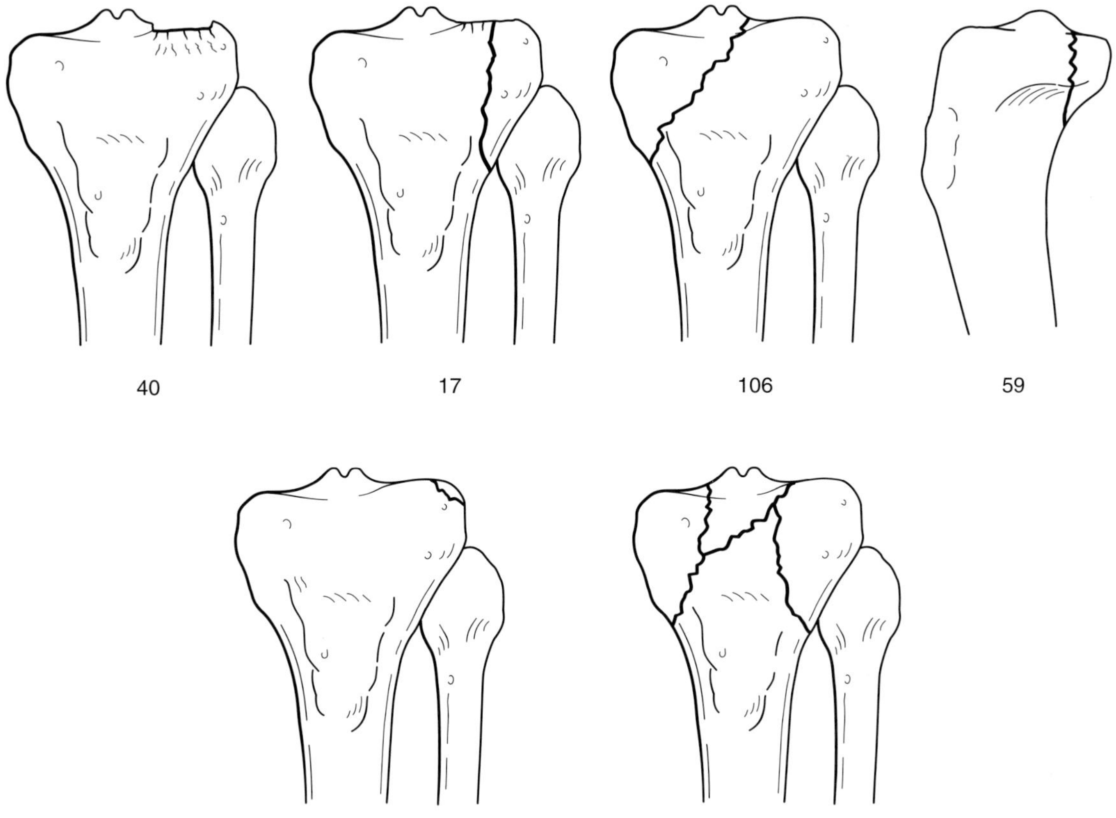

Figure 7–1. The numerical distribution of subtypes in 294 minimally displaced fractures. (The numbers of subtypes are shown.)

Table 7–1. MINIMALLY DISPLACED FRACTURES IN THE AUTHOR'S SERIES (N = 313)

Age	Average: 48	Range: 16–97
Sex	Male: 198	Female: 115
Knee	Right: 144	Left: 152
Both plateaus: (73)	Lateral: 174	Medial: 66
Depression	Average: 1 mm	Range: 0–3
Widening	Average: 1 mm	Range: 0–3
Instability >5 degrees	27%	

Fifty-eight percent of patients with minimally displaced fractures had another fracture or knee ligament injury in the same extremity. Forty-one percent of these were closed fractures, and another 11% had an open ipsilateral fracture (Table 7–2). Collateral or cruciate ligament injuries were noted in 10% of patients, some of whom also had associated ipsilateral fractures. The fibular head or neck was fractured in 34% of patients.

DIAGNOSIS

Minimally displaced fractures are by definition displaced or depressed less than 4 mm from normal anatomic position as noted by anteroposterior, plateau, and lateral x-ray views. If fracture lines are not seen clearly on these standard views, oblique projections or tomograms should be obtained. Assessment of knee stability by performing varus and valgus stress tests is essential to a complete diagnosis (see Fracture Diagnosis, Chapter 2). Stress x-ray will show whether instability is caused by torn collateral ligament or fracture movement. Twenty-seven percent of minimally displaced fractures in the author's series were 5 degrees or more unstable; about one third of the knee instability was due to collateral ligament injury.

HOW THE AUTHOR MAKES TREATMENT DECISIONS

I treat most isolated minimally displaced fractures that are stable to stress testing by closed methods. If the lateral plateau is fractured, closed treatment with plaster cast or fracture brace is adequate because such fractures rarely lose position (Fig. 7–2).

If the medial plateau or both plateaus are fractured, I advise percutaneous screw fixation supplemented by a fracture brace to provide assurance that the fracture will maintain position.[100, 238, 361, 424, 562, 663, 939, 1149]

If the knee is unstable to stress testing, I recommend percutaneous cannulated screw fixation and repeat stress testing in surgery. If the knee is then stable,

Table 7–2. INJURIES ASSOCIATED WITH MINIMALLY DISPLACED FRACTURES (N = 316)

Ligament injuries	10%
Fractures (167 patients)	
Subcondylar	27%
Tibial spine	14%
Patellar	<1%
Femoral condyle	<1%
Supracondylar	<1%
Femoral shaft	4%
Hip	1%
Tibial shaft	7%
Ankle	<1%
Multiple	5%

Total associated fractures = 215.

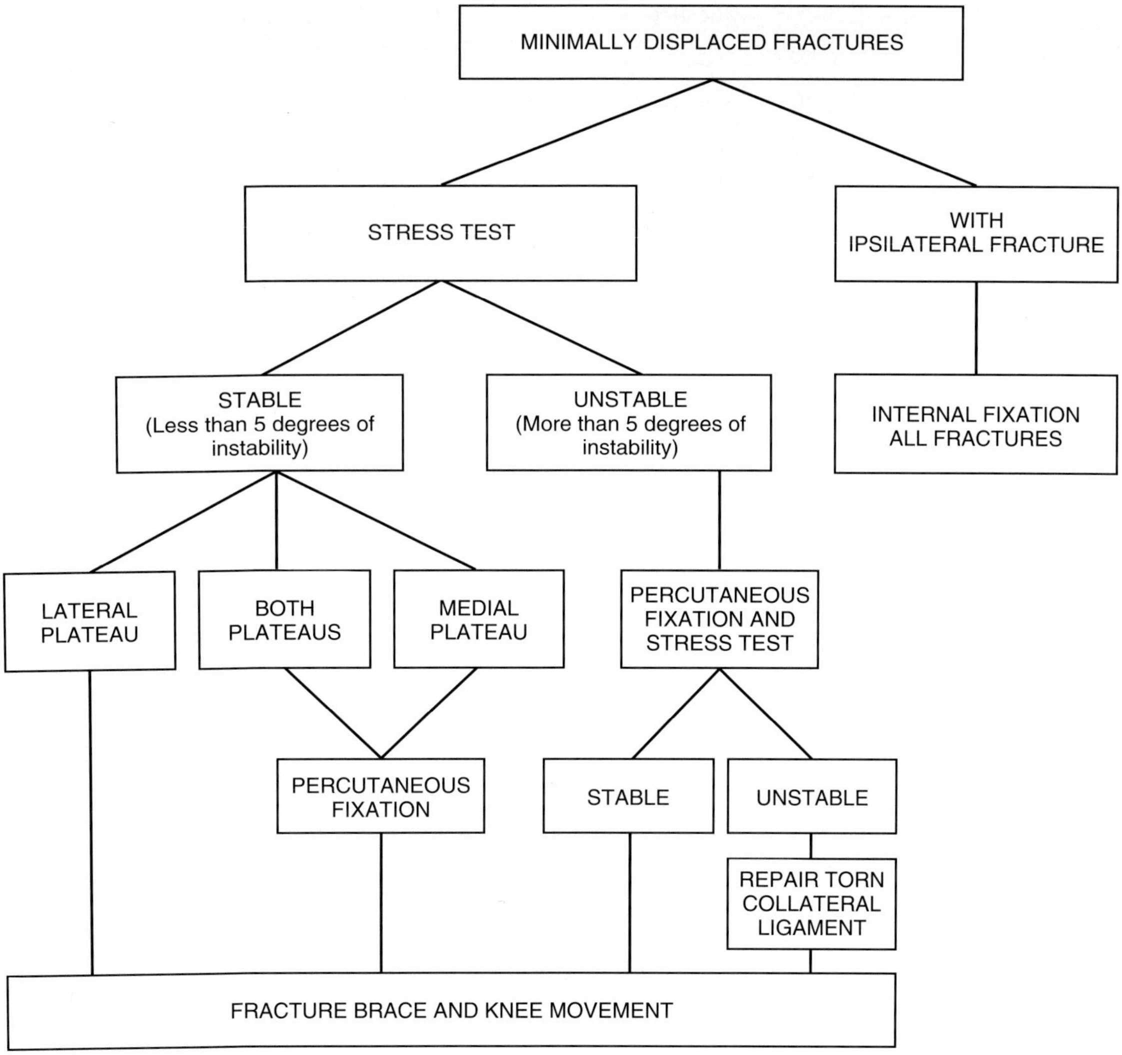

Figure 7–2. Treatment algorithm for management of minimally displaced fractures.

I use a fracture-brace. If the knee remains unstable, I repair the torn collateral ligament and use a fracture brace for postoperative support. If there is doubt about collateral ligament injury, stress x-ray in surgery will clearly indicate the cause of instability.

If there is another fracture elsewhere in the limb, I prefer to treat the minimally displaced fracture by percutaneous fixation or open reduction and the other fracture by appropriate internal fixation to hasten rehabilitation of the injured limb.

TREATMENT

In the last 20 years 84% of minimally displaced fractures in the author's series were treated by closed methods and only 16% required open management. A long-leg or thigh-to-ankle cast has been the traditional treatment, but fracture- or cast-braces are now being used more frequently because of their efficiency in controlling knee alignment and potential for allowing knee movement (Fig. 7–3). For the patient confined to bed by other injuries, traction and early passive and active knee movement are employed (Table 7–3).

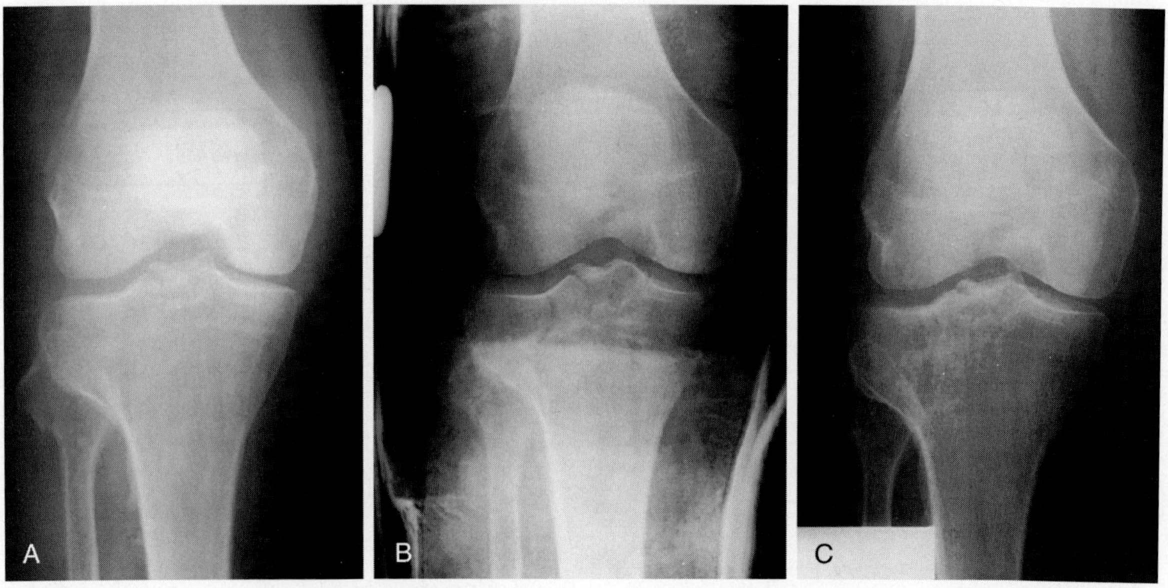

Figure 7–3. A minimally displaced lateral plateau fracture in a 56-year-old man treated in a cast-brace. *A*, Original anteroposterior view. *B*, In a cast-brace. *C*, The fracture healed after 3 months.

For minimally displaced fractures of the lateral plateau I prefer to use a cast- or fracture-brace for about 8 weeks or until fracture healing can be seen by x-ray. Since hinged braces provide knee movement as well as support, they are preferred to a cast because early movement hastens rehabilitation. Light weight-bearing with crutches is started at about 8 weeks and continued until the knee recovers strength and movement. Full weight-bearing is then begun.

Minimally displaced fractures involving the medial condyle or both condyles have a tendency to settle asymmetrically, resulting in varus deformity after healing (Fig. 7–4). Sarmiento and associates pointed out that an intact fibula promotes varus deformity by supporting only the lateral condyle.[940] These medial plateau fractures require special care in the selection and implementation of treatment. A long-leg cast does not maintain sufficient control over valgus-varus movement to prevent displacement.[564] Wedging of a long-leg cast in a direction

Table 7–3. TREATMENT METHODS USED IN THE AUTHOR'S SERIES (N = 319)

TREATMENT	1940–1973	1974–1994
Closed		
Functional	5%	5%
Fracture-brace	0	5%
Plaster cast	85%	47%
Traction	8%	10%
Closed reduction	1%	1%
Cast-brace	≤1%	16%
Total closed	(99%)	(84%)
Open		
Open—no cast	0	7%
Open—cast	<1%	5%
Open—traction	0	3%
Arthroscopic reduction	0	1%
Percutaneous fixation	0	0
External fixation	0	0
Total open	(<1%)	(16%)

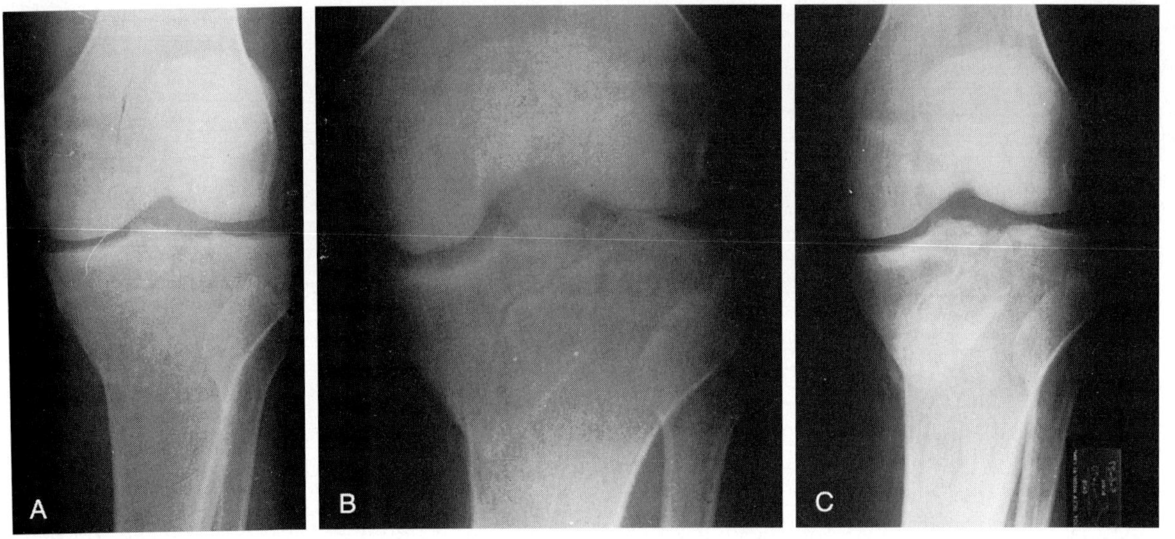

Figure 7–4. An oblique minimally displaced fracture involving the medial plateau, which was treated in a plaster cast. *A*, Note the obliquely oriented fracture line from the lateral articular surface to the medial tibial flare. *B*, After 2 months in a cast, the medial plateau has displaced. *C*, The fracture healed with a varus deformity at 5 months. (Reprinted by permission from Hohl, M.: Treatment methods in tibial condylar fractures. South. Med. J., 68:987, 1975; and from Hohl, M.: Complications of treatment of fractures and dislocations of the knee. *In* Epps, C. (Ed.): Complications in Orthopedic Surgery. Philadelphia, J. B. Lippincott, 1994, p. 546.)

opposite to the expected displacement is sometimes effective, but a more reliable method is to use a cast-brace or fracture-brace stressed opposite to the anticipated displacement as the hinges are affixed.[243] Traction protects against loss of fracture position, but may sometimes align the knee straight, eliminating normal knee valgus.[710]

Although rarely required for minimally displaced fractures, rigid internal fixation prevents loss of fracture position. Though percutaneous wire loops, multiple Kirschner wires, or threaded pins were used previously, cannulated screws provide more rigid fixation to prevent loss of reduction particularly in unstable fractures.[100, 377, 424, 884, 939] Minimally displaced plateau fractures with associated fractures about the knee (e.g., patellar, femoral condyle, subcondylar) should be rigidly fixed to minimize the likelihood of fracture healing with knee deformity and to promote early knee rehabilitation.

Regardless of the treatment method selected, x-rays should be taken weekly and compared critically with earlier views to ensure that fracture position has not changed.[454] If it has changed, an open treatment method should be used to correct the displacement.

Table 7–4. COMPLICATIONS IN MINIMALLY DISPLACED FRACTURES (N = 248)

No complication in 90%	Complication in 10%		
Complication	Treated closed (235)	Treated open (13)	Total (248)
Phlebitis	2%	8%	10%
Arterial injury	0	0	0
Compartment syndrome	0	0	0
Peroneal nerve injury	0	0	0
Wound infection	0	0	0
Fracture position loss	8%	0	8%
Avascular necrosis	0	0	0
Open fracture	1%	15%	2%
Other	<1%	0	<1%
Total	11%	8%	11%

Table 7–5. FOLLOW-UP RESULTS OF ISOLATED MINIMALLY DISPLACED FRACTURES (2–13 YEARS WITH A MEAN FOLLOW-UP OF 5 YEARS [N = 23])

Point rating	Average: 91	Range: 73–100
Pain	Barometric	None–mild
Flex deformity	None	None
Knee motion	130 Degrees	105–140
Deformity	1 Degree	0–10
Instability	1 Degree	0–10
Arthritis	None	None

COMPLICATIONS

Ten percent of the minimally displaced fractures in the author's series had complications (Table 7–4). Loss of fracture position was noted in 8% and only after closed treatment. The fractures that tended to displace usually had an oblique fracture line that involved the medial plateau (see Fig. 7–4). Fractures that involved only the medial plateau or both plateaus with an intact fibula also tended gradually to subside into a varus deformed position.[940] Another reason for loss of position may be the notion that a fracture is minimally displaced and is not a potential problem based solely on the initial appearance on x-ray. The forces that caused the fracture initially likely caused much greater displacement at the moment of injury than that seen by x-ray after the limb was placed in emergency splints. Such a fracture is predisposed to return to its original displaced position unless positive methods are used to prevent it.

If serial x-rays reveal a loss of position after closed treatment methods, open reduction with rigid internal fixation is used to restore anatomic position (see Table 7–4).

RESULTS

After follow-up of more than 2 years (mean of 5 years), twenty-three minimally displaced fractures without ligament injury or ipsilateral fracture, were found to be stable, well aligned, moved almost in a normal range without flexion contracture, and had a minimum of residual discomfort, if any. The mean point rating was 91 points (out of 100) (Table 7–5). Only 6% of minimally displaced fractures required a late surgical procedure once the fracture had healed.

Restricted movement was seldom a significant problem on follow-up evaluation in the author's series. Most authors have not commented on loss of motion after a minimally displaced fracture regardless of the method of treatment used.[29, 459, 729, 901, 905]

If there had been a collateral ligament injury in association with the fracture, the point rating result was 86, because of late knee instability and mild arthritic

Table 7–6. FOLLOW-UP RESULTS OF MINIMALLY DISPLACED FRACTURES ASSOCIATED WTH LIGAMENT OR IPSILATERAL FRACTURES (2–13 YEARS WITH A MEAN FOLLOW-UP OF 5 YEARS)

	WITH LIGAMENT INJURY (N = 3)		WITH ASSOCIATED FRACTURE (N = 27)	
Point rating	Average: 86	Range: 78–92	Average: 83	Range: 56–100
Pain	Barometric	None–Mild	Mild	None–Moderate
Flex Deformity	None	None	7 Degrees	0–15
Knee Motion	127 Degrees	125–135	118 Degrees	80–135
Deformity	None	None	2 Degrees	0–10
Instability	8 Degrees	0–15	3 Degrees	0–15
Arthritis	Mild	0–Mild	Mild	0–Mild

Table 7–7. LITERATURE RESULTS

AUTHORS	YEAR	FRACTURES	SATISFACTORY RESULTS (%)
Gylling and Lindholm[414]	1953	28	86
Apley[29]	1956	8	75
Hohl and Luck[459]	1956	29	93
Anger et al[24]	1968	17	59
Roberts[903]	1968	39	79
Porter[849]	1970	29	96
Hohl[450]	1974	50	86
Rinonapoli and Aglietti[901]	1977	42	93
Moore et al[728]	1987	69	90
Hohl (isolated)	1994	23	91

changes seen on x-ray. If there had been an ipsilateral fracture, the point rating result was 83 because of limited knee motion, including lack of full extension and mild traumatic arthritic changes (Table 7–6).

Published Results

Several authors have discussed treatment results in minimally displaced fractures. But each used his or her own definition of the term "minimally displaced," making comparisons difficult. The displacement or depression the authors discussed varied from 0 to 9 mm. Another problem was that some fractures in these series were not isolated minimally displaced fractures but were instead minimally displaced fractures with ipsilateral leg fractures.

The patients in these published series were treated predominantly by closed means and had generally good to excellent results.[24, 29, 414, 448, 459, 728, 901, 905] Immobilization for up to 2 months did not appear to affect knee movement at follow-up (Table 7–7).

SUMMARY

Minimally displaced fractures are seen in a wide variety of configurations, involving either one or both tibial plateaus with displacement or depression of less than 4 mm. References in the literature to minimally displaced tibial plateau fractures indicate that most of these fractures have satisfactory results. In the author's series, the presence of a collateral ligament injury or an ipsilateral fracture caused a significant deterioration in the result. When associated fractures are present, rigid internal fixation of both fractures is likely to produce the best results.[4, 562, 934]

CHAPTER 8

Local Compression Fractures

Local compression fractures are the most frequently encountered displaced fractures of the tibial plateau. They result from a combination of axial compression and valgus forces that push the lateral femoral condyle into the articular surface of the tibial plateau (Fig. 8–1).[538, 777, 1109] The most common type of fracture produced is a cup-shaped depression lined with fragments of articular surface. In local compression fractures, one to two thirds of the involved plateau is depressed a variable distance into the cancellous bone of the upper tibia (Fig. 8–2). A single depressed fragment is less common. Some local compression fractures also have a vertical fracture line starting just lateral to the depressed area and extending to the tibial flare.

The location of the depression and, to some extent, its depth depend on how much the knee is flexed as fracture occurs. If the knee is flexed only a few degrees, the depressed area will be in the middle of the plateau and will usually be no more than 6 to 8 mm in depth. If the knee is in greater flexion, the depressed area will be located more posteriorly with as much as 20 to 25 mm of depression.[1095] Local compression fractures tend to occur in a slightly older age group than do other plateau fractures (Table 8–1).

Ipsilateral fractures, ligament injuries about the knee, or both injuries together were present in 37% of local compression fractures. Fewer ipsilateral fractures (27%) were noted with local compression types than with other tibial

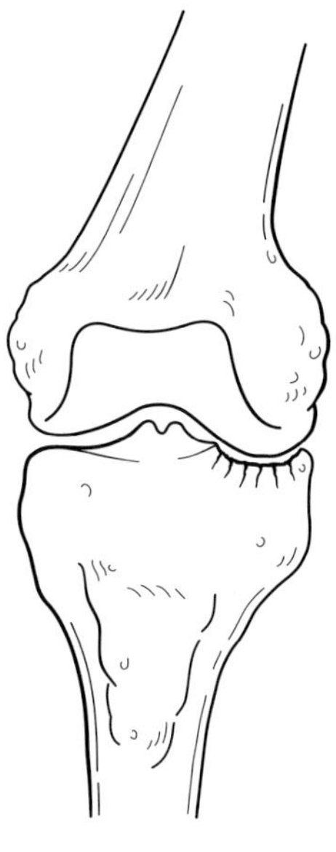

Figure 8–1. Valgus and axial loading forces have caused a local compression fracture. Note the lateral femoral condyle in the articular depression.

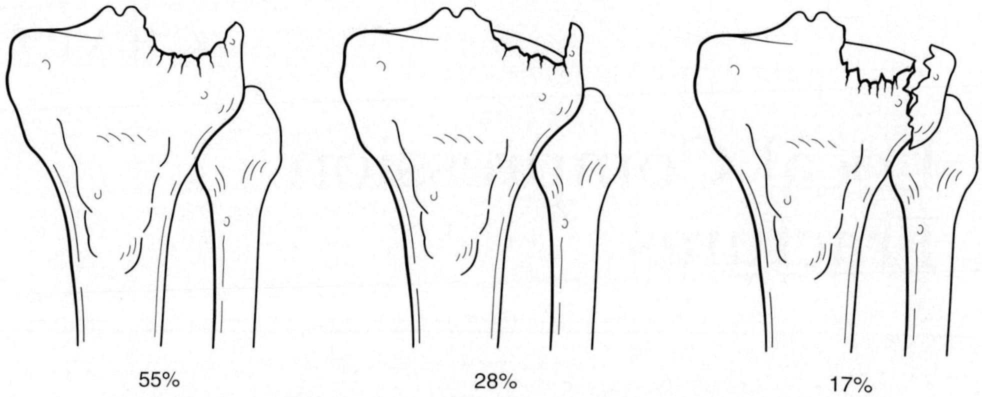

Figure 8–2. Diagrams and distribution of three subtypes of local compression fracture.

plateau fractures in the author's series. Additional fractures, especially those in close proximity to the knee, affect decision-making about treatment and have negatively affected long-term results.

Torn collateral or cruciate ligaments were noted in 12% of patients in the author's series. Ligament injuries affect treatment decisions and results; thus, their early diagnosis is important (Table 8–2).

DIAGNOSIS

An examination of the knee reveals joint swelling with tenderness over the fractured plateau. If collateral ligament injury has occurred, tenderness over the medial femoral condyle or along the course of the ligament will also be noted. Knee stability should be assessed by performing varus and valgus stress testing with the knee in extension and in a few degrees of flexion. Collateral ligament instability of 5 degrees greater than that of the normal knee is significant.[344, 457, 671, 911]

A local compression fracture can be distinguished from other plateau fractures by its radiographic appearance in anteroposterior and lateral views (Fig. 8–3). A portion of the articular surface is depressed, but the rim of the plateau is usually intact. Oblique projections provide a different view of the anterior and posterior aspects of the plateau and may show fracture lines that are not evident in the two standard views.[36] In some fractures there is a vertical split component that may produce confusion as to whether the fracture should be classified as a local or a split compression fracture. The crucial consideration is whether the split fragment has enough articular surface to support the femoral condyle when the fragment has been reduced. The author believes that the fragment should have at least 1 cm of articular surface for this support. Any fragment of this size or larger would indicate that the fracture is classified as a split compression fracture. Fractures with a smaller fragment are classified as local compression fractures.

Table 8–1. LOCAL COMPRESSION FRACTURES IN THE AUTHOR'S SERIES (N = 408)

Age	Average: 53	Range: 6–95
Sex	Male: 228	Female: 180
Knee (both 4)	Right: 170	Left: 229
Condyles	Lateral: 378	Medial: 21
Depression	Average: 10 mm	Range: 4–28
Widening	Average: 1 mm	Range: 0–8
Instability >5 degrees	75%	

Table 8–2. INJURIES ASSOCIATED WITH LOCAL COMPRESSION FRACTURES (N = 415)

Ligament injuries	12%
Fractures	
Subcondylar	12%
Tibial spine	6%
Patellar	<1%
Femoral condyle	0
Supracondylar	0
Femoral shaft	<1%
Hip	<1%
Tibial shaft	4%
Ankle and foot	1%
Multiple	4%

Total fractures in 110 patients = 119; fibular fractures in 23%.

Some local compression fractures cannot be seen, even on multiple x-ray views. If a fracture is nonetheless suspected, the knee should be aspirated under sterile conditions. Aspirate containing bloody effusion with fat globules is presumptive evidence of an articular fracture. To demonstrate such a fracture, the author obtains a magnetic resonance imaging study of the knee.[71, 711, 1144] This study will show an abnormal signal at the articular surface and in the subcondylar cancellous bone typical of a fracture.

In an unstable knee, a valgus stress x-ray demonstrates whether a fracture or a collateral ligament tear (avulsion or insubstance) is responsible for the instability.[68, 344] If a fracture is the cause of instability, the lateral femoral condyle is seen to dip into the fracture defect in the tibial plateau, but the medial cartilage space is not widened. If there is a torn ligament, the femoral condyle will dip into the articular depression and the medial cartilage space will widen even as much as 15 mm.

X-rays provide limited and often inaccurate information about the depth of articular depression because of magnification and variations in the tube angle in relation to the plane of the plateaus.[725] Several options allow accurate measurements of depressed areas: A plateau view as described by Moore and Harvey (Fig. 8–4), tomograms, or computed tomography (CT) scans.[263, 302, 316, 431, 725, 770, 844, 864, 865, 957, 1101, 1144] The author prefers CT scans to determine the number of millimeters of depression of the plateau surface in local compression fractures.

The anteroposterior position of the articular depression should be ascertained by lateral x-ray (if it can be seen) or by CT scan or lateral tomograms (Fig. 8–5).

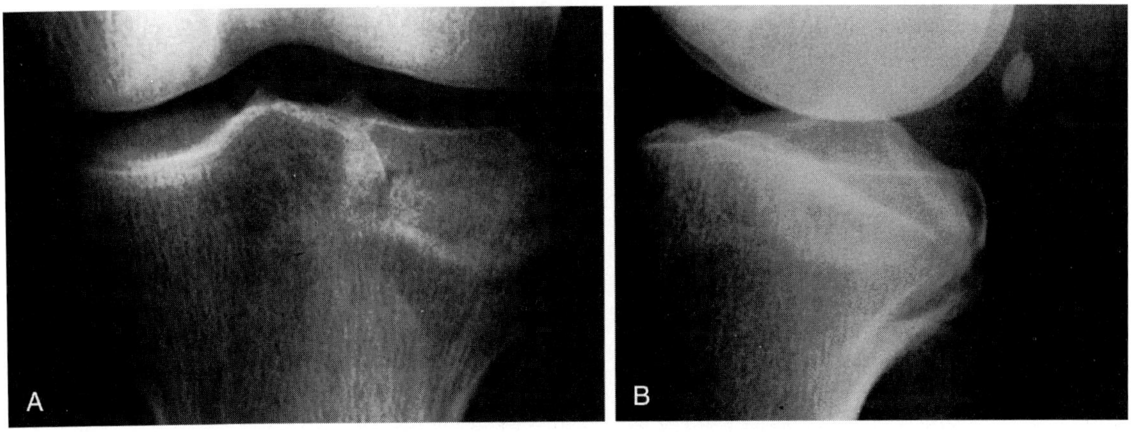

Figure 8–3. X-rays of a local compression fracture of the lateral plateau. *A*, Anteroposterior view with an articular depression. *B*, Lateral view locating the depression posteriorly.

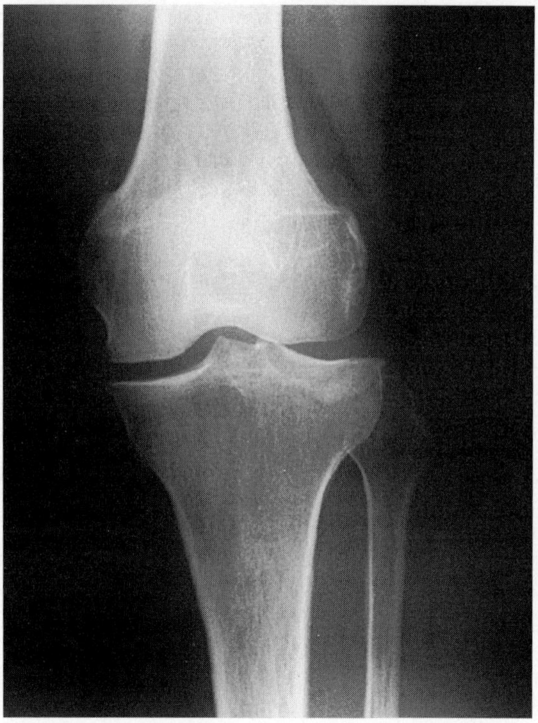

Figure 8–4. Plateau view (10 degrees caudal view). The line of vision is exactly across both plateaus.

HOW THE AUTHOR MAKES TREATMENT DECISIONS

The decision about whether to treat a particular local compression fracture by closed or operative methods is made on the basis of the amount of knee instability, the location and depth of the depression, and the presence or absence of an ipsilateral fracture (Fig. 8–6).

Functional treatment is appropriate for most patients older than 50 years of age with stable knees. This treatment could be as little as a soft dressing or a hinged brace to allow knee movement without weight-bearing until healing has occurred.

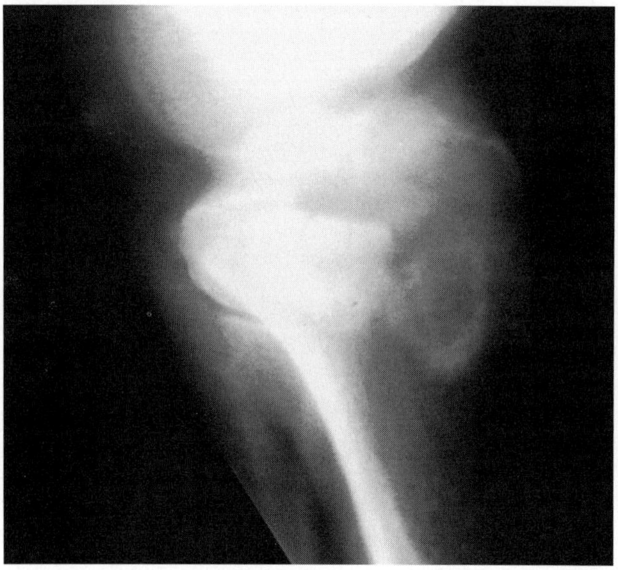

Figure 8–5. Lateral tomogram of a local compression fracture.

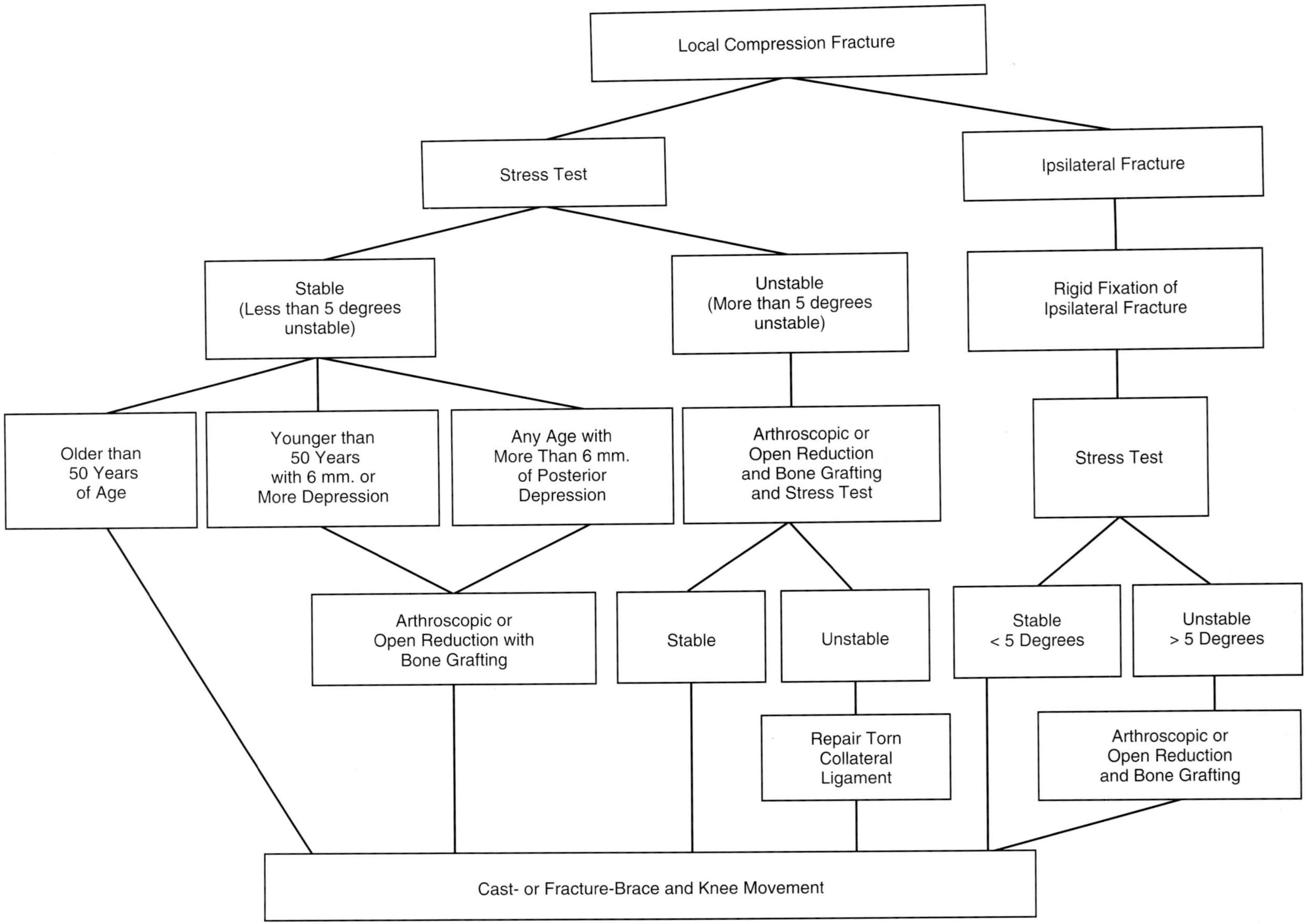

Figure 8–6. Treatment algorithm for local compression fractures.

The author usually treats stable knees by closed methods and unstable knees by surgical means.[873] There are some exceptions to this general rule however. In order to avoid articular irregularities that may lead to traumatic arthritis, patients younger than 50 years of age should have surgical reduction of a plateau depressed 6 mm or more even if the knee is stable to stress testing.[428, 848, 849] A posteriorly located depression in a patient of any age with normal knee stability should be elevated. If such a fracture is left unreduced, the knee will be unstable whenever it is in more than 40 degrees of flexion.[1095]

Knees with instability due to an uncorrected articular depression will remain unstable and during a long follow-up have a greater incidence of late traumatic arthritis than stable knees.[176, 871] The author corrects instability by surgically elevating the articular surface to a normal position.[810] Although this can be done either through an arthrotomy exposure or by arthroscopic visualization, the author prefers arthroscopic reduction in otherwise uncomplicated fractures because of the relative ease of obtaining good reductions with lesser morbidity. Instability noted on gentle stress testing after fracture reduction in surgery is caused by a torn collateral ligament. If such instability is present, the author restores knee stability by repairing the torn ligament and by using a fracture-brace postoperatively.[244, 553] Some surgeons prefer to repair lateral collateral ligaments surgically and treat torn medial collateral ligaments in a brace or cast for several weeks believing that they will heal.[879, 922, 1137, 1138]

If reduction by either arthrotomy or arthroscopic-assisted reduction is contraindicated in unstable knees, the alternative is to use a brace for long-term ambulatory support and accept some knee instability and deformity.

If there is a split fragment of bone associated with a local compression fracture, the depression can be reduced by arthroscopic or open reduction methods, and the fragment then fixed to the tibia by one or two screws with washers.

Patients with local compression and coexisting ipsilateral fractures (e.g., tibial or femoral fractures) should have all fractures reduced and fixed. Because a local compression fracture, despite an accurate reduction, can easily lose reduction, a cast- or fracture-brace is required until the fracture has healed.

TREATMENT

Closed

Local compression fractures that are treated by closed methods rarely continue to depress during the weeks required for bone healing.[873] The healing process repairs the bone. At the same time fibrocartilage grows from the fracture defects to smooth the articular surface. The amount of depression filled in by fibrocartilage is debatable.[508] If a depressed fracture is not elevated, the residual depression will cause some degree of permanent knee deformity and instability.

In the treatment of stable fractures by functional methods, aspiration of hemarthrosis, temporary splinting for comfort, knee motion as early as possible, and non–weight-bearing are used. A plaster cast is neither required nor helpful, except to protect the knee of an uncooperative patient from pain or additional injury. For patients confined to hospital for other injuries, light traction is a good choice because it decreases early fracture pain and encourages knee motion. Weight-bearing is deferred until signs of fracture healing can be seen on x-ray, usually 8 to 10 weeks after injury. Progressive weight-bearing is permitted as tolerated thereafter (Table 8–3).

Open

There are two ways to elevate articular depressions in current use. The method that is used most frequently is the arthrotomy method in which the

Table 8–3. TREATMENT METHODS USED IN THE AUTHOR'S SERIES (N = 408)

TREATMENT	1940–1973	1974–1994
Closed	N = 280	N = 128
Functional	5%	<1%
Fracture-brace	0	<1%
Cast-brace	0	9%
Plaster cast	73%	9%
Traction	7%	5%
Closed reduction	3%	2%
Total closed	88%	27%
Open		
Open—No cast	1%	20%
Open—Cast	12%	34%
Open—Traction	0	2%
Arthroscopic reduction	0	16%
Percutaneous fixation	0	0
External fixation	0	1%
Total open	13%	73%

fracture is disimpacted and reduced through a window in the tibial flare.[292, 346, 504, 848, 849, 890] The resultant defect in the metaphyseal bone is then packed tightly with bone grafts to support the elevated fragments. Cancellous screws may be used for additional support.[404, 831]

The other method is arthroscopic-assisted reduction in which the fracture is viewed using an arthroscope rather than directly. The remainder of the procedure is the same.[155, 346, 423, 456, 466–468, 491, 492, 1083] Early experience indicates that the arthroscopic method allows good reduction, is easier on the patient, and shows results that are at least as good as the arthrotomy method.[155, 346, 456, 504]

Technique of Operative Reduction

Open reduction by arthrotomy is performed through an anterolateral approach with the knee flexed 90 degrees. The fascia lata may be released partially from its tibial attachment or retracted superiorly after osteotomy of Gerdy's tubercle to expose the joint capsule. An incision through the meniscotibial ligament exposes the tibial plateau (see Chapter 6, pp. 44–45). The knee is stressed into varus by an assistant or by a femoral distractor that is applied anterolaterally across the knee. The extent of articular damage is assessed. A 1- to 2-cm window is made on the lateral tibial flare (some surgeons prefer the medial flare).[890] The fracture is reduced by carefully and systematically disimpacting and elevating the depressed fragments from the window using curved impactors or elevators to loosen fracture fragments and pushing or gently pounding these fragments to articular level. Image intensification is helpful to monitor the position of the impactors and progress of plateau elevation. Care must be taken to avoid separating cancellous bone from the articular surface or penetrating into the knee joint (Fig. 8–7). If the surface is unstable, two or three Kirschner wires may be inserted to hold the major fragments in position until bone grafting and supplementary fixation have been accomplished. Reduction of articular fragments leaves a defect in the cancellous bone of the proximal tibia that must be filled, preferably by bone grafts, to prevent redepression of the articular surface. Intraoperative plateau and lateral x-rays should be taken before closure to ensure that reduction has been accomplished.

Bone grafting is used to pack the defect created after elevation of the depressed articular surface. The iliac crest is the traditional source and gold

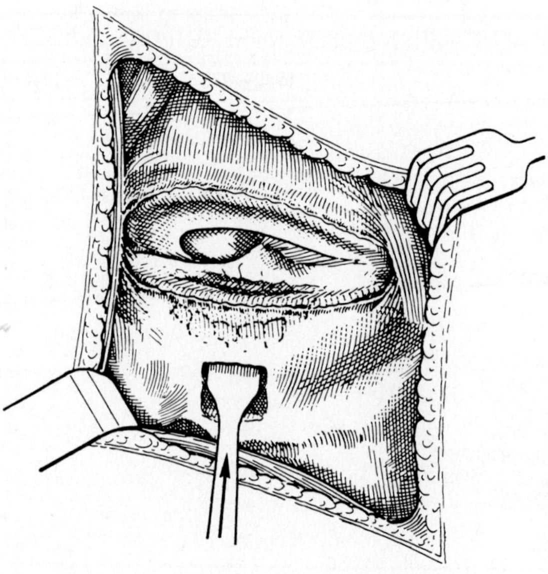

Figure 8–7. Elevating fragments through a tibial flare window and observing reduction of the articular surface. (From Laurin, C. A., Riley, L. H., and Roy-Camille, R. (Eds.): Atlas of Orthopedic Surgery, Vol. 3. Paris, Masson, 1992, p. 371.)

standard for bone grafts. Bone is packed tightly under the elevated surface so that it will resist pressure from the opposing femoral condyle.[810, 848, 849] Often during the several weeks required for bone healing, cancellous bone softens and compacts, and this may result in some loss of fracture reduction (Fig. 8–8).

Off-the-shelf bank cancellous grafts are being used increasingly instead of iliac bone, especially in older patients, because of ease of use and decreased morbidity from harvesting bone graft from the iliac crest.[272, 810, 1147] Bone substitutes of coral or other calcified materials are also being used successfully to fill bone defects.[127, 492, 691] Results after use of off-the-shelf and coral-based bone grafts are similar to those after use of iliac bone.[181, 492, 755] Under investigation currently is a biologically compatible injectable calcific material that solidifies and also provides fracture support.

When bone is osteoporotic or the fracture is very comminuted, cortical bone, used either as prop grafts or as a sheet beneath the articular surface is recommended because it provides nearly incompressible support for the plateau.[290, 571, 633, 819, 1131] These grafts are especially useful in osteoporotic bone because of their strength and durability. Allografts of cortical bone are almost universally available now and are used in preference to harvesting autologous grafts from the patient's own tibia. If allografts are not available, cortical struts can be harvested from the proximal tibia by extending the skin incision 3 or 4 inches down the tibial shaft. Appropriately sized and shaped grafts are then cut from the tibial cortex by a motor saw and inserted through slots made in the proximal tibia 1 cm distal to the lateral articular surface and into cancellous bone of the intact medial plateau to provide incompressible support for the elevated fragments (Fig. 8–9).

In elderly and infirm patients with osteoporotic bone, consideration can be given to filling the subarticular defect with acrylic cement for immediate strength to allow more rapid mobilization of the patient.[539]

In single fragment depressions or in normal quality bone, metallic internal fixation using Kirschner wires or preferably cancellous screws inserted under the elevated fragments can be used to help maintain reduction.[831]

Rarely the articular surface is so comminuted and destroyed that the best efforts to elevate and reduce fragments fail to produce a stable articular surface. In these instances, the surgeon may have to consider using an articular substitute. A bicortical iliac graft, fibular head, and patella have been used successfully for this purpose.[348, 494, 495, 601, 988, 1085]

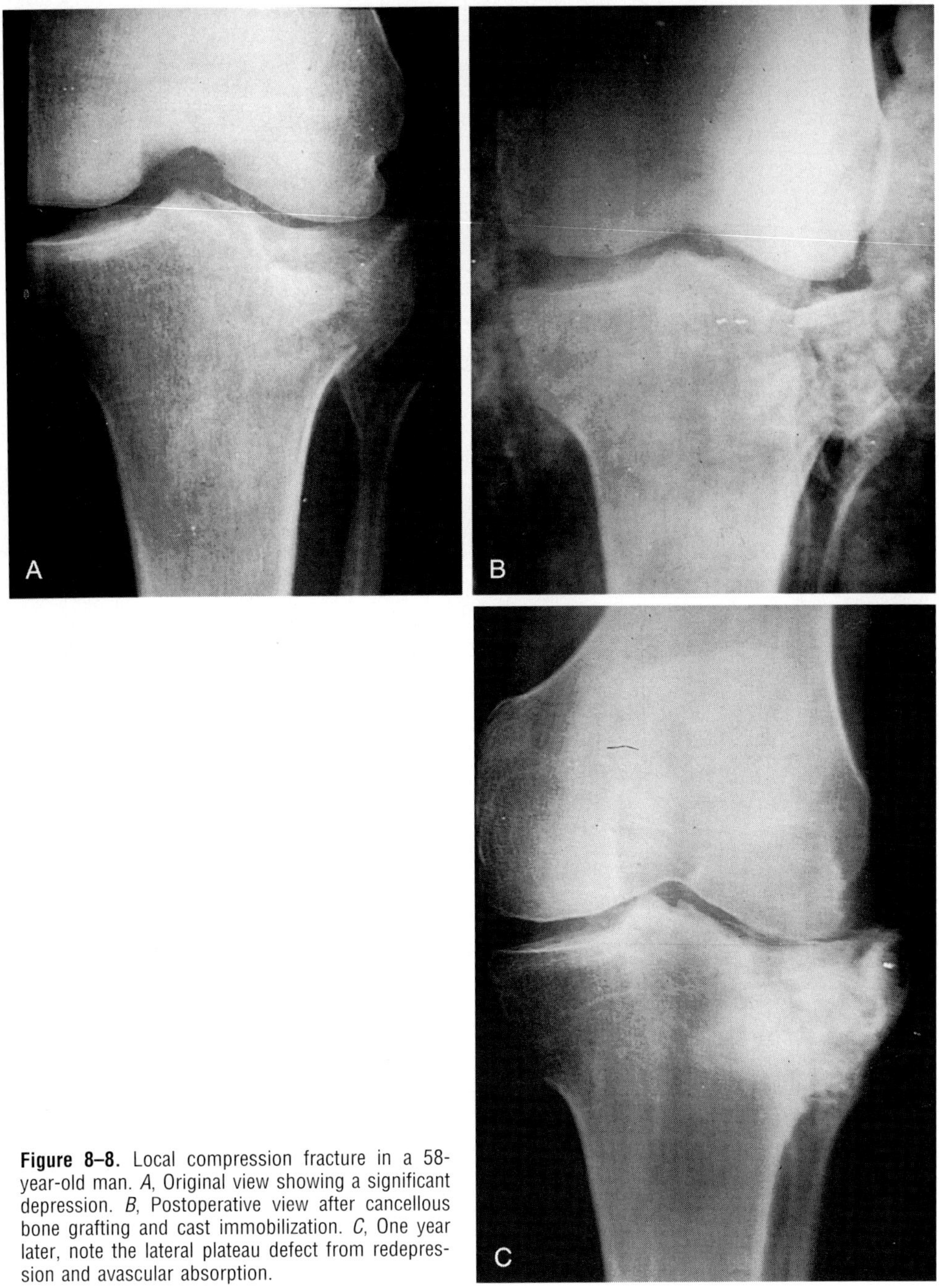

Figure 8–8. Local compression fracture in a 58-year-old man. *A*, Original view showing a significant depression. *B*, Postoperative view after cancellous bone grafting and cast immobilization. *C*, One year later, note the lateral plateau defect from redepression and avascular absorption.

Iliac substitution is the most convenient and least destructive of knee function.[348] In this technique a wedge-shaped piece of bicortical iliac bone is harvested and cleaned of soft tissue. Either the inner or outer surface has a shape that closely matches normal articular contours. The narrow end of the iliac graft is driven into cancellous bone beneath the intercondylar eminence. The graft is rigidly fixed by a plate and screws with cancellous grafts to fill the defect beneath the iliac graft (Fig. 8–10). Many good results have been reported with this method.[348]

Other articular substitutes, including the patella and the fibular head, have

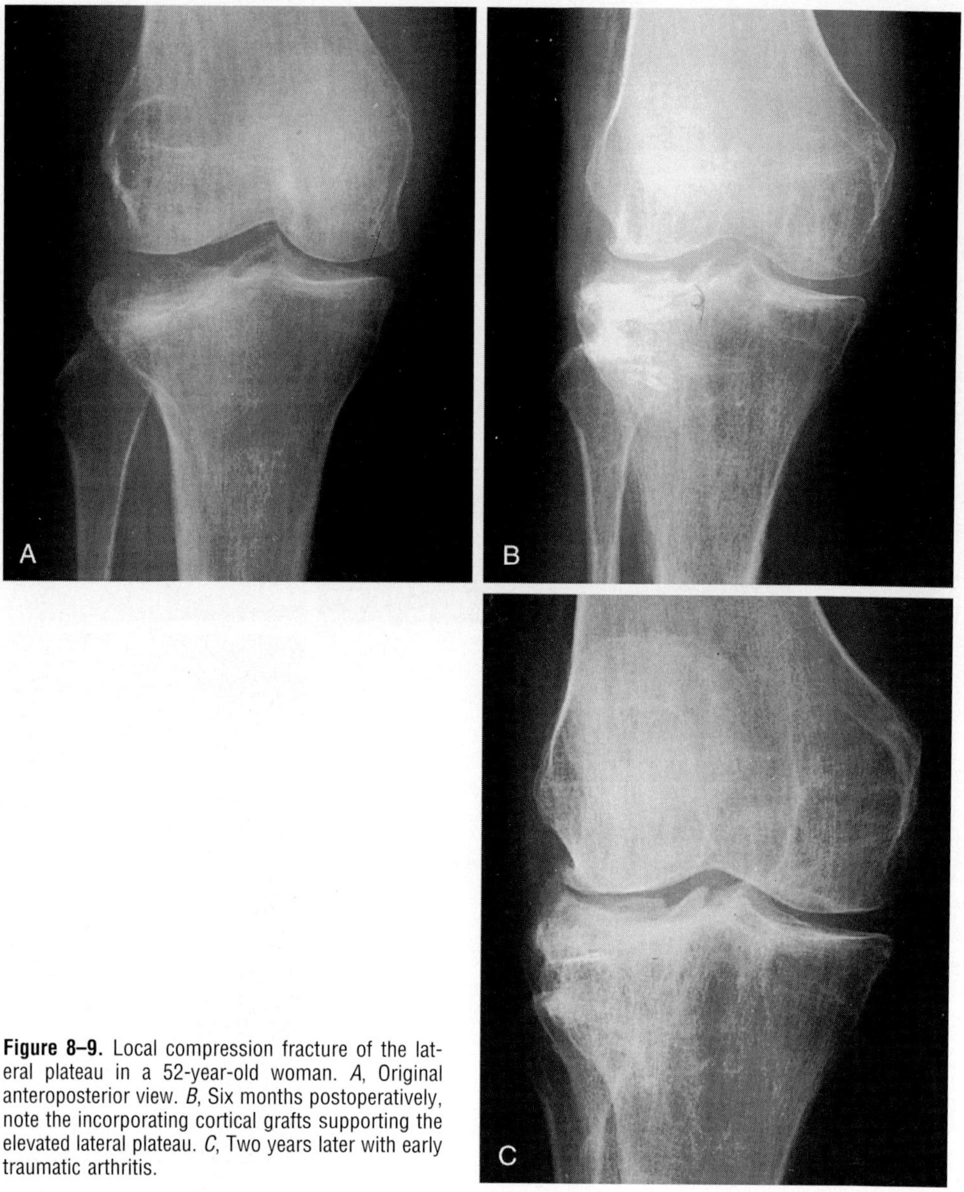

Figure 8–9. Local compression fracture of the lateral plateau in a 52-year-old woman. *A*, Original anteroposterior view. *B*, Six months postoperatively, note the incorporating cortical grafts supporting the elevated lateral plateau. *C*, Two years later with early traumatic arthritis.

been used.[494, 495, 843, 988] The advantage of these grafts is that articular cartilage is already present. The author prefers not to sacrifice the patella considering the potential loss of strength in the knee considering the satisfactory results from use of the ilium. In the infirm or very elderly, a unicompartmental knee replacement or a total knee replacement offers a reasonable early or late treatment alternative.[99, 352, 523, 592]

Technique of Arthroscopic Reduction

Arthroscopic-assisted reduction techniques have been used increasingly for more than a decade. The following suggestions come from the author's experience with such techniques.

The lateral tibial flare is exposed, and a 1- to 2-cm window is created well distal to the joint surface. This wound is temporarily packed for hemostasis. Parapatellar arthroscopic portals are created, and a suprapatellar drain is inserted. The use of a tourniquet for hemostasis has not been necessary in most

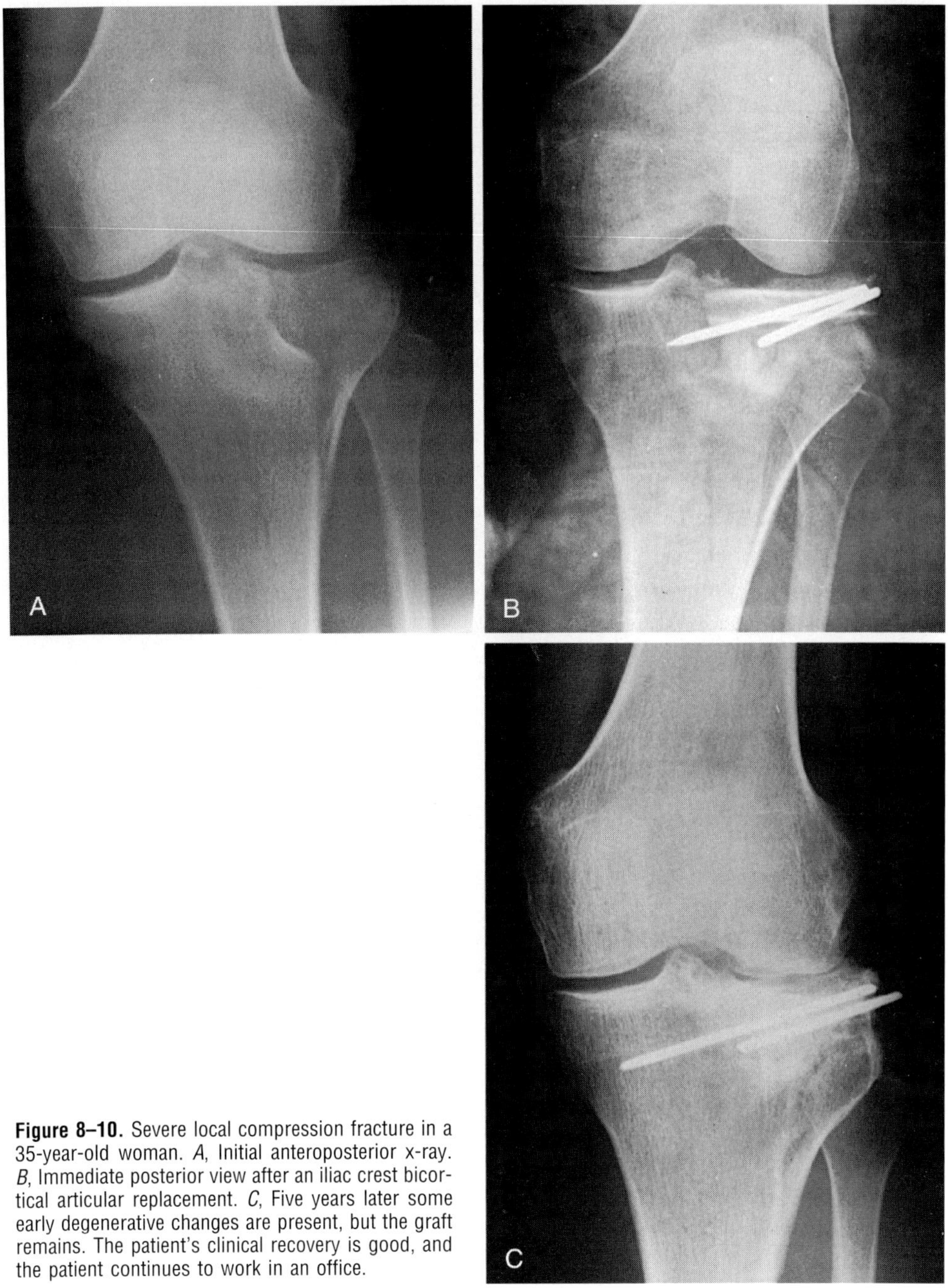

Figure 8–10. Severe local compression fracture in a 35-year-old woman. *A*, Initial anteroposterior x-ray. *B*, Immediate posterior view after an iliac crest bicortical articular replacement. *C*, Five years later some early degenerative changes are present, but the graft remains. The patient's clinical recovery is good, and the patient continues to work in an office.

patients. A pump is not used because of the likelihood of fluid escaping into the surrounding tissues. The arthroscope is inserted through either the medial or the lateral portal. Irrigation and débridement of debris and clots from the joint are carried out using a shaver. The fracture, menisci, and ligaments are evaluated. The lateral meniscus provides a reliable guide to the normal position of the articular surface (Fig. 8–11). The intact posterior rim of the tibial plateau is immediately distal to the meniscus. In a depressed fracture the meniscus will appear located well above the depressed surface. Disimpaction of the fracture is accomplished using various sizes and shapes of curved impactors. These im-

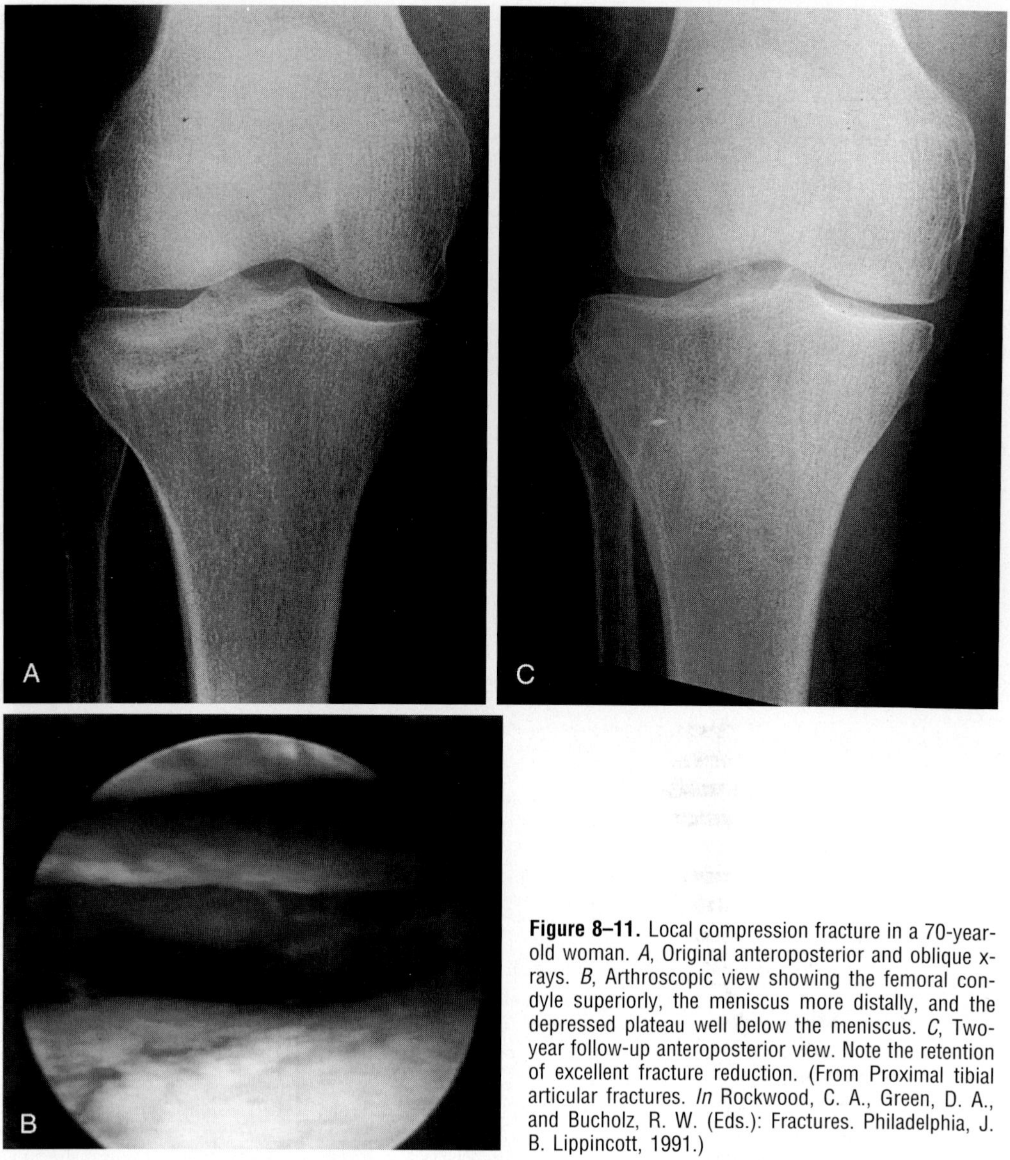

Figure 8–11. Local compression fracture in a 70-year-old woman. *A*, Original anteroposterior and oblique x-rays. *B*, Arthroscopic view showing the femoral condyle superiorly, the meniscus more distally, and the depressed plateau well below the meniscus. *C*, Two-year follow-up anteroposterior view. Note the retention of excellent fracture reduction. (From Proximal tibial articular fractures. *In* Rockwood, C. A., Green, D. A., and Bucholz, R. W. (Eds.): Fractures. Philadelphia, J. B. Lippincott, 1991.)

pactors are inserted through the tibial flare window and tapped upward under the depressed fragments until a normal articular level has been achieved. The impactor will need to be moved about frequently to ensure that all fragments are elevated uniformly and gradually. Overreduction of articular fragments is readily corrected by straightening the knee and allowing the femoral condyle to push them into position. Intraoperative plateau and lateral x-rays should be taken to ensure adequacy of reduction. The previously obtained iliac bone grafts (or bank bone grafts) are then packed tightly under the fragments, and the window is replaced. A cancellous screw or Kirschner wires may be inserted percutaneously if additional stability is required. A fracture- or cast-brace is used postoperatively to resist redepression of elevated fragments.

Another arthroscopic method involves drilling a guide wire through the tibial flare proximalward into the middle of the articular depression to more accurately and exactly elevate the depressed surfaces. First, a cruciate guide is used to insert a guide pin into the most depressed area of the plateau. Once the guide pin is in place, a large cannulated drill makes the entry hole into the tibial flare. Cannulated impactors then follow the guide pin directly to the depressed area, and the depressed area is gently elevated. The guide pin is then removed, and final elevation using various impactors is carried out to secure a uniform articular surface.[504] Bone grafts are finally packed under the elevated plateau through the drill hole as with previous techniques.

LIGAMENT INJURIES

One in nine local compression fractures has an associated medial collateral ligament injury. In patients older than 50 years of age, the medial collateral ligament usually avulses from its femoral origin rather than tearing through its substance. Ligament avulsions heal readily after a few weeks of immobilization, but some heal with ligament lengthening and cause late knee instability. Because of the uncertainty of knowing whether there is an avulsion injury or insubstance tearing of the ligament, the author recommends that both torn and avulsed collateral ligaments be repaired. If a torn ligament is not repaired, more than one half of the knees that had torn ligaments will be 10 degrees or more unstable 2 years or more after injury. Knees with repaired collateral ligaments showed less than 5 degrees of instability.[244]

Technique of Ligament Repair

Medial collateral ligament injuries are repaired either through a medial utility incision or a midline approach. Deep tissue ecchymosis often helps to localize the site of injury. Sufficient dissection is done to clearly expose the site of superficial and deep injury. Staples or sutures are used to fix avulsions to bone and sutures for midsubstance tears (Fig. 8–12). Postoperative support in a plaster cast for 5 or 6 weeks is usually advocated; however, studies of ligament healing suggest that some protected knee movement may enhance healing and eventual ligament strength.[1137, 1138] The author uses a fracture- or cast-brace after collateral ligament repairs and has not noted increased instability as a result.

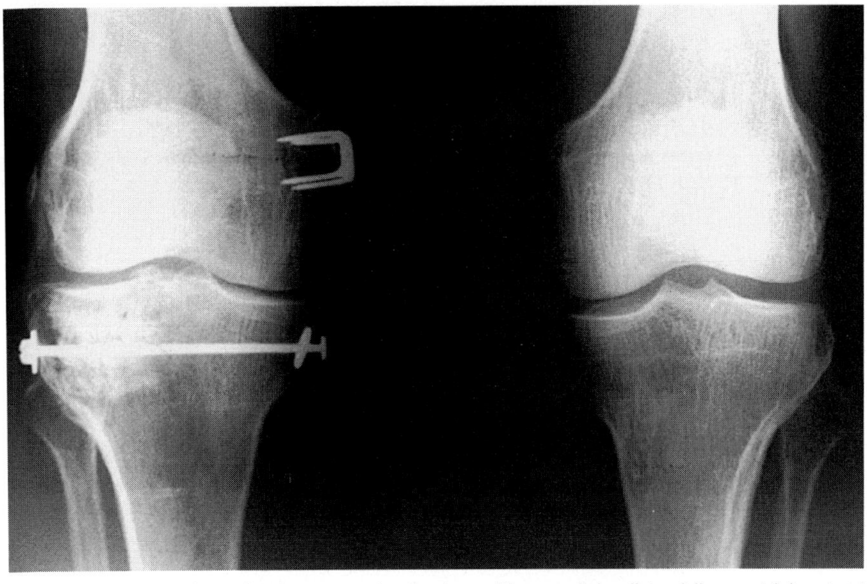

Figure 8–12. Two years after a local compression fracture with a medial collateral ligament injury treated by open reduction, cortical bone grafting, and stapling of the avulsed medial collateral ligament to the medial femoral condyle, this 47-year-old man had a stable and almost normally functional knee. (From Delamarter, R., and Hohl, M.: Ligament injuries associated with tibial plateau fractures. Clin. Orthop., 250:96, 1990.)

Postoperative Care

Pressure from the femoral condyle will cause redepression of an elevated tibial plateau unless measures are taken in the postoperative period to prevent it. Years ago it was shown that a long-leg cast, even stressed into varus position, does not sufficiently limit valgus-varus movement to prevent pressure on elevated plateau surfaces.[564] Either leg traction or a brace can be used to hold joint surfaces apart. The brace should be applied within a few days of surgery after the initial knee swelling has subsided. If a cast-brace is to be used, the surgeon should take part in its application to protect against valgus stresses as the quadrilateral thigh socket cast and the below-knee casts are applied. Then, as the surgeon applies varus stress, the hinges are fixed temporarily by hose clamps to the casts (see Fig. 7–3). Knee motion is then tested to ensure proper hinge alignment. Finally, the hinges are secured permanently by plaster or fiberglass. X-rays taken in the brace should show a slightly widened lateral cartilage space.

An important advantage of bracing is that knee movement can take place while the articular reduction is protected. At least 8 weeks of protection of the elevated joint surface is necessary to allow revascularization and healing of fracture fragments. Light weight-bearing begins at about 8 weeks, and full weight-bearing at 12 weeks. X-rays are taken every 10 to 14 days during the first 4 to 6 weeks to ensure that loss of reduction is not occurring.

Complications

Complications were encountered in 13% of local compression fractures, 5% after closed treatment and 23% after open treatment (Table 8–4). After closed treatment, 98% of fractures in the author's series did not develop additional depression.[874] In the unlikely event that the amount of depression should increase 3 mm or more before fracture healing, a change of treatment, most likely open reduction with grafting and fixation, is indicated to restore and maintain the articular surface.

One half of the postoperative complications were related to a loss of fracture reduction. The more rigid the grafting material used, the fewer knees suffered significant loss of reduction. Ten of 17 iliac grafted fractures lost some reduction as did only 3 of 14 fractures grafted with cortical bone. Half of 45 elevated surfaces in the author's series treated by any open method did not depress any further. Six of 45 surfaces depressed 6 mm or more. If a fracture heals after redepression of more than 3 to 5 mm, some type of reconstructive procedure, osteotomy, or articular replacement may be necessary to correct the resultant deformity.

Table 8–4. COMPLICATIONS IN LOCAL COMPRESSION FRACTURES (N = 346)

COMPLICATION (%)	CLOSED (N = 231)	OPEN (N = 115)	TOTAL (N = 346)
Phlebitis	<1%	<1%	<1%
Arterial injury	0	<1%	<1%
Compartment syndrome	<1%	<1%	<1%
Peroneal nerve injury	0	2%	<1%
Wound infection	0	4%	1%
Fracture position loss	2%	12%	5%
Causalgia	<1%	0	<1%
Open fracture	2%	1%	1%
Avascular necrosis	0	2%	<1%
Total	5%	23%	13%

Table 8–5. FOLLOW-UP RESULTS OF ISOLATED LOCAL COMPRESSION FRACTURES (MEAN FOLLOW-UP OF 7 YEARS [2–13 YEARS])

	AVERAGE	RANGE
Point rating	84	36–100
Pain	Occasional	None–Mild
Flex deformity	9 Degrees	None–10 Degrees
Knee motion	128 Degrees	50–140 Degrees
Deformity	7 Degrees	None–15 Degrees
Instability	5 Degrees	None–15 Degrees
Arthritis	Minimal	None–Moderate

No associated fractures or ligament injuries.
Total number of fractures = 97.

Results

Functional results, in general, after local compression fractures have been satisfactory.[149, 428, 462, 848, 849, 874] It is rare to observe much loss of motion in patients treated by closed methods; however, after operative reduction, especially if the knee was immobilized for more than 6 weeks, there may be permanent loss of at least a few degrees of motion. Early movement with the protection of a knee brace has largely resolved this problem (Table 8–5).

In the author's series, the mean point rating after a local compression fracture was 84, and many patients had flexion deformity and restriction of knee motion at a mean follow-up of 7 years. Patients who underwent surgical elevation of the depressed fracture had a point rating of 87 and had a lesser incidence of deformity and instability. Patients treated by closed methods rated 82 and had somewhat more deformity and instability (Table 8–6).

Collateral ligament injuries had a significant effect on outcome. If a torn ligament was diagnosed but unrepaired, the point rating was 62. Although some of these patients had open elevation of the depressed plateau, the majority were treated by closed methods with a plaster cast. If the torn ligament was repaired along with elevation of the plateau, the point rating was 86 and knee stability considerably improved. Traumatic arthritic changes were present in more than half of those with unrepaired ligament injuries and only 13% of those with repaired ligaments (Table 8–7).

If a ligament injury or an ipsilateral fracture was present, the point ratings were 72 and 75, respectively, with a greater restriction of knee motion and instability (Table 8–8).

The long-term problems most frequently noted have been knee deformity and instability. Valgus deformity and instability tend to go together and are

Table 8–6. FOLLOW-UP RESULTS BY CLOSED AND OPEN TREATMENT (MEAN FOLLOW-UP OF 6 YEARS [2–29 YEARS])*

	CLOSED TREATMENT	OPEN TREATMENT
	Average	Average
Point rating	82	87
Pain	Mild	Mild
Flex deformity	1 Degree	1 Degree
Knee motion	128 Degrees	130 Degrees
Deformity	7 Degrees	5 Degrees
Instability	6 Degrees	5 Degrees
Arthritis	Mild	Mild

*No associated fracture or ligament injury. Closed treatment used in 56 cases; open treatment used in 41 cases.

Table 8–7. RESULTS AFTER COLLATERAL LIGAMENT INJURIES (MEAN FOLLOW-UP OF 5 YEARS)

	COLLATERAL LIGAMENT INJURIES			
LIGAMENT	**Number**	**Point Rating**	**Mean Stability (Degrees)**	**Arthritis (%)**
Repaired	8	86	3	13
Unrepaired	11	62	10	55

Table 8–8. FOLLOW-UP RESULTS OF LOCAL COMPRESSION FRACTURES ASSOCIATED WITH LIGAMENT OR IPSILATERAL FRACTURES (MEAN FOLLOW-UP OF 7 YEARS [2–13 YEARS])

	LIGAMENT INJURY	**IPSILATERAL FRACTURE**
	Average	**Average**
Point rating	72	75
Pain	Barometric ache	Mild
Flex deformity	4 Degrees	8 Degrees
Knee motion	115 Degrees	123 Degrees
Deformity	7 Degrees	7 Degrees
Instability	7 Degrees	6 Degrees
Arthritis	Moderate	Mild

Patients with ligament injury = 19; patients with ipsilateral fractures = 30.

Table 8–9. POINT RATING IN ISOLATED LOCAL COMPRESSION FRACTURES BY DEPRESSION REMAINING AFTER FRACTURE HEALING

FINAL DEPRESSION (MM)	DEFORMITY (DEGREES)	POINT RATING	%
0	0	97	2
1	1	95	4
2	3	93	7
3	4	92	8
4–5	6	91	20
6–8	8	84	7
9–11	10	79	28
>12	11	68	24

usually caused by residual articular depression. The degree of deformity depends on the number of millimeters of depression that remain in the mid to anterior portion of the tibial plateau (Table 8–9).

Initial fracture depression also bears some relationship to the result. In the author's series, fractures with less than a 5-mm depression (all treated by closed means) had an average point rating of 86 at follow-up and showed a minimum of valgus deformity and instability. Regardless of whether treated closed or operatively, fractures that were depressed between 7 and 9 mm had a point rating of 80. However, fractures depressed 10 to 12 mm treated closed rated 76, and those treated operatively rated 82. With a depression of more than 13 mm, there was little difference between closed or operative treatment. The mean point rating for stable local compression fractures followed for more than 2 years was 95. Unstable fractures that were treated closed averaged 81 points, and those treated operatively averaged 84 points. Traumatic degenerative changes at more than 5 years' follow-up were noted in 36% of fractures, less than the average in most other plateau types (42%). Fractures with final instability of 5 degrees or less had 13% moderate to severe arthritis and a point rating average of 87. Fractures with more than 5 degrees of instability had 28% moderate to severe arthritis and an average point rating of 67.

Thirteen percent of local compression fractures required a later surgical procedure to correct residual problems after a fracture or to remove metallic implants.

SUMMARY

Local compression fractures recover knee motion readily but have residual problems of instability and deformity in a significant number of patients treated either by closed or operative methods. Postoperative knee support is exceptionally important to the retention of fracture position after open or arthroscopic reduction.

CHAPTER 9

Split Compression Fractures

Split compression fractures (23% of displaced tibial plateau fractures) consist of a wedge-shaped articular fragment and a depressed fracture of some of the remaining articular surface (Fig. 9–1). Valgus and axial forces produce this predominantly lateral plateau fracture.[538] These forces, exerted through the femoral condyle, split off a tibial articular fragment, drive the femoral condyle into the remaining joint surface, and depress that surface (Fig. 9–2).

This type of fracture should not be confused with one variety of local compression fracture that has a small split fragment in addition to a depressed area on the remaining tibial plateau (see Fig. 8–10A). The treatment of each type is quite different, because the split fragment in local compression fractures has so little articular surface that it cannot be relied on to provide support for the femoral condyle when reduced to its normal position. Split fragments in split compression fractures have enough articular cartilage to support the femoral condyle (Fig. 9–3).

If the split fragment can be reduced and made to heal in its normal position, the femoral condyle will be supported and knee alignment restored. Although satisfactory reduction of the split fragment can often be accomplished by closed reduction, the depressed articular surface cannot be elevated except by surgical means. Most surgeons prefer to do open reduction with internal fixation so that the articular depression can be elevated and the split fragment fixed in anatomic position. A significant advantage of internal fixation is that early movement and rehabilitation of the knee can help to minimize late knee stiffness. Ninety percent of split compression fractures in the author's series were surgically treated during the last 20 years (Table 9–1).

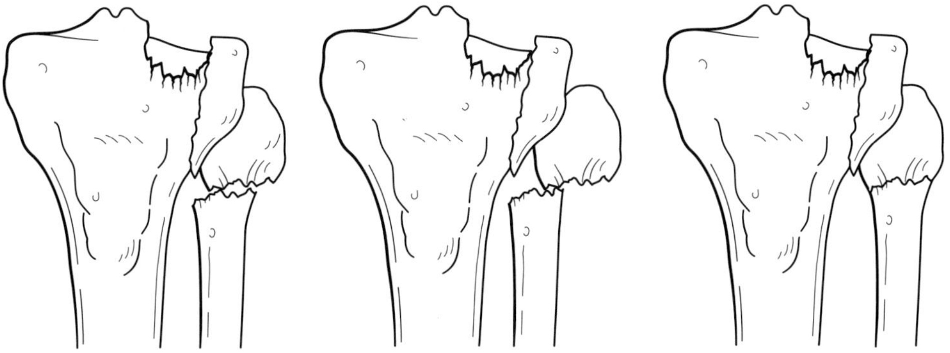

Figure 9–1. Split compression fracture subtypes and their frequency.

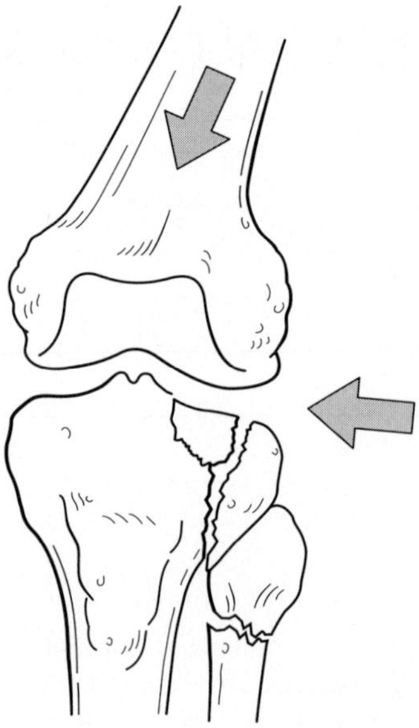

Figure 9–2. Valgus and axial compression forces create a split compression fracture.

DIAGNOSIS

Knee examination reveals swelling and effusion with tenderness over the fractured plateau. If there is also tenderness over the course of the medial collateral ligament, a ligament injury must be suspected.[68, 244, 457, 1122] Stress testing in valgus and varus directions should be done to assess knee stability. If stress testing with the knee in extension or in a few degrees of flexion indicates more

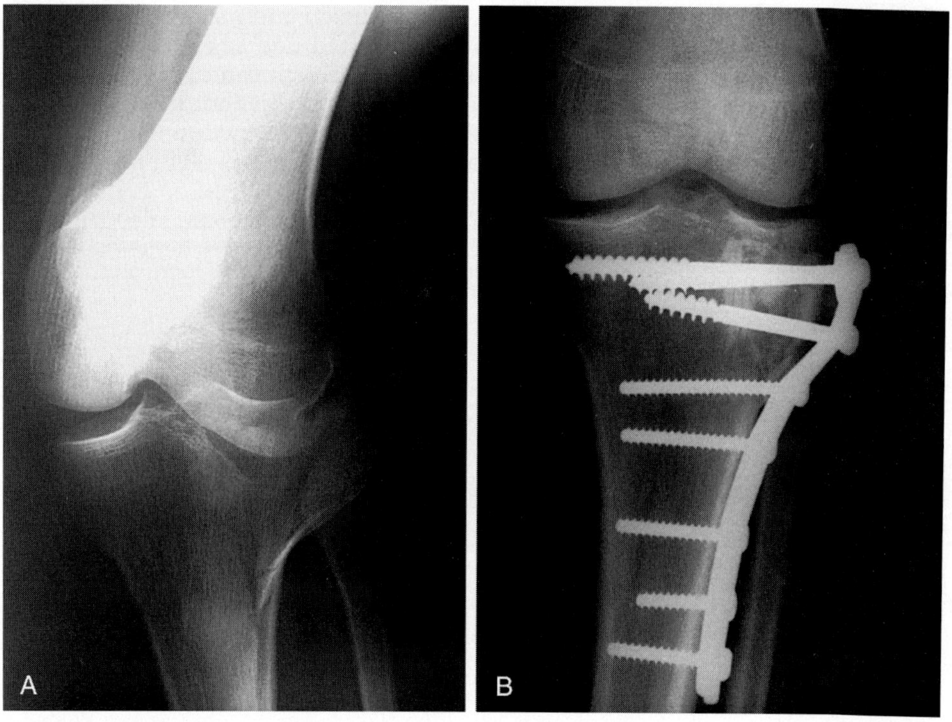

Figure 9–3. Split compression fracture with a marked depression. *A*, Anteroposterior view. *B*, Postoperative view after bone grafting and buttress plating.

Table 9–1. SPLIT COMPRESSION FRACTURES IN THE AUTHOR'S SERIES (N = 283)

Age	Average: 48	Range: 15–86
Sex	Male: 170	Female: 105
Knee	Right: 107	Left: 172
Plateau	Lateral: 268	Medial: 11
Depression	Average: 11 mm	Range: 4–30
Widening	Average: 5 mm	Range: 0–20
Instability >5 degrees	87%	

than 5 degrees of laxity compared with the opposite knee, instability is present.

Anteroposterior and lateral x-ray views show the size of the split fragment, its lateral displacement (tibial widening), and its depression below normal articular level. These views also show a depressed fracture in the remaining articular surface and its anteroposterior location. Standard x-ray views give variable and inaccurate measurements of the depth of depression because of magnification and the normal posterior tilt of the tibial plateaus. More accurate measurements can be made from Moore's[725] plateau view, anteroposterior and lateral tomograms,[770] or computed tomography (CT) scans[263, 864] (Fig. 9–4A and B).

The cause of knee instability, whether from fracture movement or ligament injury, is easily determined with stress x-rays. Valgus stress reproduces the mechanism of injury, temporarily further displacing the split fragment and causing the lateral femoral condyle to dip into the depressed tibial plateau. Permanent displacement of the split fragment has not been observed; instead it returns to a prestress position when the force is stopped. If there is a torn medial collateral ligament, the medial cartilage space will be significantly widened[671] (see Fig. 9–4C). If there is no collateral ligament injury, the medial cartilage space remains normal. Collateral ligament tears have been reported in 19% of split compression fractures.

Forty-two percent of split compression fractures in the author's series were associated with other injuries in the same extremity. Ipsilateral fractures were found in 32% (2% were open fractures) and ligament injuries in 20% (Table 9–2).

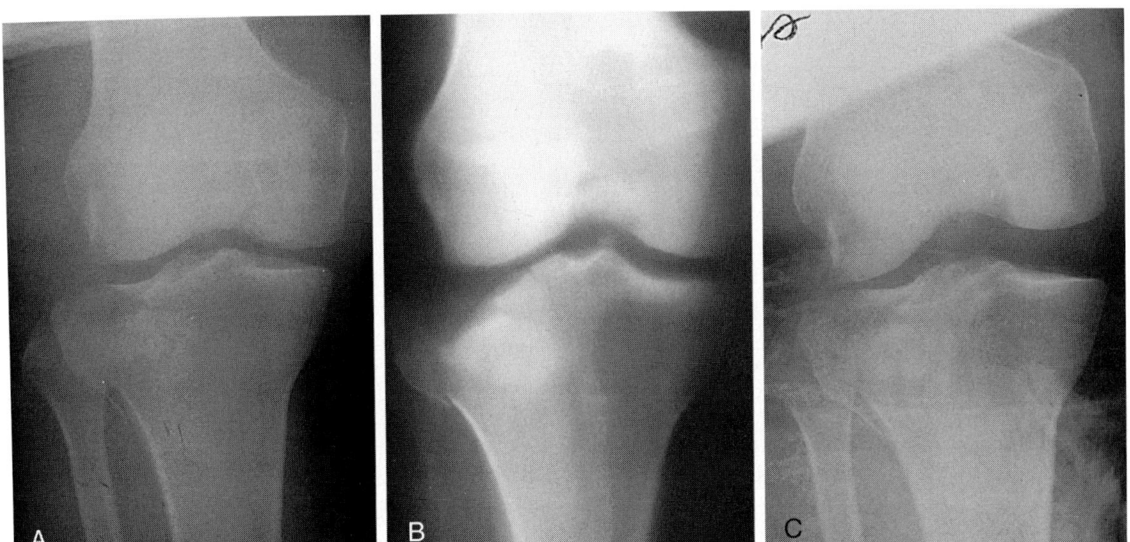

Figure 9–4. Split compression fracture in a 27-year-old man. *A*, Original anteroposterior view. *B*, Tomogram showing the depressed lateral articular surface. *C*, Valgus stress showing a medial collateral ligament injury.

Table 9–2. INJURIES ASSOCIATED WITH SPLIT COMPRESSION FRACTURES (N = 271)

INJURY	%
Ligament injury	20
Fractures	
Subcondylar	14
Tibial spine	10
Patellar	<1
Femoral condyle	<1
Supracondylar	0
Femoral shaft	0
Hip	0
Tibial shaft	4
Ankle	3
Multiple	2

Total fractures in 87 patients = 93; fibular fractures in 56%.

If internal fixation is planned, stress testing of the knee can be deferred until just after rigid fracture fixation has been accomplished; then both valgus and varus stress is applied. If the fixation has not restored knee stability, either the reduction was not anatomic or there is a torn collateral ligament. If torn, ligament repair is carried out to ensure optimum long-term knee stability.

HOW THE AUTHOR MAKES TREATMENT DECISIONS

The author uses operative treatment (usually open but occasionally arthroscopic-assisted reduction) in most split compression fractures in the belief that articular reduction is more accurate and the results significantly better than when closed methods are used with similarly displaced fractures. The author performs stress testing on isolated split compression fractures (Fig. 9–5).

If the knee is stable and the x-ray demonstrates less than 3 mm of tibial widening, the author uses a cast- or fracture-brace and takes x-rays during the initial few weeks to ensure retention of position. If there is 3 mm or more of tibial widening, the author uses open or arthroscopic-assisted reduction with a buttress plate and encourages early knee movement.

The author uses open reduction and rigid internal fixation for unstable split compression fractures. Once the fracture has been internally fixed, the author again performs stress testing, and if the fracture is stable, early knee movement is begun. If the knee remains unstable, the author repairs the torn collateral ligament and uses a fracture-brace postoperatively.

Plateau fractures and any associated ipsilateral fractures are treated by operative means along with the ipsilateral fracture in order to hasten rehabilitation of the leg.

TREATMENT

Some form of open (or in selected cases, arthroscopic-assisted) reduction and internal fixation is used in the majority of split compression fractures due to the relative ease of the procedure and the satisfactory results obtained (Table 9–3).

Split compression fractures with little lateral displacement of the split fragment and with depression of 6 mm or less have been treated by plaster cast, cast-brace, traction, closed reduction, or percutaneous fixation. Plaster cast treatment is not recommended, because it provides insufficient support to maintain fracture position and often results in knee stiffness from immobilization of 2 months or more[224, 564] (Fig. 9–6). Cast-bracing has the advantage of controlling angular knee stresses to prevent loss of fracture position while still allowing

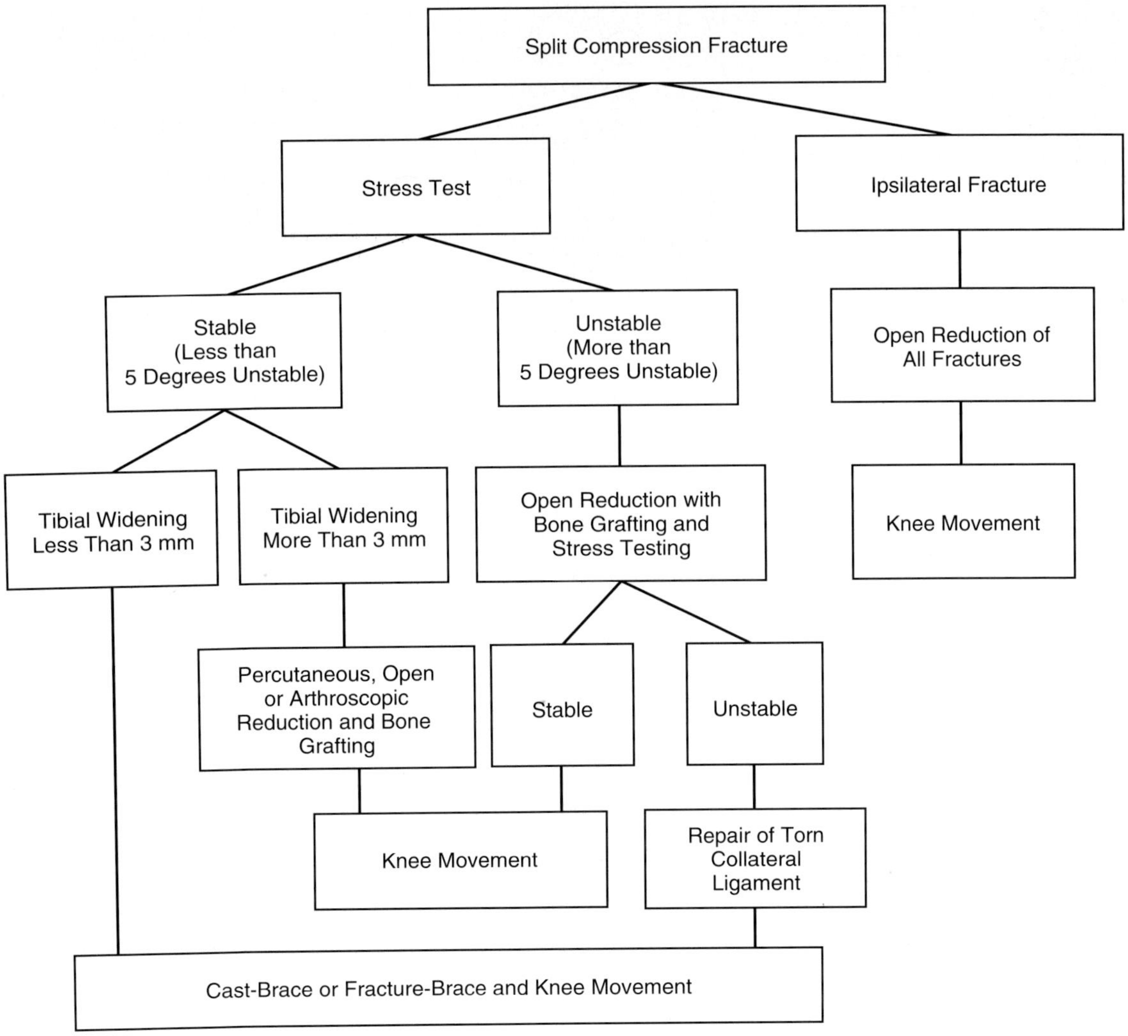

Figure 9–5. Treatment algorithm for split compression fractures.

movement of the joint.[122, 243, 289, 721, 972] Skeletal traction, although acceptable in terms of the aforementioned conditions, requires several weeks of hospitalization. When closed reduction under anesthesia is used, the split fragment can be reduced accurately but the articular depression remains.

Open Reduction

Since these fractures almost always involve the lateral tibial plateau, an anterolateral approach provides adequate visualization of both the split fragment and the depressed articular area. After the skin and subcutaneous tissues have been opened, the anterior fracture gap of the split fragment is identified. The coronary ligament is divided at the anterior meniscotibial interval. This inframeniscal approach to the joint permits inspection of the lateral meniscus for peripheral or insubstance tears. If no insubstance meniscal tear is found, the meniscus is preserved for later resuture (see Chapter 6). Only essential soft tissue stripping of the split fragment should be done to avoid delayed healing or necrosis because of devitalization of the fragment. Once the fracture site has been identified, cleaned, and irrigated, the depressed articular fragment is visualized by gently hinging the split fragment outward (Fig. 9–7). This open

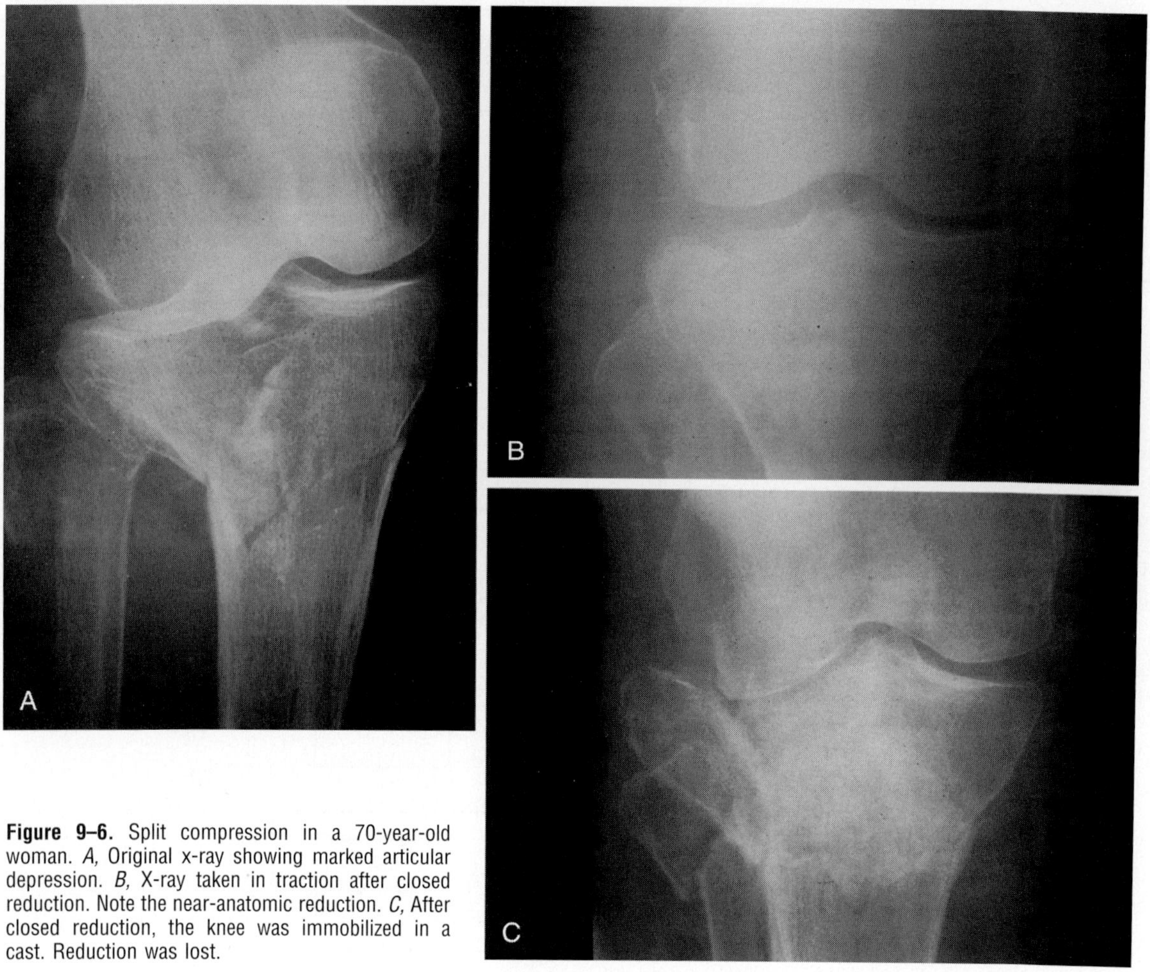

Figure 9–6. Split compression in a 70-year-old woman. *A,* Original x-ray showing marked articular depression. *B,* X-ray taken in traction after closed reduction. Note the near-anatomic reduction. *C,* After closed reduction, the knee was immobilized in a cast. Reduction was lost.

Table 9–3. TREATMENT USED IN SPLIT COMPRESSION FRACTURES (N = 283)

TREATMENT	1940–1973 (N = 165)	1974–1994 (N = 118)
Closed Treatment		
Functional	3%	<1%
Fracture-brace	0	0
Cast-brace	0	3%
Plaster cast	43%	3%
Traction	4%	3%
Closed reduction	12%	0
Cast-brace	0	0
Total closed	62%	10%
Open Treatment		
Open—No cast	3%	42%
Open—Cast	34%	42%
Open—Traction	1%	3%
Arthroscopic reduction	0	3%
Percutaneous fixation	0	0
External fixation	0	<1%
Total open	38%	90%

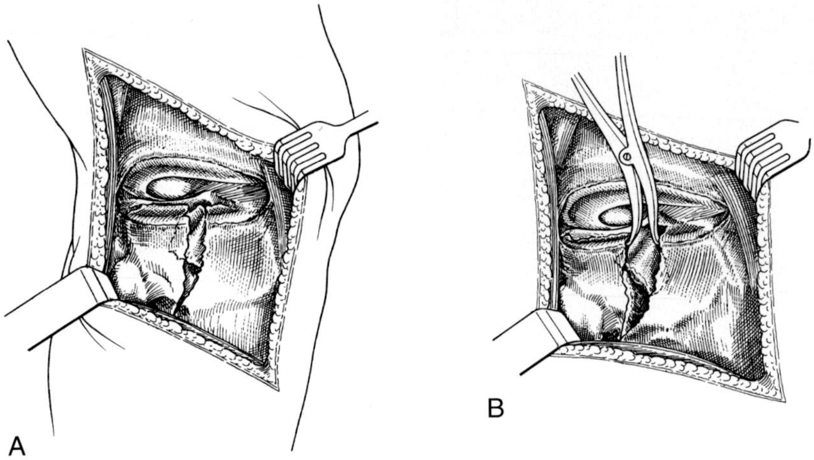

Figure 9–7. Inframeniscal approach to a split compression fracture. *A*, Note the split fracture line. *B*, Split fragment spread open to expose the depressed area. (From Laurin, C.A., Riley, L.H., and Roy-Camille, R. (Eds.): Atlas of Orthopedic Surgery, Vol 3. Paris, Masson, 1992, p. 372.)

position is held by a small interlaminar spreader, while the impacted and depressed articular fragments are gently disimpacted and pushed uniformly up to normal articular level using osteotomes, periosteal elevators, or impactors. These disimpacted fragments must be supported by grafts of cancellous bone obtained from the proximal tibia, iliac crest, or bone bank. The split fragment is then reduced, closing the anterior fracture line while visualizing articular cartilage alignment. Periosteal elevation along the anterior fracture gap distally from the joint surface allows accurate interdigitation of the fracture. Temporary fixation with Kirschner wires permits intraoperative plateau and lateral x-ray views to confirm reduction. A decision is then made with regard to the type of internal fixation to be used (Fig. 9–8).

The internal fixation device should fix the split fragment with sufficient rigidity to withstand active and passive movement without the need for external support. In general, when there is no comminution of the fragment or of the proximal tibia and an accurate fit has been obtained in good quality bone, two or three cancellous screws with washers engaging the medial cortex provide rigid fixation. If there is fragment comminution or osteoporosis, a contoured T or L buttress plate or tibial plateau plate, fixed to the proximal tibia with two or three cancellous screws and cortical screws distally, is needed to provide optimal rigidity of fixation. The plate is contoured during surgery or prebent before surgery using an anteroposterior x-ray as a guide to the shape of the tibial flare. The advantage of using a plate is the buttressing effect on the split fragment. Final intraoperative x-rays are done to confirm reduction and adequacy of fixation.

Arthroscopic-Assisted Reduction

Arthroscopic inspection of the freshly injured knee joint can be done after evacuation of hemarthrosis. The status of menisci, cruciate ligaments, and the articular surface is easily evaluated (Fig. 9–9). A small incision is made over the tibial flare. If the split fracture is in this location, it is levered apart sufficiently to permit insertion of a small impactor to gently disimpact and elevate the depressed articular surface. One can also use the technique of making a window in the flare and then insert impactors through that window to elevate the depressed fragments. Once the depression has been corrected and the underlying defect grafted, the split fragment is reduced manually and fixed with either

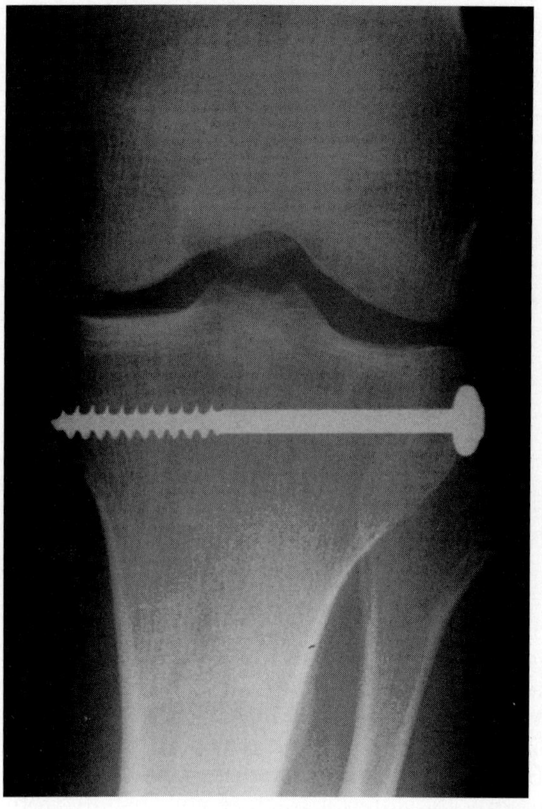

Figure 9–8. Split compression fracture treated by open reduction, reduced anatomically and fixed by single screw.

percutaneous screws or a side plate. Although reduction is monitored arthroscopically, x-rays should be taken intraoperatively to document the accuracy of articular restoration.

Closed Methods

Closed techniques for the treatment of split compression fractures involve closed reduction under anesthesia. The goal of reduction is to reposition the split fragment to its anatomic position. Of course, the articular surface depression cannot be corrected by closed reduction. As long as the depression is 6 mm or less, the knee adapts to it because the split fragment fully supports the femoral condyle. As long as the split fragment has been reduced and heals in a position

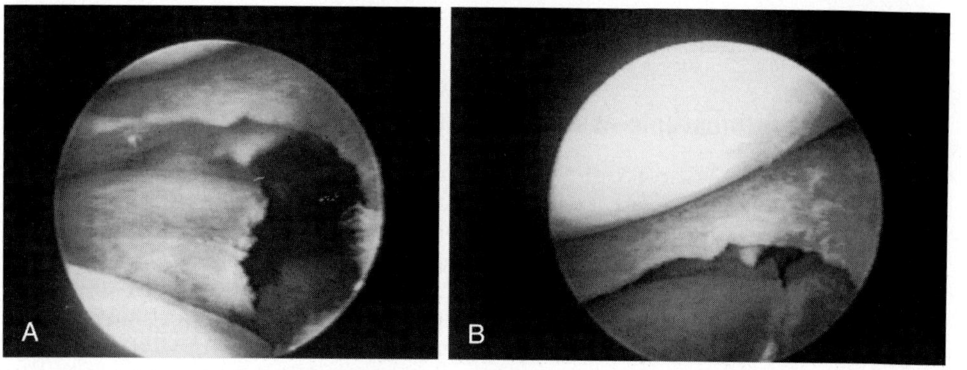

Figure 9–9. Arthroscopic view of split compression fracture. *A*, Note depressed fragment well below lateral meniscus. *B*, After reduction and screw fixation.

to support the femoral condyle at a normal articular level, the result should be acceptable. Reduction is carried out on a fracture table utilizing skeletal traction.

A technique of reducing the split fragment is the Ilfeld traction-compression method.[482] This technique utilizes skeletal traction of 60 to 70 lb, aspiration of hemarthrosis, and x-rays to monitor fracture position. If the split fragment remains below normal articular level despite traction, it is pounded upward with a padded mallet. Care is taken not to injure the peroneal nerve. Once the fragment is at normal articular level, the fracture is impacted using a Bohler clamp or giant nutcracker. X-rays should then show that the split fragment is anatomically located to provide support for the femoral condyle. Percutaneous screw fixation is the best method for maintaining reduction. Guide wires are placed under x-ray control, and two or more cannulated screws are inserted to fix the split fragment. Comminution of the split fragment is a contraindication to screw fixation and provides an indication for buttress plating.

A cast or cast-brace should not be used after closed reduction unless percutaneous fixation has been used. If percutaneous fixation cannot be used, skeletal traction of about 20 lb can be used to maintain reduction and permit passive and later active knee movement. The patient is transferred in traction from the fracture table to a bed and maintained with gradually decreasing traction weights for approximately 4 weeks. By this time there is usually sufficient stability to permit application of a cast-brace or a fracture-brace until bone healing is evident.

LIGAMENT INJURIES

Knee stability should be tested after internal fixation of the fracture. If instability remains, collateral ligament injury must be suspected. Stress x-rays show medial collateral ligament injury by demonstrating joint space widening. Surgical exposure of the medial ligament and repair of the deep and superficial divisions of that ligament have been shown to improve joint stability.[244, 457, 553]

For a torn or avulsed collateral ligament, the author recommends operative repair with stapling of ligament avulsion into its bed or suturing of insubstance tears. After ligament integrity has been restored, the knee should remain more stable than if the ligament had not been repaired.[244, 553] Some knees with unrepaired medial collateral ligaments are found to be stable on long-term follow-up, but the majority will be unstable.[244, 727] Most unrepaired ligament avulsions from bone heal well, but insubstance tears heal with scar tissue and relative lengthening and thus leave some knee instability.

Post ligament-repair support for the knee has traditionally been a long-leg cast for 6 to 8 weeks. Because of improved repairs and increased basic scientific knowledge about the ligamentous weakening that occurs with immobilization, the trend is to allow some knee movement early after the repair in the protection of a fracture-brace or cast-brace.[243, 1137, 1138] Knee movement is restricted at first and is increased gradually over a period of 6 weeks.

Post Reduction Management

Postoperative care depends on the type of treatment used; however, if possible, the knee should be moving within 3 or 4 weeks. If a cast has been used, some alternate means of support, such as a cast-brace or traction, should be used within 3 or 4 weeks to avoid the prolonged rehabilitation required after dense intra-articular adhesions develop.

Aftercare of split compression fractures treated by open reduction and rigid internal fixation is much like that for a minimally displaced fracture. Wound healing is the main priority. If the wound seems at all questionable it is better to rest the knee for a few days and start movement when healing is proceeding normally. Continuous passive motion is helpful in starting movement soon after

Table 9–4. COMPLICATIONS IN 238 SPLIT COMPRESSION FRACTURES

COMPLICATION	CLOSED TREATMENT (N = 88)	OPEN TREATMENT (N = 150)	TOTAL (N = 238)
Phlebitis	5%	3%	3%
Arterial injury	0	1%	<1%
Compartment syndrome	<1%	1%	1%
Peroneal nerve injury	2%	4%	3%
Wound infection	0	3%	2%
Fracture position loss	3%	15%	11%
Avascular necrosis	0	3%	2%
Open fracture	2%	2%	2%
Other	<1%	3%	2%
Total	13%	35%	26%

surgery and seems to reduce postoperative pain. Though normally not required for compliant patients, a cast, traction, or brace should be used for noncompliant patients. Prolonged immobilization results in some degree of permanent impairment of knee motion and thus should be avoided. X-rays are taken postoperatively at approximately monthly intervals to check for a change in fracture position. Light weight-bearing is started at about 2 months after surgery, and full weight-bearing is started at 3 months if x-rays demonstrate fracture healing.

Complications

The complication rate for closed treatment of split compression fractures was 13%, and the complication rate for open treatment was 35%. Most of the complications involved loss of fracture reduction, phlebitis, or wound infection (Table 9–4). Regardless of the treatment used, fracture position needs to be checked by x-rays during the time period when relatively easy correction of position loss by rereduction, either closed or open, can be effected. Fracture position loss of 2 mm or more occurred in 3% of patients treated by closed methods and in 13% of patients treated by open methods. Of those treated open, loss of position was much less frequent when the fractures had been fixed with buttress plates. Many fractures that lost position had been fixed by one or two screws or bolts without a sideplate. Phlebitis and pulmonary embolism occur unpredictably and may be related to immobilization of the knee, which suggests that early knee movement would probably be beneficial.

Wound infection was another complication of operatively treated split compression fractures. In the postoperative period, unusual or persistent knee effu-

Table 9–5. FOLLOW-UP RESULTS IN ISOLATED SPLIT COMPRESSION FRACTURES TREATED BY ALL METHODS SINCE 1940 (MEAN FOLLOW-UP OF 8 YEARS [2–45 YEARS])

	AVERAGE	RANGE
Point rating	78	42–100
Pain	Mild	None–moderate
Flex deformity	1 Degree	0–15 Degrees
Knee motion	122 Degrees	90–140 Degrees
Valgus deformity	5 Degrees	0–15 Degrees
Instability	5 Degrees	0–15 Degrees
Arthritis	Minimal	None–Severe

No associated fractures or ligament injury. Total number of fractures = 57.

Table 9–6. RESULTS OF SPLIT COMPRESSION FRACTURES TREATED CLOSED OR OPEN (MEAN FOLLOW-UP OF 8 YEARS)

	CLOSED TREATMENT	OPEN TREATMENT
	Average	Average
Point rating	76	80
Pain	Mild	Occasional
Flex deformity	2 Degrees	2 Degrees
Knee motion	116 Degrees	120 Degrees
Deformity	6 Degrees	5 Degrees
Instability	6 Degrees	5 Degrees
Arthritis	Mild	Mild

Fractures treated closed = 20; fractures treated open = 37. Total number of fractures = 57.

sion accompanied by elevation of body temperature signals the advisability of aspiration, smear, and culture of knee fluid. A positive smear or culture indicates infection, which must be treated aggressively by arthrotomy or arthroscopic débridement. Arthroscopic débridement and irrigation can be used when infection is confined only to the joint; however, in most cases, the surgical wound is also involved.

Results

After a mean follow-up period of 8 years, the average point rating of knees with isolated split compression fractures in the author's series was 78 (Table 9–5). Traumatic arthritis was observed in 25% of fractures that were followed for 6 years or more. Knee motion averaged near normal in isolated split compression fractures but was noted to be more restricted after a ligament injury or an ipsilateral fracture (Table 9–7).

Treatment by nonoperative methods produced an average point rating of 76, whereas operative treatment yielded an average of 80 points. The more displaced fractures were operated on with greater frequency than were those with lesser displacements (Table 9–6). The average point rating result deteriorated to 72 when there was also an ipsilateral fracture and to 69 when there was a collateral ligament injury (Table 9–7).

When the proximal tibia healed with normal width, the result was a point rating of 80.[915] When there was widening of 5 mm or more, the average result deteriorated to 68 points (Table 9–8).

Twenty percent of split compression fractures required late surgery, usually for removal of metallic fixation materials.

Table 9–7. RESULTS OF SPLIT COMPRESSION FRACTURES WITH LIGAMENT OF IPSILATERAL FRACTURE (MEAN FOLLOW-UP OF 6 YEARS [2–15 YEARS])

	WITH LIGAMENT INJURY (N = 19)	WITH IPSILATERAL FRACTURE (N = 26)
	Average	Average
Point rating	69	72
Pain	Mild–moderate	Mild
Flex deformity	4 Degrees	3 Degrees
Knee motion	106 Degrees	102 Degrees
Deformity	6 Degrees	7 Degrees
Instability	7 Degrees	6 Degrees
Arthritis	Moderate	Moderate

Table 9–8. TIBIAL WIDENING AND POINT RATING

POST REDUCTION WIDENING	POINT RATING
0 mm (62)	80
1–4 mm (34)	71
5–10 mm (8)	68

SUMMARY

Stable split compression fractures with only a minimum of split fragment displacement do well with closed treatment; however, most fractures are unstable and tend to do better with operative treatment. Closed reduction under anesthesia is useful when operative methods cannot be used.

CHAPTER 10

Total Depression Fractures

Total depression fracture lines begin near the intercondylar eminence and pass obliquely distalward to the medial or lateral tibial cortex. Although displaced distally and angulated as a whole, the articular surface is relatively undamaged except for the cartilage overlying the fracture line (Fig. 10–1). There are two basic configurations of total depression fractures. In the first, the fracture line begins on the articular surface of a compartment and passes to the tibial flare on that same side. In the second, the fracture line begins on the articular surface of a compartment and passes under the intercondylar eminence to the tibial flare on the opposite side. The latter variety, called the "entire plateau fracture-dislocation" by Moore,[724] has greater displacement and higher incidence of collateral ligament injury than has the former.

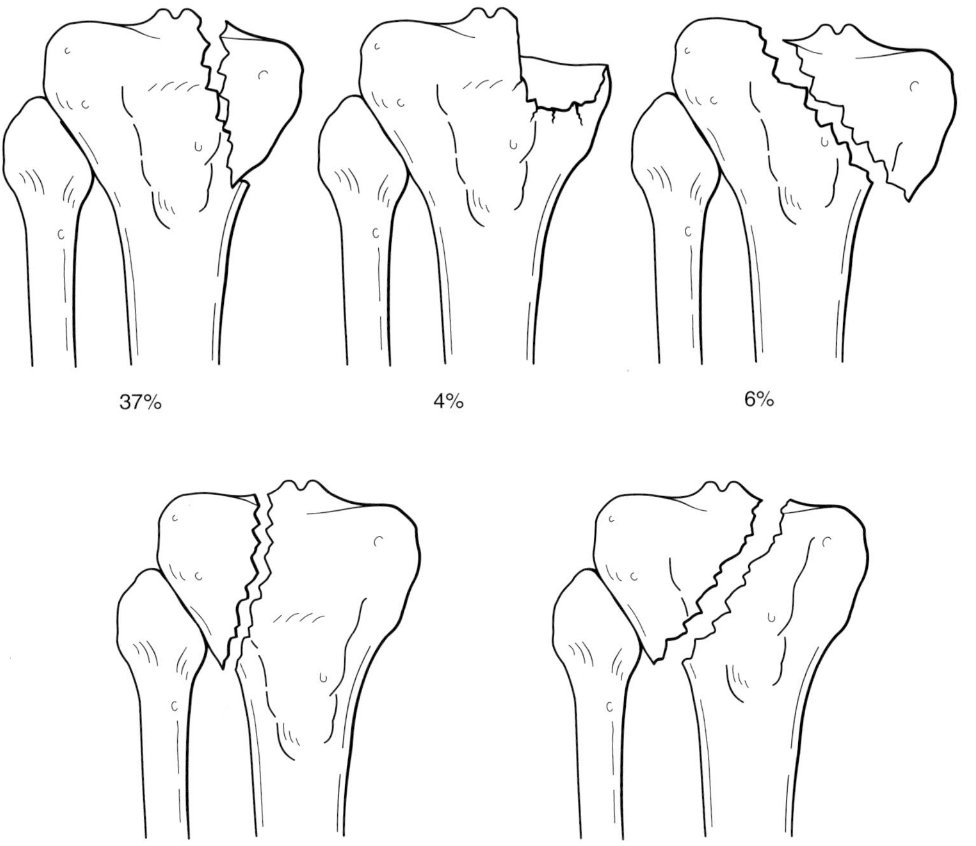

Figure 10–1. Total depression subtypes and distribution.

Table 10–1. TOTAL DEPRESSION FRACTURES IN THE AUTHOR'S SERIES (N = 200)

Age	Average: 47 yr	Range: 16–84 yr
Sex	Male: 126	Female: 74
Knee (both = 10)	Right: 91	Left: 89
Plateau	Lateral: 103	Medial: 97
Depression	Average: 7 mm	Range: 4–23
Widening	Average: 5 mm	Range: 1–25
Instability >5 degrees	63%	

Total depression fractures account for 17% of displaced proximal tibial articular fractures in the author's series. Fifty-two percent of these involve the lateral tibial plateau, and 48% involve the medial tibial plateau (Table 10–1).

Sixty-four percent of patients with total depression fractures had associated injuries. Fifty-four percent had ipsilateral fractures (6% were open fractures), and 30% had ligament injuries (Table 10–2).

DIAGNOSIS

Where fracture lines begin and end as well as their direction on anteroposterior x-rays make the diagnosis of a total depression fracture. Fracture lines originate near the intercondylar eminence and pass distally and obliquely to either the medial or the lateral tibial cortex (Figs. 10–1 and 10–2). Knee stability should be tested with the knee in extension and in a few degrees of flexion. Instability of 5 degrees or more indicates either fracture movement, collateral ligament injury, or both. The cause of knee instability can be confirmed by stress x-rays.

Thirty percent of patients with total depression fractures in the author's series had associated ligament injuries. Initial x-rays may show avulsion fractures at ligament attachments or cartilage space widening in the knee compartment opposite the fracture.

HOW THE AUTHOR MAKES TREATMENT DECISIONS

I have employed open reduction and rigid internal fixation in more than two thirds of total depression fractures treated during the last 20 years. I determine stability in isolated total depression fractures by stress testing (Fig. 10–3).

Stable fractures that involve the lateral plateau are managed in a cast-brace

Table 10–2. INJURIES ASSOCIATED WITH 197 TOTAL DEPRESSION FRACTURES

INJURY	%
Ligament injury	30
Ipsilateral fractures	
Subcondylar	17
Tibial spine	21
Patellar	2
Femoral condyle	1
Supracondylar	2
Femoral shaft	1
Hip	1
Tibial shaft	5
Ankle and foot	2
Multiple	6

112 fractures in 98 patients. The fibula was fractured in 23%.

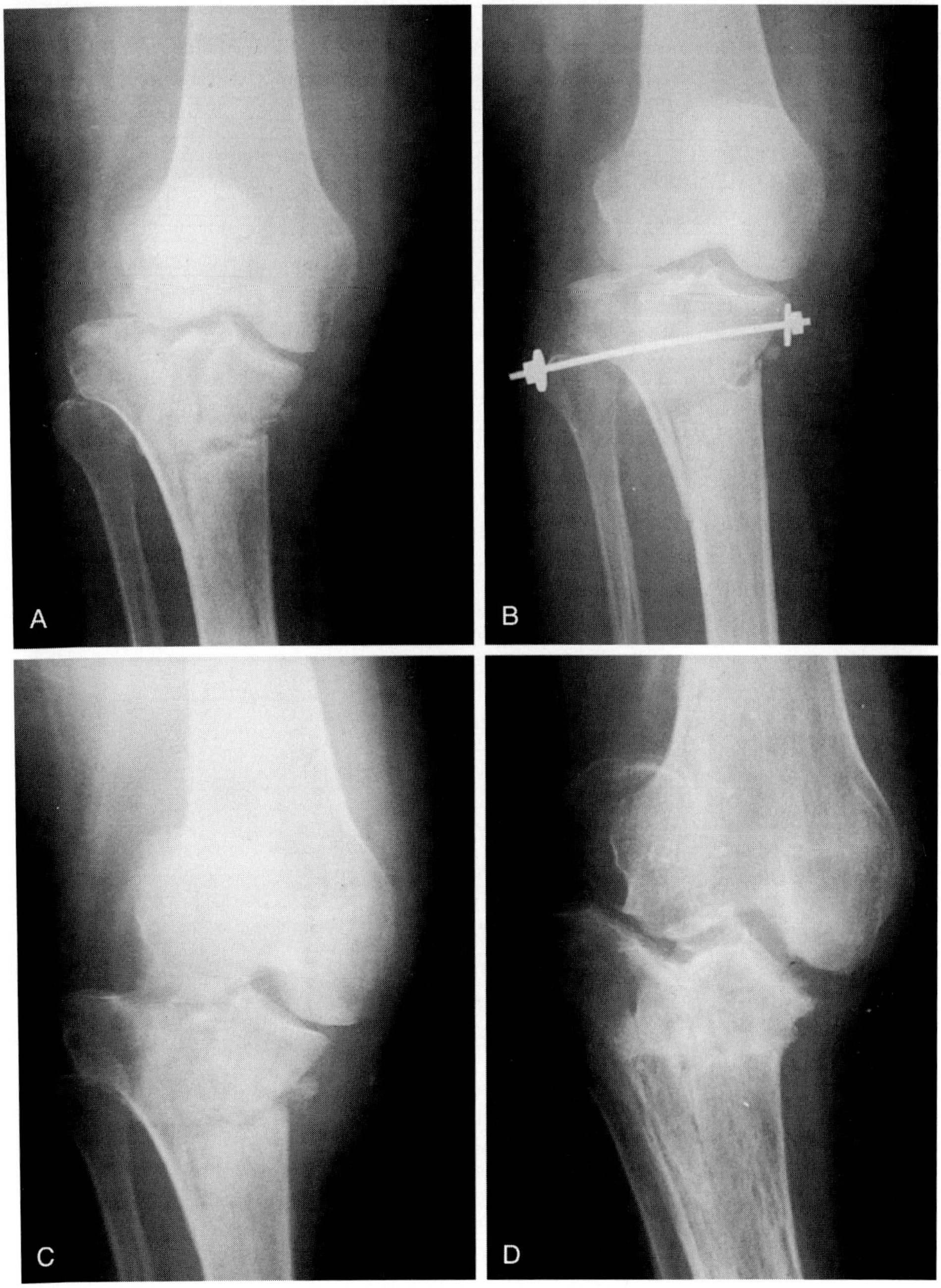

Figure 10–2. Total depression fracture in a 61-year-old woman. *A,* Note the fracture displacement. *B,* After operative treatment and inadequate internal fixation. Note the malreduction. *C,* One month after surgery, the bolt was removed and the medial tibial condyle became displaced. *D,* Three months after the injury, total knee replacement was performed.

or a fracture-brace. X-rays should be taken at least weekly in the first weeks after an injury to check for loss of fracture position.

Stable fractures that involve the medial plateau are much more likely to lose position in the first few weeks after an injury than are those involving the lateral plateau. I therefore employ internal fixation with a buttress plate and thus encourage early restoration of function.

Unstable fractures are rigidly fixed with buttress plates after accurate reduction. Stress testing is carried out after internal fixation. Knees with fractures that

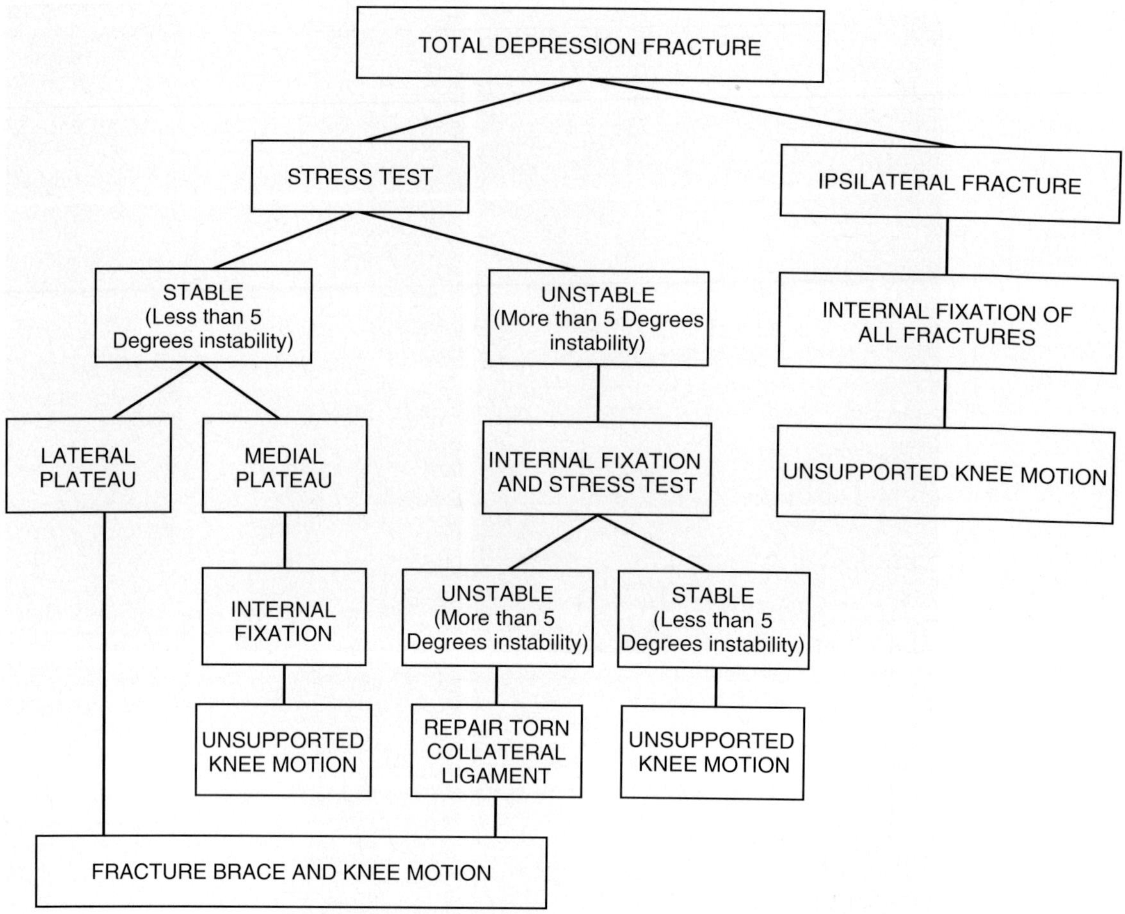

Figure 10–3. Treatment algorithm for total depression fractures.

are then stable are encouraged to move early. Knees that remain unstable have their torn collateral ligaments repaired and are managed postoperatively in a fracture brace.

Total depression fractures repaired with ipsilateral fractures are treated by open reduction of all fractures to aid restoration of function in the limb.

TREATMENT

The objectives of treatment are to reduce the fracture to its anatomic position and to maintain this position until healing has occurred. Reduction is often as simple as bringing the injured limb into alignment. In doing this, tension is placed on capsular structures that will often restore total depression fractures to anatomic position. When seen in an emergency room splinted, total depression fractures often appear to be undisplaced by x-ray but tend to redisplace if appropriate treatment is not utilized.

Successful closed reduction of a medial plateau fracture is almost always possible because the fracture fragment has strong capsular and collateral ligament attachments. When placed under stress, these attachments "pull" the plateau back into position. Successful closed reduction of a lateral plateau fracture is not so likely because the capsular attachments are less substantial. This plateau may need to be pushed or "pounded" up to normal articular level.[482] The challenge after successful closed reduction is to maintain the reduction until healing takes place.

Most total depression fractures, especially those involving the medial plateau, are currently treated by open reduction and internal fixation because postreduction management is easier and late results are better than with closed methods (Table 10–3). It is almost always possible, however, to use closed treatment when skin loss or systemic problems preclude open reduction. If a closed method such as a cast, cast-brace, or fracture-brace is used to maintain reduction, monitoring of fracture position by frequent x-rays to detect redisplacement early enough to effect rereduction becomes especially important.

Open Treatment

Arthroscopic examination and débridement of the knee allow for assessment and correction of meniscal lesions prior to fracture fixation. Arthrotomy of the knee is seldom helpful and should be avoided. Internal fixation of total depression fractures begins with exposure of the proximal tibia. The anterior and distal fracture margins are cleared of soft tissue attachments and clots. The fracture is then reduced manually by angulating the knee and applying direct pressure to interdigitate fracture margins. Temporary fracture fixation with smooth guide or Kirschner wires allows assessment of reduction by intraoperative x-ray. Then an internal fixation device, cannulated or cancellous screws or buttress plate, is chosen. If the fracture interdigitates perfectly with no comminution, two or three screws with washers will be sufficient for fixation. If the fragment is comminuted, buttress plate fixation is best because it provides the most rigid fixation (Fig. 10–4). Bone grafting is seldom indicated unless a substantial defect persists after reduction and fixation. Small bony voids can be adequately filled from locally obtained cancellous bone.

Once fixation has been achieved, knee stability is again tested. In the absence of collateral ligament injury, the knee should be stable. If instability persists after fixation, an intraoperative stress x-ray should be used to document the site and the extent of the instability. Collateral ligament repair is then recommended to restore knee stability.

Closed Treatment

I treat stable total depression fractures with no more than 4 or 5 mm of depression below normal articular level by closed means. I make especially certain that fractures of the medial plateau are reduced so that permanent varus

Table 10–3. TREATMENT USED IN TOTAL DEPRESSION FRACTURES (N = 198)

TREATMENT	1940–1973 (N = 121)	1974–1994 (N = 77)
Closed Treatment		
Functional	1%	1%
Fracture brace	0	3%
Cast-brace	0	8%
Plaster cast	48%	10%
Traction	12%	4%
Closed reduction	22%	4%
Total closed	83%	30%
Open Treatment		
Open—no cast	3%	26%
Open—cast	14%	35%
Open—traction	<1%	0
Arthroscopic reduction	0	2%
Percutaneous fixation	0	3%
External fixation	0	4%
Total open	17%	70%

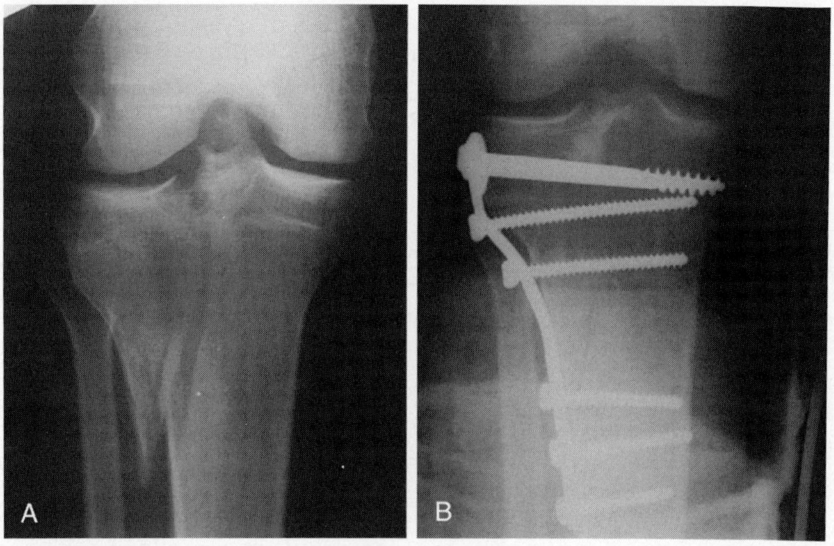

Figure 10–4. Total depression fracture in a 28-year-old man. *A*, Note the large lateral condylar fragment. *B*, Excellent reduction and fixation with a buttress plate.

deformity of the knee is avoided. Some fractures, especially those involving the medial plateau, tend to gradually redisplace in the early weeks after injury and thus must be carefully monitored by serial x-rays until fracture healing is ensured. Fracture-bracing or cast-bracing provides more protection against redisplacement than does a plaster cast but internal fixation, such as percutaneous fixation, is used more often today. Fractures that displace further should be strongly considered for percutaneous fixation or open reduction and internal fixation rather than being rereduced by closed means.

I do not hesitate to employ closed reduction of total depression fractures, even those with as much as 15–20 mm depression, if open reduction is contraindicated. The reduction is accomplished with the leg in traction by applying valgus stress to a medial fracture or varus stress to a lateral fracture. This maneuver usually restores the plateau to its normal articular level. If the reduction is less than anatomic, the depressed plateau is gently pounded upward with a padded mallet.[482] The problem is to maintain reduction. Although traction is an option it entails hospitalization for several weeks and may cause some loss of normal knee valgus in medial condylar fractures.[728, 940] Cast-bracing, another option, should be applied with stress to unweight the injured plateau.[122, 243, 720, 972] Periodic x-rays are required during the healing phase since a small but significant number of these fractures redisplace. Percutaneous fixation after closed reduction is an attractive option if skin condition permits.[126, 361, 424, 540, 562, 663, 1149] It should be supplemented by a fracture-brace or cast-brace until the fracture has healed.

POST TREATMENT CARE

I advocate early knee movement without bracing or external support after open reduction with rigid internal fixation. Continuous passive motion for a few days after surgery adds to patient comfort while promoting knee movement. Care should be taken to ensure that knee movement is consistent with normal and rapid wound healing. In noncompliant patients fractures are best protected in a cast-brace or fracture-brace. Weight-bearing is deferred for 2 to 3 months until x-ray demonstrates fracture union.

After closed treatment, x-rays should be taken every week or 10 days to ensure continued maintenance of fracture reduction. A minimum of 8 weeks of

Table 10–4. COMPLICATIONS IN TOTAL DEPRESSION FRACTURES (N = 170)

COMPLICATION	CLOSED TREATMENT (N = 104)	OPEN TREATMENT (N = 66)	TOTAL (N = 170)
Phlebitis	2%	3%	2.4%
Arterial injury	0	3%	1%
Compartment syndrome	0	0	0
Peroneal nerve injury	1%	6%	3%
Wound infection	0	3%	1%
Fracture position loss	22%	18%	21%
Avascular necrosis	0	0	0
Open fracture	4%	11%	6%
Other	2%	5%	3%
Total	31%	49%	37.4%

fracture immobilization is required for healing. Weight-bearing is begun as union occurs at 6 to 8 weeks post injury.

COMPLICATIONS

In the author's series the complication rate after total depression fractures was 37%. Thirty-one percent of fractures treated with closed methods and 49% of openly treated fractures had a complication (Table 10–4). Loss of fracture reduction was the main complication encountered after either closed or open management. Serial x-rays taken during the weeks after fracture allow early detection of a change of position. If there is a significant loss of fracture position after closed treatment, early open reduction is usually indicated. Surgically treated fractures that lost reduction had usually been internally fixed by tibial bolts or pre-1970 screws. Rarely was loss of reduction noted after the use of a buttress plate.

Other complications after open reduction are problems of wound healing and infection. Antibiotics are used routinely for 2 days postoperatively or longer if required.

RESULTS

In the author's series, the average follow-up point rating for total depression fractures without ligament injury or ipsilateral fracture was 76 (Table 10–5). Patients treated by closed methods had an average point rating of 73, whereas patients treated by open methods had a point rating of 79.

If there was collateral ligament injury, the average point rating was 84, which is probably attributable to both the open reduction and ligament repair in these patients. If there was an ipsilateral fracture, there was an average point

Table 10–5. FOLLOW-UP RESULTS IN ISOLATED TOTAL DEPRESSION FRACTURES (N = 20)

	AVERAGE	RANGE
Point rating	76	(36–95)
Pain	Mild	None–mild
Flex deformity	2 Degrees	0–15 Degrees
Knee motion	126 Degrees	0–145 Degrees
Deformity	4 Degrees	0–10 Degrees
Instability	2 Degrees	0–8 Degrees
Arthritis	Mild	None–severe

The mean follow-up time was 6 years. There were no associated fractures or ligament injuries.

Table 10–6. RESULTS AFTER LIGAMENT INJURY OR IPSILATERAL FRACTURE

	Ligament Injury (N = 17) Average	**Associated Fracture (N = 33)** Average
Point rating	84	74
Pain	Mild	Mild
Flexion contracture	1 Degree	0–10 Degrees
Knee motion	126 Degrees	110 Degrees
Deformity	2 Degrees	2 Degrees
Instability	3 Degrees	2 Degrees
Arthritis	Mild	Mild

Mean follow-up time of 6 years.

rating of 74; these patients had limited knee motion compared with those with isolated plateau fractures (Table 10–6).

Late traumatic arthritis was noted in 1 of 20 knees (5%) after rigid fixation in anatomic position and was observed in 17 of 45 knees (38%) with more than 2 mm of articular malalignment. Eleven of 23 knees that healed with 5 degrees or more deformity developed moderate to severe arthritis. Six of 27 knees that were stable at follow-up had arthritic changes. Twelve of 38 knees that were unstable at follow-up had arthritic changes. Twenty-six percent of total depression fractures required hardware removal or an osteotomy.

SUMMARY

Total depression fractures have a particular fracture configuration that is notable because of the limited damage to the articular surface and great potential to heal with angular deformity. The major goal of treatment is to reduce the fractured plateau to its normal articular level so as to prevent angular deformity of the knee. For this reason, the trend has been to use open reduction with rigid fixation, thus allowing early knee motion without the need for rigid external support.

CHAPTER 11

Split Fracture-Dislocations

Split fracture-dislocation consists of a coronal plane fracture with a wedge-shaped fragment displaced from the posterior third of either plateau or, less often, from the anterior portions of either plateau (Fig. 11–1*A, B*). Intercondylar eminence fractures or cruciate ligament tears are frequently associated (Table 11–1).

Split fracture-dislocations make up only 3% of proximal tibial articular fractures. Moore classified this fracture as a fracture-dislocation because of its high incidence of associated soft tissue injuries.[724] Some posteriorly located split fractures may be reduced under anesthesia by extending the knee. Other split fractures, however, cannot be reduced adequately by knee extension and require operative reduction and internal fixation. Functional results at long-term follow-up have not been favorable compared with those for other unicondylar fractures, partly because of the frequent association of split fracture with intercondylar eminence fractures or cruciate ligament injury.[852, 1071]

DIAGNOSIS

Examination usually reveals a swollen knee flexed about 30 degrees. Tenderness is present directly over the fracture site. The knee cannot be extended passively. Stress testing often demonstrates collateral or cruciate ligament instability.

The diagnosis of split fracture is based on the fracture's appearance on anteroposterior and lateral x-ray views. A characteristic double horizon or double plateau shadow is seen in the anteroposterior view (see Fig. 11–1*A*). The lateral view demonstrates the split fragment displaced distally from either the anterior or posterior margin of the plateau. Although oblique views are seldom helpful in diagnosis, tomograms or computerized tomograms clearly delineate the fracture and its displacement (Fig. 11–1*B*). When a tibial spine or intercondylar eminence fracture is also present, these additional studies are helpful.

A careful evaluation of the neurovascular function of the leg is important, because split fracture-dislocations have a high incidence of soft tissue injuries compared to other plateau fracture types.

Ipsilateral injuries were associated with 67% of split fractures in the author's series. Other fractures were noted in 54% (open fractures were 2%) and ligament injuries in 27% (Table 11–2).

HOW THE AUTHOR MAKES TREATMENT DECISIONS

I perform internal fixation on anteriorly located fractures, either percutaneously or by open reduction. Fractures that are stable after internal fixation are supported in a fracture-brace. In those that remain unstable the torn collateral ligament should be repaired and cruciate stability restored, if possible (see Fig. 11–2).

Most split fractures are located on the posterior margin of either plateau. I

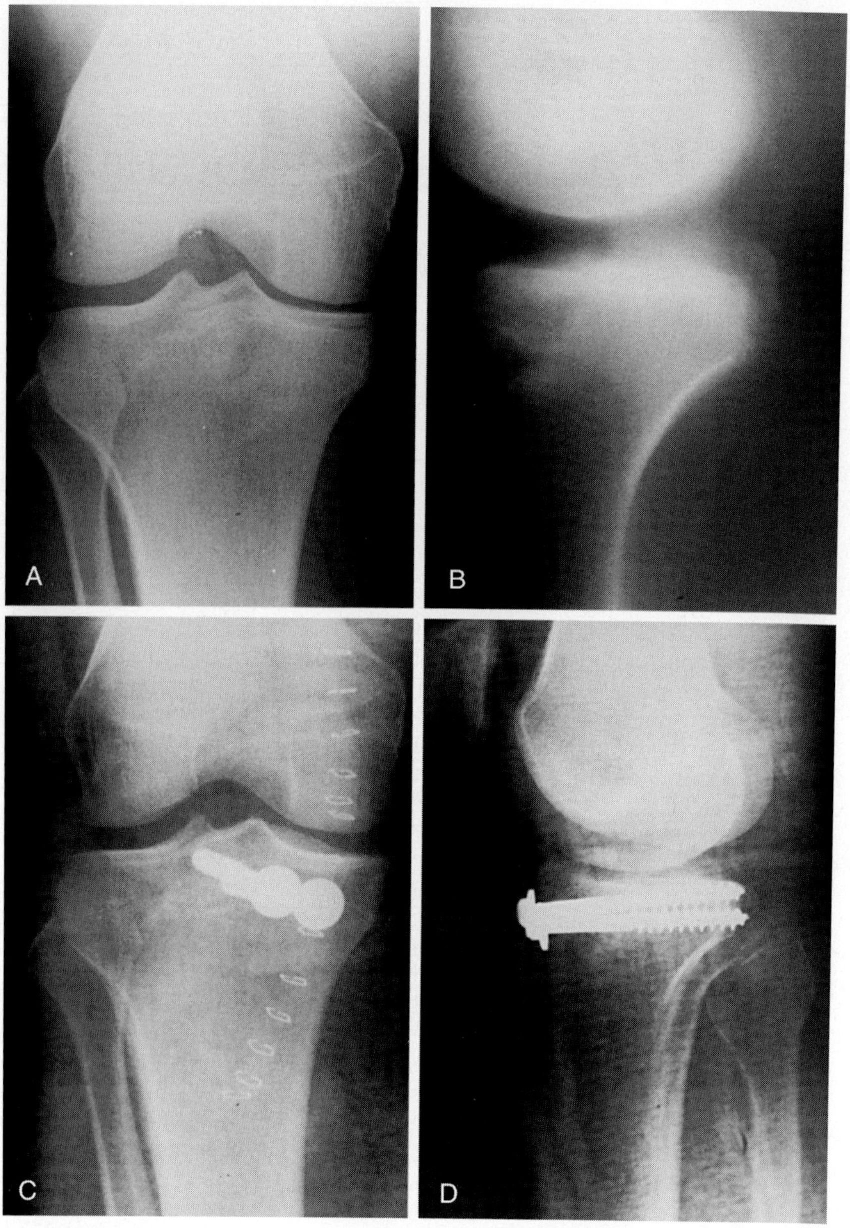

Figure 11–1. Split fracture-dislocation of the medial plateau in a 27-year-old man. *A,* An anteroposterior view. Note the medial double horizon. *B,* A lateral tomogram. The anterior third of the plateau is depressed. *C,* A postoperative anteroposterior view. *D,* A postoperative lateral view.

Table 11–1. SPLIT FRACTURES IN THE AUTHOR'S SERIES (N = 48)

Age	Average: 42	Range: 16–82 yr
Sex	Male: 32	Female: 11
Knee	Right: 32	Left: 16
Plateau (Both = 3)	Lateral: 25	Medial: 20
Location	Anterior: 6	Posterior: 42
Depression	Average: 7 mm	Range: 1–14 mm
Widening	Average: 4 mm	Range: 0–17 mm
Instability >5 Degrees	50%	

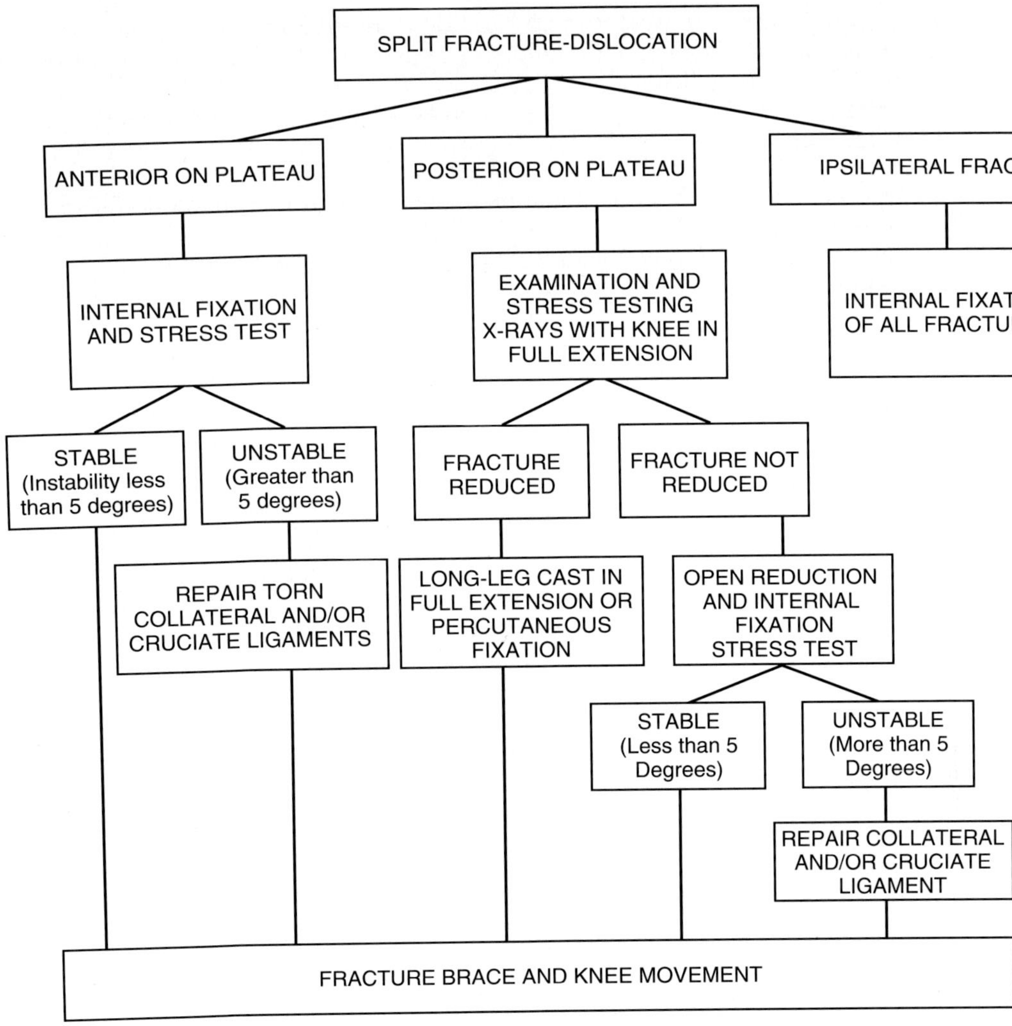

Figure 11–2. Treatment algorithm for split fractures.

examine knees with such fractures under anesthesia to test collateral ligament stability and especially to ascertain by x-ray whether the displaced posterior fragment returns to normal articular level when the knee is fully extended. If the fragment reduces, I insert guide pins for temporary fixation and then lag

Table 11–2. INJURIES ASSOCIATED WITH 48 SPLIT FRACTURES

Ligament injuries	27%
Fractures (33)	
Subcondylar	21%
Tibial spine	25%
Patellar	0
Femoral condyle	4%
Supracondylar	0
Femoral shaft	0
Hip	4%
Tibial shaft	13%
Ankle and foot	2%
Multiple	2%

The total number of fractures in 26 patients is 33. The fibula was fractured in 38%.

screws from anterior to posterior to provide definitive fixation. If percutaneous fixation is contraindicated, I maintain the knee in full extension in a long-leg cast until the fracture heals.

If the fracture fails to reduce as the knee is fully extended, open reduction and internal fixation are used. Once the fracture has been fixed rigidly, the knee is tested for stability. If the knee is stable, a fracture-brace is used until the fracture has healed. If the knee remains unstable, the torn collateral and cruciate ligaments are repaired.

More than 50% of split fracture-dislocations have associated ipsilateral fractures. Half of these involve the intercondylar eminence, including the attachments for cruciate ligaments. I reduce intercondylar eminence fractures and fix them by screw or wires. Other ipsilateral fractures should also be treated operatively to rapidly restore function to the injured leg.

TREATMENT

Closed Reduction

If closed reduction restores anatomic position of the fractured posterior fragment, cast immobilization is used with the knee in full extension. The knee is immobilized until the fracture has healed (approximately 6 to 8 weeks). X-rays should be taken weekly in the first 3 weeks to ensure that reduction is being maintained. If the fragment displaces more than 2 mm, open reduction with internal fixation should be carried out without delay.

Closed reduction of anteriorly located fractures can only rarely be accomplished by direct upward pressure on the fragment, and open reduction is usually required (Table 11–3).

Open Reduction

After successful closed reduction, percutaneous fixation using pins or screws is readily accomplished. Two guide pins are drilled across the fracture, and if x-rays show reduction, cannulated screws are inserted over the guide pins to engage the posterior cortex as verified by x-ray or image intensifier.

Open reduction and internal fixation give assurance that reduction will be maintained. A posteromedial fracture can be exposed through a vertical capsular

Table 11–3. TREATMENT METHODS USED IN THE AUTHOR'S SERIES (N = 48)

TREATMENT	1940–1973 (N = 28)	1974–1994 (N = 20)
Closed		
Functional	7%	5%
Fracture-brace	0	0
Cast-brace	0	0
Plaster cast	46%	5%
Traction	11%	0
Closed reduction	11%	0
Total closed	75%	10%
Open		
Open—No cast	7%	30%
Open—Cast	18%	40%
Open—Traction	0	0
Arthroscopic reduction	0	5%
Percutaneous fixation	0	0
External fixation	0%	15%
Total open	25%	90%

incision parallel to the posterior edge of the medial collateral ligament (see Chapter 6). Soft tissue attachments to the fragment should be preserved and only enough of the fracture edges exposed to ensure accurate reduction of the fragment into its bed. The joint surface and reduction are viewed through an arthrotomy made by horizontally dividing the meniscotibial ligament, which is repaired later. Temporary fixation with Kirschner wires allows lag screws to be inserted from anterior to posterior. A minimum of two screws is used (see Fig. 11–1*C* and *D*). Another surgical approach is through the popliteal space, partially severing the medial gastrocnemius tendon and exposing the posteromedial upper tibia. When this approach is used either screws or a buttress plate provides fixation.[233]

If there is an associated displaced intercondylar eminence fracture, it should be replaced in its bed to restore knee stability. Cruciate ligament tears from the femoral origin or tibial insertion should be repaired if possible. Insubstance tears are considered irreparable. Late cruciate reconstruction should be considered if there is persistent instability.

POST REDUCTION CARE

After closed treatment and cast immobilization with the knee in full extension, x-rays are taken weekly to ensure that reduction is maintained. Immobilization is continued until bony callus can be seen clearly on x-ray, usually after 8 weeks. Weight-bearing should not be permitted until healing has begun and knee motion has been restored.

After percutaneous fixation with pins, some form of support for the knee is advisable to allow soft tissue injuries to heal and to protect the reduction. Fracture- or cast-bracing provides optimal support while allowing early knee movement. After open reduction with rigid fracture fixation, the knee should be mobilized within a week or two to prevent the development of stiffness. In the period between exercise sessions, a fracture-brace is advised until the fracture has demonstrably healed, usually at about 8 weeks after surgery.

If an intercondylar eminence fracture is also present, cast-brace protection of the knee is advisable for 6 to 8 weeks. If a cruciate ligament has been repaired, cast-bracing that limits knee movement between 30 and 60 degrees is used for 6 weeks.

COMPLICATIONS

In the author's series there were 17% overall complications in the treatment of split fractures; 20% after open treatment. The more serious complications seen after split fracture-dislocation treatment were arterial injury and loss of fracture reduction (Table 11–4).

Table 11–4. COMPLICATIONS AFTER SPLIT FRACTURES (N = 38)

COMPLICATION	CLOSED TREATMENT (N = 17)	OPEN TREATMENT (N= 21)	TOTAL (N = 38)
Phlebitis	0	5%	3%
Arterial injury	0	5%	3%
Compartment syndrome	0	5%	3%
Peroneal nerve injury	0	0	0
Wound infection	0	0	0
Fracture reduction loss	6%	5%	5%
Avascular necrosis	0	0	0
Open fracture	6%	0	3%
	0	0	0
Total	12%	20%	17%

Table 11–5. RESULTS OF FOLLOW-UP IN SPLIT FRACTURES (N = 6)

	AVERAGE	RANGE
Point rating	72	37–92
Pain	Mild	Minor to moderate
Flex deformity	2 Degrees	0–5 Degrees
Knee motion	88 Degrees	50–135 Degrees
Deformity	3 Degrees	0–15 Degrees
Instability	6 Degrees	0–10 Degrees
Arthritis	Mild	None to moderate

The mean follow-up time was 5 years. There were no associated fracture or ligament injuries.

Arterial injury requires early diagnosis and repair. Since arterial repair requires popliteal exposure, a posterior fracture can easily be visualized, reduced, and fixed using a buttress plate after circulation has been restored.

The other complication, loss of fracture reduction, occurred after closed reduction or after less than rigid internal fixation. If more than 2 mm of redisplacement occurs, open reduction and internal fixation are indicated.

RESULTS

In the author's series treatment of split fractures produced few good or excellent results. The mean result in isolated split fractures was 72 points (Table 11–5). There were several reasons for inferior results, including late knee instability and limited knee movement. Patients treated by closed methods averaged a point rating of 75 points, and those treated by open reduction averaged 72 points.

If a cruciate or collateral ligament injury was associated with the split fracture, the result averaged 77 points. If there was an ipsilateral fracture, the average was 76 points.

The main late sequelae were instability and loss of knee motion. Patients treated operatively were often noted to have less than ideal reductions and seldom with rigid fixation. Without rigid fixation, knee rehabilitation was delayed and knee stiffness resulted. Later surgical procedures were required in 17% of split fractures.

SUMMARY

Most split fractures occur on the posterior margin of the tibial plateau and are characterized by a double horizon appearance on the initial anteroposterior x-rays. Reduction in posterior fractures can often be achieved by fully extending the knee; maintaining this reduction is difficult to accomplish. Therefore, the best treatment is open reduction with internal fixation and early knee movement. Despite this, results are often disappointing. Injuries to the intercondylar eminence or cruciate ligaments cause intra-articular scarring and knee stiffness. The knee quite often remains unstable.

CHAPTER 12

Rim Avulsion and Rim Compression Fracture-Dislocations

Rim compression and rim avulsion fracture-dislocations are combined bone and ligament injuries that render the knee markedly unstable and characterized by either avulsion of the plateau margin, depressed fracture of the plateau rim, or a combination of both. They result from valgus, varus, or twisting forces that, by stretching and tearing of capsular ligaments, may avulse a marginal articular fragment or cause a compression fracture on the margin of the tibial plateau. Failure to appreciate and treat the instability that accompanies these fractures will result in an unstable knee and an inferior result (Table 12–1).

Rim compression fracture is initiated by a rupture of the collateral ligament and capsule with or without avulsion of an articular margin. Then the combination of continuing force and the loss of ligament integrity allows marked angulation between the femur and the tibia to occur. This causes the femoral condyle to strike the plateau rim instead of the central articular surface and produce a depressed rim fracture. The mechanism of injury is easily visualized and documented on stress x-rays (Fig. 12–1*A*, *B*).

Sixty-seven percent of rim fractures in the author's series were associated with significant knee ligament injuries or ipsilateral fractures. Ipsilateral fractures were noted in 30% (3% were open fractures), and ligament injuries in 54% (Table 12–2).

Moore classified rim fractures as fracture-dislocations of the knee because of pronounced knee instability.[724] The object of treatment is to restore stability. Rim fractures make up 6% of displaced articular fractures.

DIAGNOSIS

Anteroposterior and lateral x-ray views may demonstrate rim avulsion, rim compression, or both; however, special studies may also be required. Larger avulsions are clearly visible. A lighter x-ray exposure or oblique projections are

Table 12–1. RIM FRACTURES IN THE AUTHOR'S SERIES (N = 73)

Age	Average: 39	Range: 10–82
Sex	Male: 46	Female: 27
Knee	Right: 40	Left: 33
Plateau (Both: 4)	Lateral: 47	Medial: 22
Depression	Average: 5 mm	Range: 0–14
Widening	Average: 2mm	Range 2–15
Instability >5 degrees	48%	

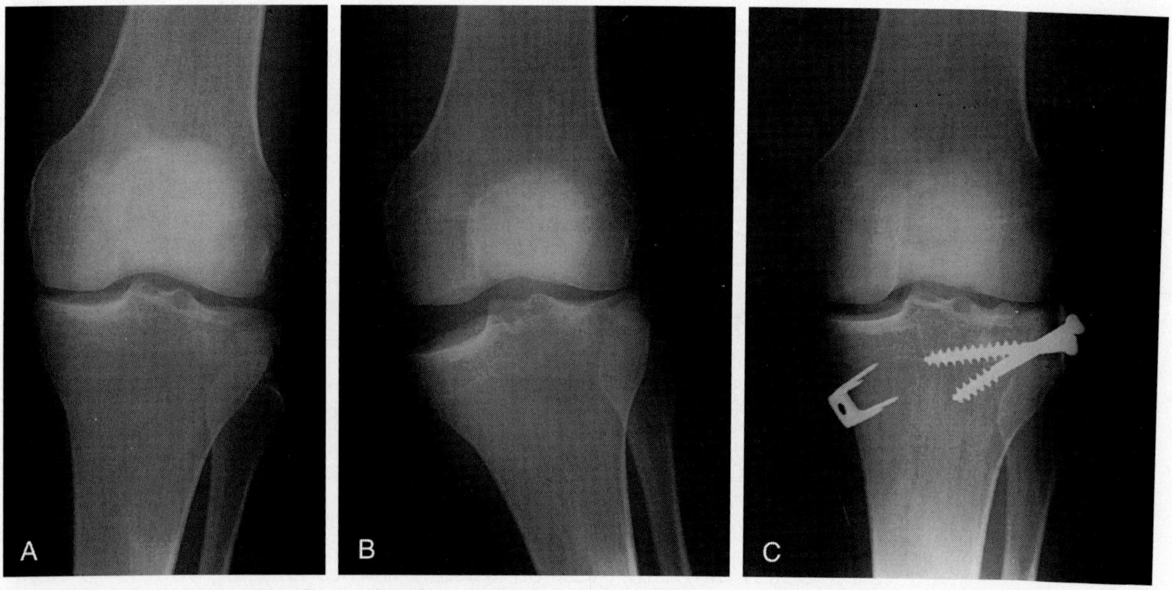

Figure 12–1. A rim compression fracture in a 31-year-old man. *A*, The original x-ray shows an injury to the margin of the lateral plateau. *B*, A stress x-ray reproduces the mechanism of injury. Note the torn medial collateral ligament. *C*, A postoperative view 3 months later showing stapling of the medial ligament tear to the tibia and elevation and support of the rim fracture.

needed to allow the fragments to be seen. A rim compression fracture may also not be easy to see on the two standard views but should be evident on oblique projections (Fig. 12–2). Stress x-rays should be taken to document the degree of knee instability. These x-rays can sometimes be done in the emergency room. If pain relief is required, a local anesthetic can be left in the knee after it is aspirated.

HOW THE AUTHOR MAKES TREATMENT DECISIONS

I test knees with rim fractures for stability (Fig. 12–3). Rim compression fractures with less than 6 mm of depression, as measured by x-ray or tomogram, are treated by closed methods unless the stress x-ray shows opening of the contralateral cartilage space. If the stress x-ray confirms a torn collateral ligament, the ligament and the capsule should be repaired to restore knee stability. I surgically elevate depressed rim fractures with 6 mm or more depression, place bone grafts under the elevated fragment, and repair the contralateral capsule and collateral ligament.

Table 12–2. INJURIES ASSOCIATED WITH 73 RIM FRACTURES

Ligament injuries	54%
Fractures	
Subcondylar	1%
Tibial spine	16%
Patellar	0
Femoral condyle	1%
Supracondylar	0
Femoral shaft	1%
Hip	3%
Tibial shaft	4%
Ankle	1%
Multiple	5%

Total fractures in 22 patients = 25; fibula fractured in 32%.

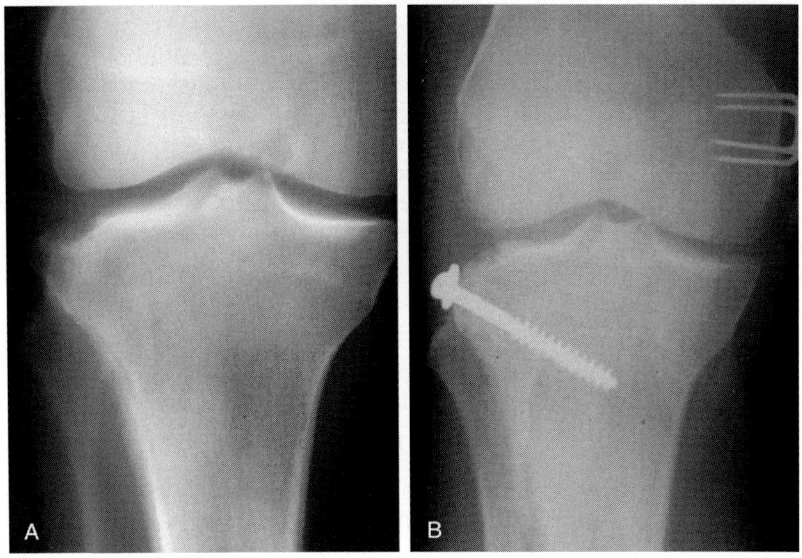

Figure 12–2. Typical rim compression fracture of the lateral plateau. *A*, Note the "divot" at the margin of the plateau. *B*, A postoperative view after repair of the avulsed medial ligament from the medial femoral condyle and repair of the rim compression.

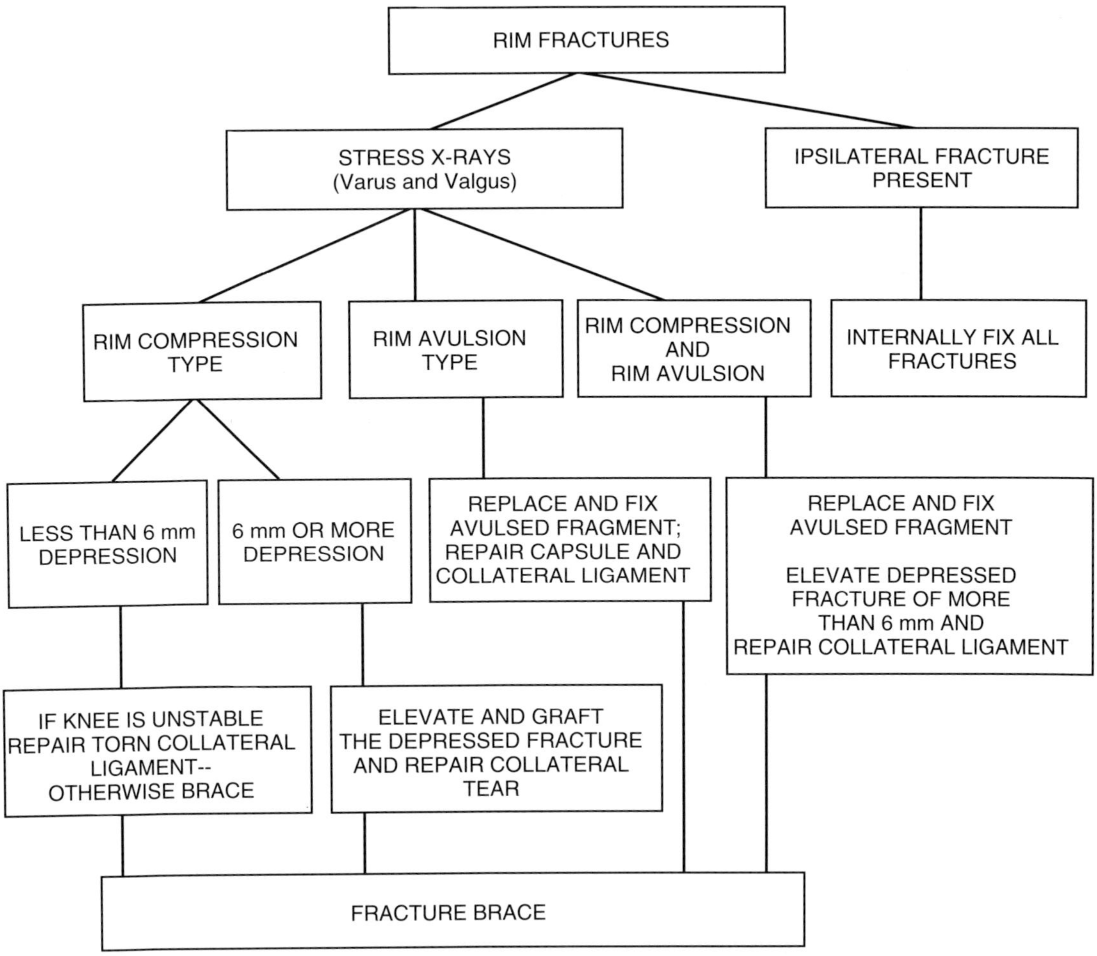

Figure 12–3. Treatment algorithm for rim fractures.

I replace avulsed fragments and fix them with screws or pins. If the collateral ligament on the same side is torn, it is repaired along with the knee capsule.

Combined rim compression and avulsion fractures are treated surgically by reduction and bone grafting of the depressed fracture and replacement and fixation of the avulsed fragment. After repair of torn capsular and collateral ligaments, the knee is protected for several weeks in a fracture brace.

Ipsilateral fractures in the same extremity as rim fractures should be reduced and internally fixed. The rim fracture and associated soft tissue injuries are treated by open reduction with capsular and collateral ligament repair.

TREATMENT

Avulsed fragments are surgically exposed with care to protect their capsular attachments and blood supply. The bed from which the fragment came is cleaned of clots, and then the fragment is reduced into it and fixed with one or two screws (Fig. 12–4; Table 12–3).

Rim compression fractures can only be reduced by operative means. The compressed area is exposed through a submeniscal approach. An osteotome, driven through the cortex below the depressed area, is levered upward to restore articular level. Bone grafts obtained locally by scooping out cancellous bone from the tibial metaphysis are used to fill the defect under the elevated area and provide support for it. The opposite collateral ligament and capsule are then repaired.

POSTOPERATIVE CARE

Cast- or fracture-brace support is used for about 6 weeks until the soft tissues and bone have healed. There is little possibility of loss of reduction of a surgically elevated rim fracture because the femoral condyle should not articulate directly with this area. Knee movement is begun gradually in a fracture-brace.

COMPLICATIONS

There were 16% complications from the treatment of rim fractures in the author's series (Table 12–4). Peroneal nerve injury was present in only three

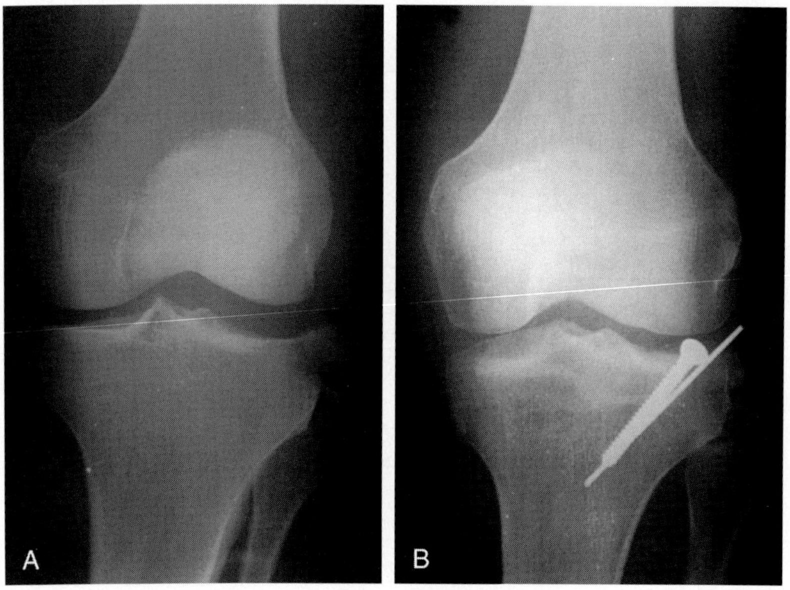

Figure 12–4. A rim avulsion fracture of the lateral plateau. *A*, An original anteroposterior view with widening of the lateral cartilage space. *B*, After fixation of the avulsed fragment and repair of the torn lateral capsule.

Table 12–3. TREATMENT METHODS USED IN THE AUTHOR'S RIM FRACTURES (N = 69)

TREATMENT	1940–1973 (N = 43)	1974–1994 (N = 26)
CLOSED		
Functional	7%	3%
Fracture-brace	0	4%
Cast-brace	0	12%
Plaster cast	72%	15%
Traction	7%	4%
Closed reduction	2%	0
Total closed	88%	38%
OPEN		
Open—No cast	5%	27%
Open—Cast	7%	31%
Open—Traction	0	0
Arthroscopic reduction	0	4%
Percutaneous fixation	0	0
External fixation	0	0
Total open	12%	62%

Table 12–4. COMPLICATIONS IN 57 RIM FRACTURES

COMPLICATION	CLOSED TREATMENT (N = 40)	OPEN TREATMENT (N = 17)	TOTAL (N = 57)
Phlebitis	3%	0	2%
Arterial injury	0	0	0
Compartment syndrome	0	0	0
Peroneal nerve injury	5%	6%	5%
Wound infection	0	0	0
Fracture position loss	3%	6%	4%
Avascular necrosis	0	6%	2%
Open fractures	5%	0	3%
Other	0	0	0
Total	16%	18%	16%

Table 12–5. FOLLOW-UP RESULTS OF RIM FRACTURES WITHOUT IPSILATERAL FRACTURE OR LIGAMENT INJURY (2–17 YEARS WITH A MEAN FOLLOW-UP OF 6 YEARS [N = 5])

Average point rating	85
Pain	None
Lack of extension	3 Degrees
Range of motion	80 Degrees
Deformity	1 Degrees
Instability	5 Degrees
Arthritis	None

Table 12–6. FOLLOW-UP RESULTS WITH A MEAN FOLLOW-UP OF 6 YEARS

	WITH LIGAMENT INJURY (N = 15) Average	WITH ASSOCIATED FRACTURE (N = 11) Average
Point rating	73	80
Pain	None	Minimum
Flex deformity	1 Degrees	2 Degrees
Knee motion	90 Degrees	125 Degrees
Deformity	1 Degree	None
Instability	3 Degrees	7 Degrees
Arthritis	Minimum	Minimum

patients despite the extreme distortion of the knee at the moment of injury. Knee immobilization in a cast was likely a factor in the two patients who developed thrombophlebitis. Loss of fracture position occurred twice as often after open reduction as after closed treatment.

RESULTS

In the author's series isolated rim fractures, whether treated nonoperatively closed or operatively, had an average point rating of 85 points (Table 12–5). With diagnosed ligament injury, the rating was 73 (Table 12–6).

If a diagnosed collateral ligament injury went unrepaired, the average rating declined to 69 points. Repaired collateral ligament injuries had an average rating of 86 points. If there was an ipsilateral fracture combined with the rim fracture, the average result was 80 points (Table 12–6).

Even after ligament repair, only 60% of knees were stable within 5 degrees or less at follow-up. Closed treatment resulted in 35% of patients with stable knees. If the ligament was repaired but a rim compression fracture with depression of greater than 6 mm was not reduced, knee instability was noted in 50%.

Later surgery was required in 27% of rim fractures. Three patients had four ligament reconstructions; three had hardware removal; one each had meniscectomy, manipulation to gain motion, osteotomy, or total knee replacement.

SUMMARY

Rim compression and rim avulsion fracture-dislocations are very complex injuries because of combined bone and ligament injuries that make the knee markedly unstable. The object of treatment is to restore stability. This makes bony stabilization combined with ligament and capsular repair desirable.

CHAPTER 13

Bicondylar Fractures

Bicondylar fractures (15% of displaced plateau fractures) are seen in a wide variety of configurations in which both tibial plateaus are disrupted (Fig. 13–1). Articular surfaces are typically depressed and widened (Table 13–1).

Associated injuries were noted in 76% of patients with bicondylar fractures. Ipsilateral fractures were noted in 74% (4% were open fractures), and ligament injuries were found in 15%. Subcondylar fractures, which made up more than half of ipsilateral fractures, increased the complexity of treatment (Table 13–2).

The incidence of neurovascular injuries is especially high in bicondylar fractures.[724] Early knee movement is imperative to prevent late knee stiffness. Despite the best management, traumatic arthritis has been observed in the majority of knees with bicondylar fractures that were monitored for more than 10 years.[176, 871, 967]

In the treatment of these fractures, it is difficult to achieve a well-aligned,

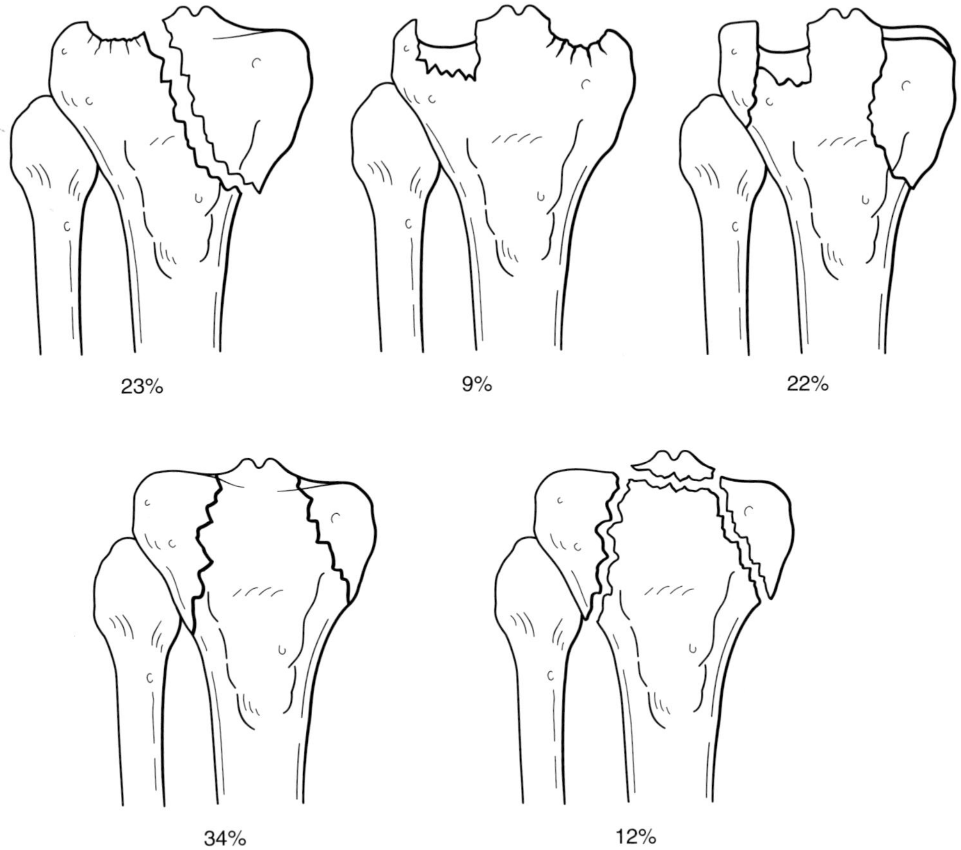

Figure 13–1. Incidence of bicondylar fracture subtypes encountered in the author's series.

Table 13–1. DEMOGRAPHICS OF BICONDYLAR FRACTURES (N = 186)

Age	Average = 47; range = 18–78
Sex	Male = 138; female = 48
Knee	Right = 89; left = 96
Both plateaus	186
Depression	Average = 9 mm; range = 2–29
Widening	Average = 6 mm; range = 0–18
Instability >5 degrees	67%

strong, stable, and moveable knee. Despite modern techniques, there has been only modest improvement in results over the years.[65, 214, 915, 921, 941, 1091] Thus, bicondylar fractures continue to present a difficult challenge.

DIAGNOSIS

Diagnosis of a bicondylar fracture is made after review of anteroposterior x-rays that show fracture lines involving both tibial plateaus (see Fig. 13–1). Oblique projections add information about the degree and direction of fracture displacement, but computed tomography (CT) scans with reconstructions in other planes are of much greater value in making treatment decisions[263, 865, 1100] (Fig. 13–2). Three-dimensional reconstructions can be especially valuable in demonstrating depression and displacement in more severely displaced fractures. I recommend use of CT scans, especially in bicondylar fractures that are to be treated by internal or external fixation.

Circulation and nerve function should be evaluated early and for several days after a fracture. Stress testing is seldom valuable because bony instability is the rule in bicondylar fractures, and ligament injury is noted in only 15%. When present, ligament injury is usually evident on the initial x-rays.

HOW THE AUTHOR MAKES TREATMENT DECISIONS

I utilize CT scans to evaluate bicondylar fractures. Because these fractures are seen in so many configurations, it is vital to ascertain the location and the extent of fracture displacement in order to make appropriate treatment decisions (Fig. 13–3).

If the CT scan and x-rays show multiple small articular fragments, I use skeletal traction, which frequently realigns the fragments satisfactorily by pulling on capsular ligamentous structures. If reduction is within 2 to 3 mm of anatomic position, I recommend that traction be continued as the definitive treatment or

Table 13–2. INJURIES ASSOCIATED WITH BICONDYLAR FRACTURES (N = 186)

Ligament injuries	15%
Fractures	
Subcondylar	55%
Tibial spine	36%
Patellar	0
Femoral condyle	0
Supracondylar	<1%
Femoral shaft	1%
Hip	2%
Tibial shaft	5%
Ankle and foot	3%
Multiple	3%

Total number of ipsilateral fractures in 137 patients is 196. Of these fractures, the fibula was fractured in 76%.

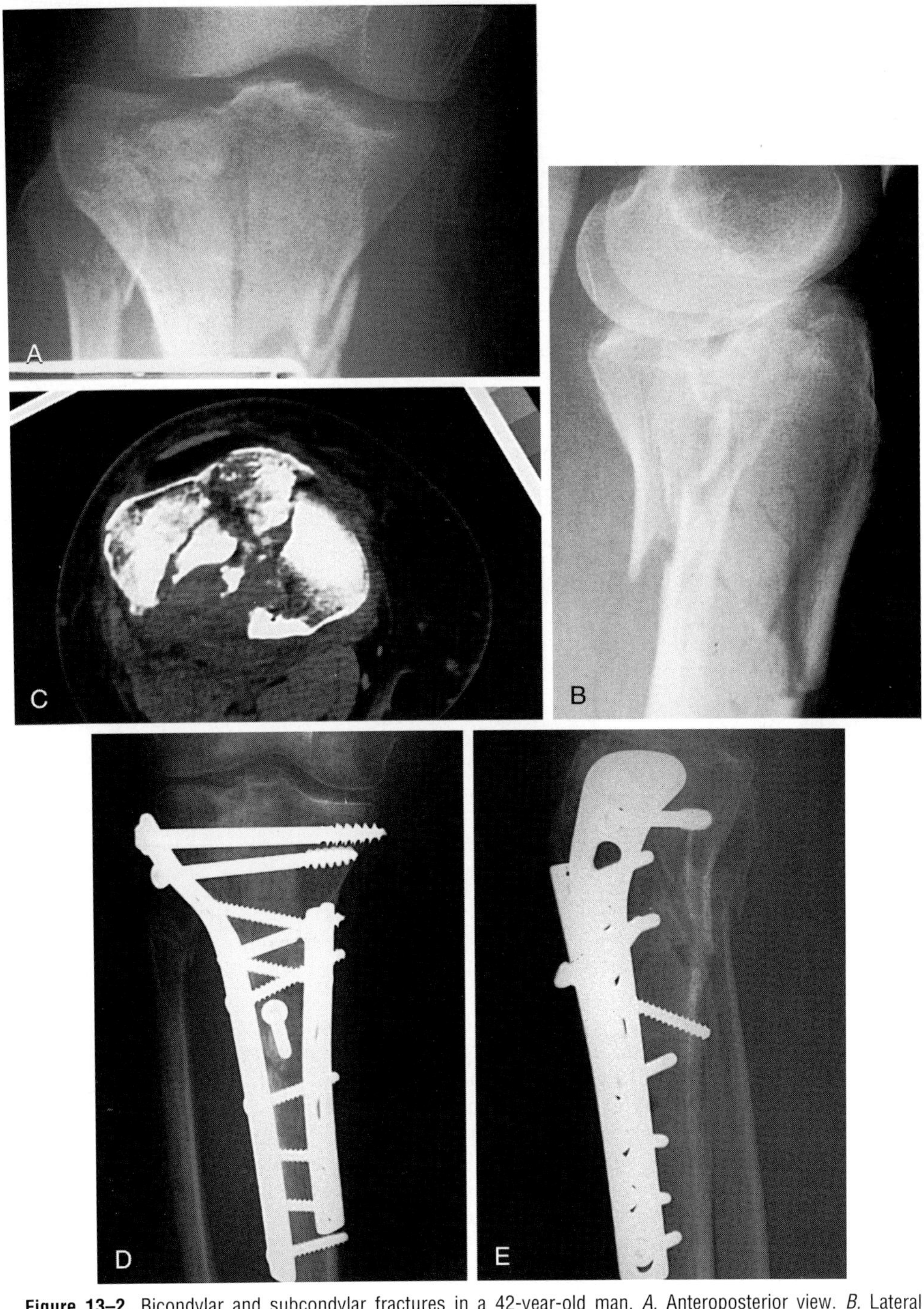

Figure 13–2. Bicondylar and subcondylar fractures in a 42-year-old man. *A*, Anteroposterior view. *B*, Lateral view. *C*, Axial computed tomography (CT) scan. Note the marked articular disruption. *D*, Postoperative anteroposterior view. Note the fixation by the tibial plateau plate and the smaller medial plate. *E*, Postoperative lateral view.

that a small pin external fixator be used and early knee movement started. If articular reduction obtained by traction leaves more than 4 to 5 mm of displacement, I try to reduce the fracture displacement by applying an external fixator and by doing a limited open reduction and fragment fixation by screws, pins, or plate.[126, 934, 1010, 1063]

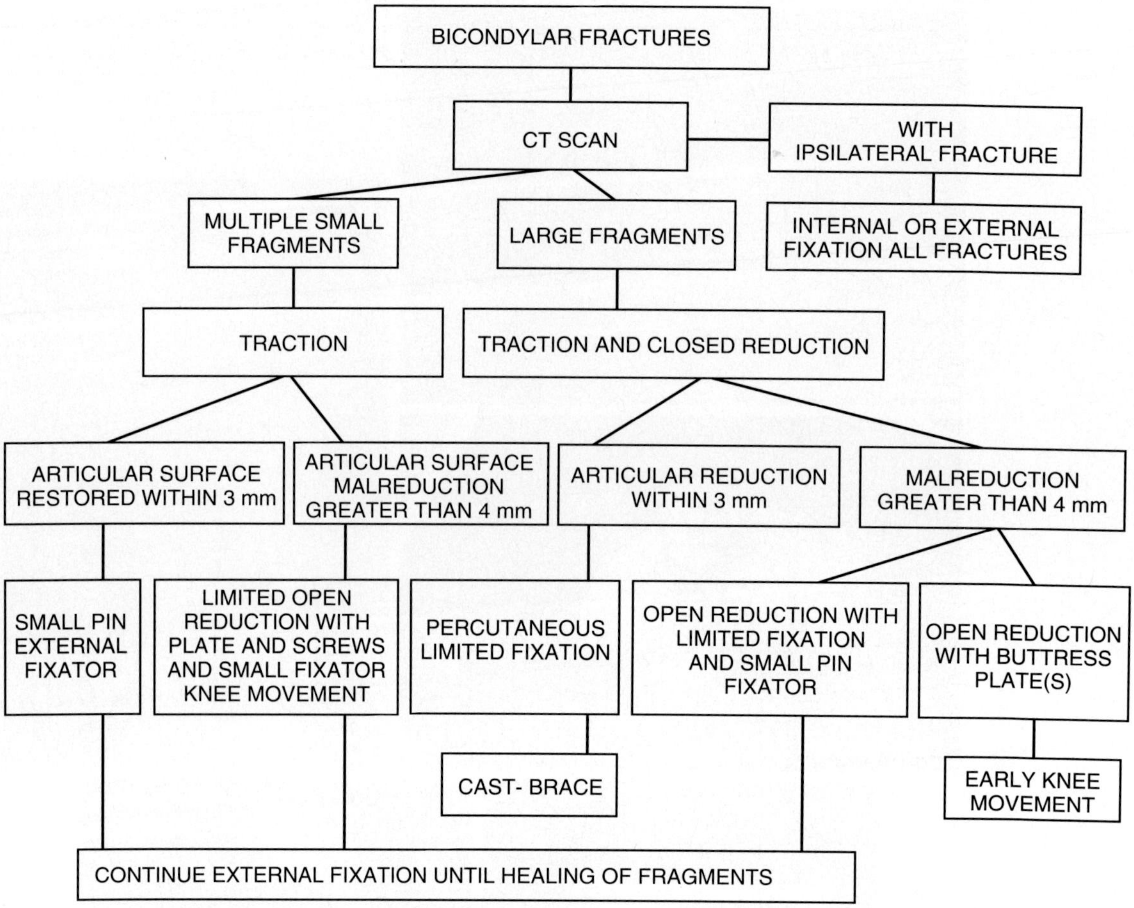

Figure 13–3. Treatment algorithm for bicondylar fractures. (CT = computed tomography.)

If imaging studies show large fragments, closed reduction using heavy traction is used.[482] Although reductions within 2 or 3 mm of anatomic position can be maintained in traction, I prefer to perform percutaneous screw or plate fixation followed by cast-bracing until callus develops.[126] Small pin external fixators should be considered because of their potential for maintaining reduction and allowing knee movement in some patients.[85, 214, 729, 760, 1063]

If malreduction remains after traction and closed fracture manipulation, I prefer open reduction with internal fixation by screws and plates. Frequently, fixation is sufficiently rigid that early knee motion can be used. An alternative method now being tested is the use of a small pin fixator with olive wires to reduce and hold the fracture.

If ipsilateral fractures are present, I favor stabilization of all fractures by open reduction and internal fixation or the use of a small pin external fixator to maintain fracture position.

In general I favor closed treatment methods, such as skeletal traction and early mobilization, when there is doubt about the likelihood of obtaining rigid internal fixation. Traction remains the best option because knee function can be maintained and late reconstructive procedures can correct malalignment. The use of a closed method also avoids the high incidence of operative complications.

TREATMENT

A wide variety of options must be considered in the treatment of bicondylar fractures (Table 13–3).

Table 13–3. TREATMENT METHODS USED IN THE AUTHOR'S SERIES (No. = 186)

TREATMENT	1940–1973 (N = 99)	1974–1994 (N = 87)
Closed		
Functional	0	0
Fracture-brace	0	2%
Cast-brace	0	5%
Plaster cast	55%	8%
Traction	13%	9%
Closed reduction	12%	6%
Total closed	80%	30%
Open		
Open—no cast	3%	33%
Open—cast	14%	31%
Open—traction	3%	2%
Arthroscopic reduction	0	1%
Percutaneous fixation	0	2%
External fixation	0	1%
Total open	20%	68%

Most bicondylar fractures are very unstable and as such become candidates for open reduction. Over the last 20 years more than two thirds of bicondylar fractures in my series have been operated on, but the long-term results obtained have not been encouraging. Schatzker and others have demonstrated the benefits of rigid fracture fixation of tibial plateau fractures.[947, 949, 950] If less than rigid fixation is all that can be obtained and a cast is used, an inferior result with knee stiffness can be expected. The additional insult and dissection required by open reduction make stiffness likely unless early knee movement can be instituted. Implantation of multiple metallic fixation devices increases the risk of postoperative wound problems, and problems are highest by far with this fracture type.[608, 1091, 1146] Thus, if the skin condition is not optimal, if operating conditions are not ideal, or the surgeon is not experienced in the method of rigid fixation of such difficult fractures, the outcome of treatment is likely to be better when appropriate closed methods or limited open reduction are used.

Rigid fixation of comminuted fractures can have many advantages. If an unstable fracture can be stabilized, it can be treated thereafter as an undisplaced fracture with the expectation of a reasonably good functional result.[910] This permits early knee mobilization, thus reducing intra-articular adhesions and maintaining muscle strength.

Acceptable reduction after closed fracture manipulation may be stabilized by plate and screws by exposing only the tibial condyle(s) without exposing the joint surface.[65] The advantage of this technique is less scar tissue and easier return of knee motion. Percutaneous screw or plate fixation of the major fragments followed by external support in a cast-brace is another alternative.[100, 126, 424, 540] This method has the advantage of simplicity but requires large bicondylar fragments to be effective.

Another alternative after closed reduction is external fixation with pins and frames to maintain reduction and still allow knee motion.[85, 214, 663, 1063] Wires with bulges on them (olive wires) can exert reduction force against condylar fragments and thus maintain reduction. External fixation involves less risk of postoperative complications than does major open surgery but rarely provides the accuracy of open reduction.

Various treatment methods are discussed in relation to their effectiveness in fracture reduction, maintenance of reduction, and restoration of knee function.

Cast

The use of a plaster cast as primary treatment for bicondylar fractures is the simplest but least reliable method of management because it is well known that valgus-varus or flexion-extension movement occurs in a cast.[564] A fracture that is initially in acceptable position in a cast may progressively deform into back knee, front knee, valgus, or varus position (Fig. 13–4). Sarmiento pointed out that when the fibula is intact, bicondylar fractures that are treated by a closed method tend to settle medially, but not laterally, resulting in varus deformity.[940]

Even if a cast maintains fracture position, immobilization results in intra-articular adhesions that leave some permanent knee stiffness. In general, fractures that were treated successfully in a cast had been impacted or had little initial displacement (Fig. 13–5).

Traction

Skeletal traction, utilizing a pin through the distal tibia or os calcis and pulling through capsular and ligamentous attachments, tends to reduce many

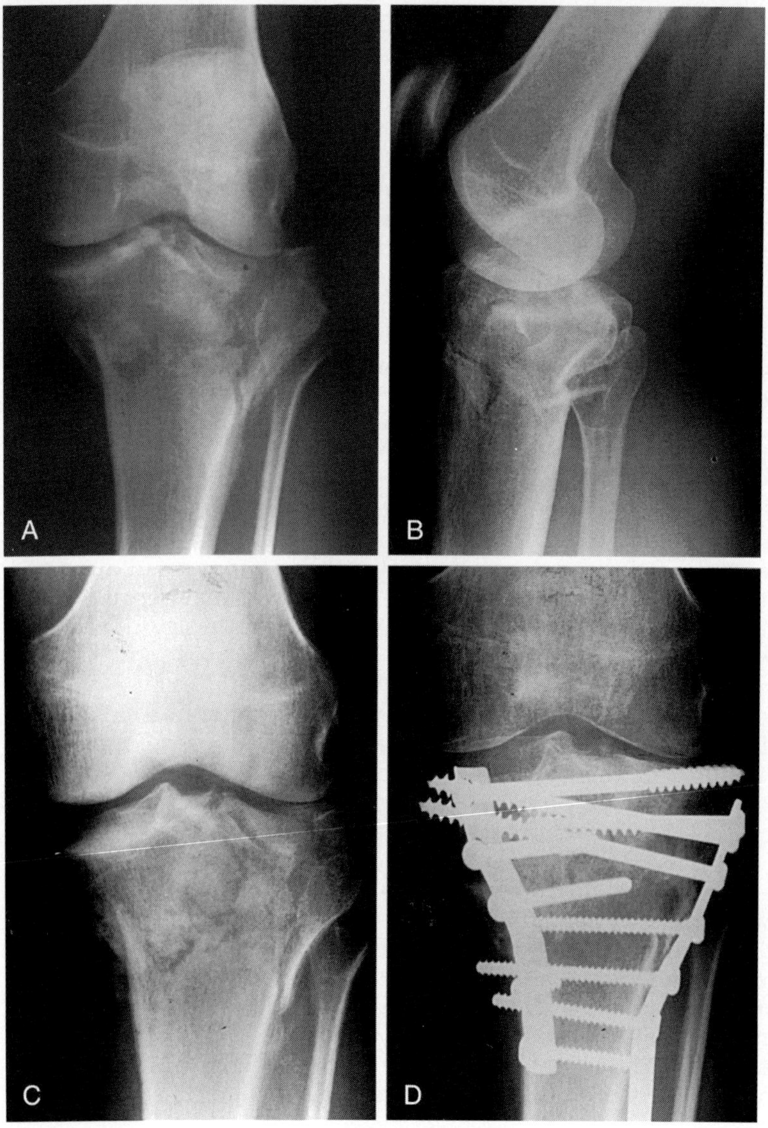

Figure 13–4. Bicondylar fracture in a 34-year-old motorcyclist who was treated initially in a plaster cast. *A*, Anteroposterior view. Note the tibial widening. *B*, Lateral view showing fracture comminution. *C*, Note the further displacement of the medial plateau 8 weeks after injury. *D*, Late open reconstruction with less than optimal articular restoration.

displaced fracture fragments to near-anatomic position. Continuing treatment in traction helps to prevent fracture redisplacement and allows knee movement.[482] Traction does, however, tend to pull the limb into a straight position, thus eliminating normal knee valgus alignment. Modified Badgley's traction, using thigh and calf plaster cuffs to maintain a constant valgus angle, tends to minimize late angular deformity while still fostering knee movement.[39, 728]

If traction is used as the primary treatment, knee movement is started within the first few days after injury and increased to 90 degrees of movement within the initial 2 weeks. Until fracture fragments solidify, they displace temporarily during knee movement; during rest, however, traction restores them to their original position. Permanent flexion contracture can usually be avoided by having the knee return to full extension whenever the knee is not being moved.

Closed Reduction

Closed reduction procedures are carried out ideally on a fracture table using skeletal traction.[78, 275, 289, 424, 482] The position of the fragments improves considerably with capsular pull on the fractured condyles as traction weight of up to 50 to 60 lb is used. The position of both condyles is determined by an x-ray, which is taken after traction has been applied. One or both condyles may remain depressed below the normal articular level. Closed manipulation will often reduce these fragments quite well. If required, gentle mallet pounding upward on the padded flare of a depressed plateau will often elevate it to normal level, which is confirmed by x-ray. An x-ray at this time, although revealing correct articular level, most often will show that there is still widening of the proximal tibia with significant fracture gaps. This is corrected by impacting the fracture from side to side using a giant nutcracker or Bohler clamp. Impaction and reduction are confirmed by x-ray.[343, 1105] Although fracture stability is improved after the fracture has been impacted, it is important to use continuous traction in the first weeks after fracture, rather than a cast or cast-brace, to prevent loss of reduction.[482] Post-reduction traction should be started using 20 lb of weight; the weight should be gradually reduced to 10 lb during the next month. Knee flexion to 90 degrees can be obtained in traction but the joint should thereafter rest in full extension. Special techniques utilizing splints (e.g., modified Badgley's traction, which is used by T.M. Moore) help to preserve the normal valgus knee alignment in traction by the use of a fixed angle between thigh and calf plaster cuffs while still permitting knee movement.[39, 728] Percutaneous fixation techniques with cannulated screws may shorten the time required in traction and hasten transfer to a cast-brace.[100, 238, 540, 562]

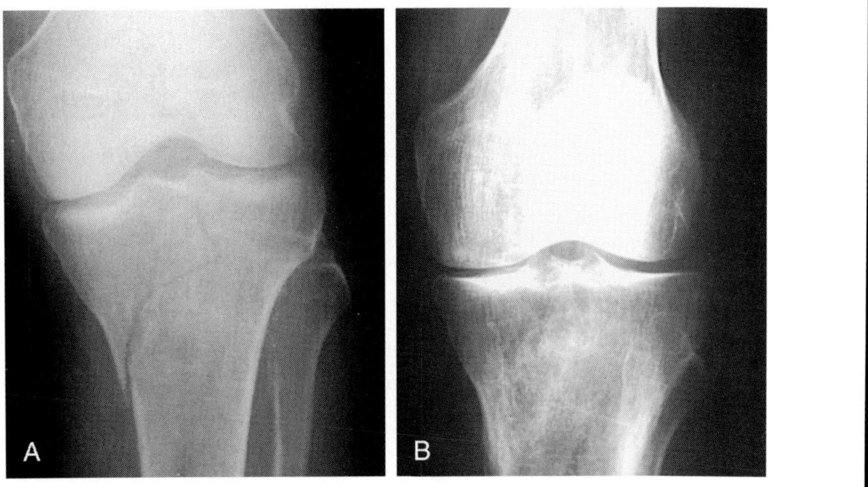

Figure 13–5. A bicondylar fracture in a 64-year-old man who was treated by "knock-knee" plaster cast for 9 weeks. *A*, Anteroposterior view showing little displacement. *B*, All fractures are consolidated in x-rays at 6 months.

Percutaneous and External Fixation

Percutaneous pinning or wiring techniques are being used increasingly after closed reduction to maintain condylar alignment.[100, 540, 562] Wire loops or cancellous screws can be used if there is no associated subcondylar fracture.

Fracture displacement can be reduced by closed means in traction as outlined earlier. After reduction has been obtained, percutaneous fixation by cannulated screws or plate is used to provide stability. After percutaneous fixation, a cast-brace is used to protect the fracture for the several weeks required for healing.[289] An external fixator is now being used for the same purpose, especially when there is an associated subcondylar fracture.

The newest treatment is external fixation, which has the advantage of holding fracture fragments in alignment while permitting the knee to move[85, 214, 641] (Fig. 13–6). This is especially useful when there are associated comminuted fractures of the proximal tibia. The main concerns are the ability to reduce the articular fragments adequately to reconstitute an articular surface and the danger of pin tract infection that ultimately might involve the fracture and the knee joint. Fracture reduction is facilitated by skeletal traction using 20 to 50 lb and by manually pushing and manipulating fragments under x-ray control until articular surfaces are level. Lateral compression can then be exerted by a "C" or Bohler clamp, or olive wires can be used with a small pin fixation system to aid in fragment reduction. Once reduction has been obtained, the fixation device must be used for sufficient time to allow fragments to heal. Premature removal of this device may lead to articular collapse, often into varus position.

Open Reduction

The goals of open reduction are accurate restoration of articular surfaces and rigid fracture fixation. The type and placement of fixation materials should be carefully planned in advance by studying plain x-rays and CT scans. Most bicondylar fractures require at least one T-, L-buttress, or plateau plate that should be placed on the side where the most fracture instability is anticipated. Two plates occasionally are required, one on either side, to secure rigid fracture fixation. Two buttress plates are bulky, and it is best to use a smaller plate on one side to avoid excessive tension on the skin during closure.

To accomplish open reduction, surgical exposures should be individualized in each case. It is necessary to see the fracture and insert internal fixation devices. In some less displaced fractures separate medial and lateral approaches may suffice. Two incisions are easier and safer to use than one long incision when there is a medial coronal plane fracture and a comminuted lateral plateau fracture. A midline incision does not allow ready access to the posterior aspect of the tibia with the knee in extension, and this makes reduction of coronal fracture very difficult to accomplish. A medial utility approach, which exposes the medial fracture, does allow reduction and fracture fixation.

In most severely displaced fractures, one large midline approach is preferable. Though popular for many years the "Y" skin incision is now rarely used because of the frequency of skin slough at the apex.[455, 519, 958] The midline approach, also used for knee replacement, permits simultaneous visualization of both condyles, the tibial shaft, and the knee joint (see Chapter 6). Osteotomy of the tibial tubercle or division of the patellar tendon with proximal reflection of the patellar mechanism provides optimal exposure.[327, 416, 792, 947] Rigid reattachment of an osteotomized tubercle fragment may prove difficult in fractures with comminution in the proximal tibia and thus should be avoided in that situation.

After exposure, and with a minimum of soft tissue stripping, fracture fragments are reduced piece by piece and temporarily fixed with Kirschner wires. Reduction is facilitated and is more likely to be accurate if femoral distractors are inserted both laterally and medially. The adequacy of reduction

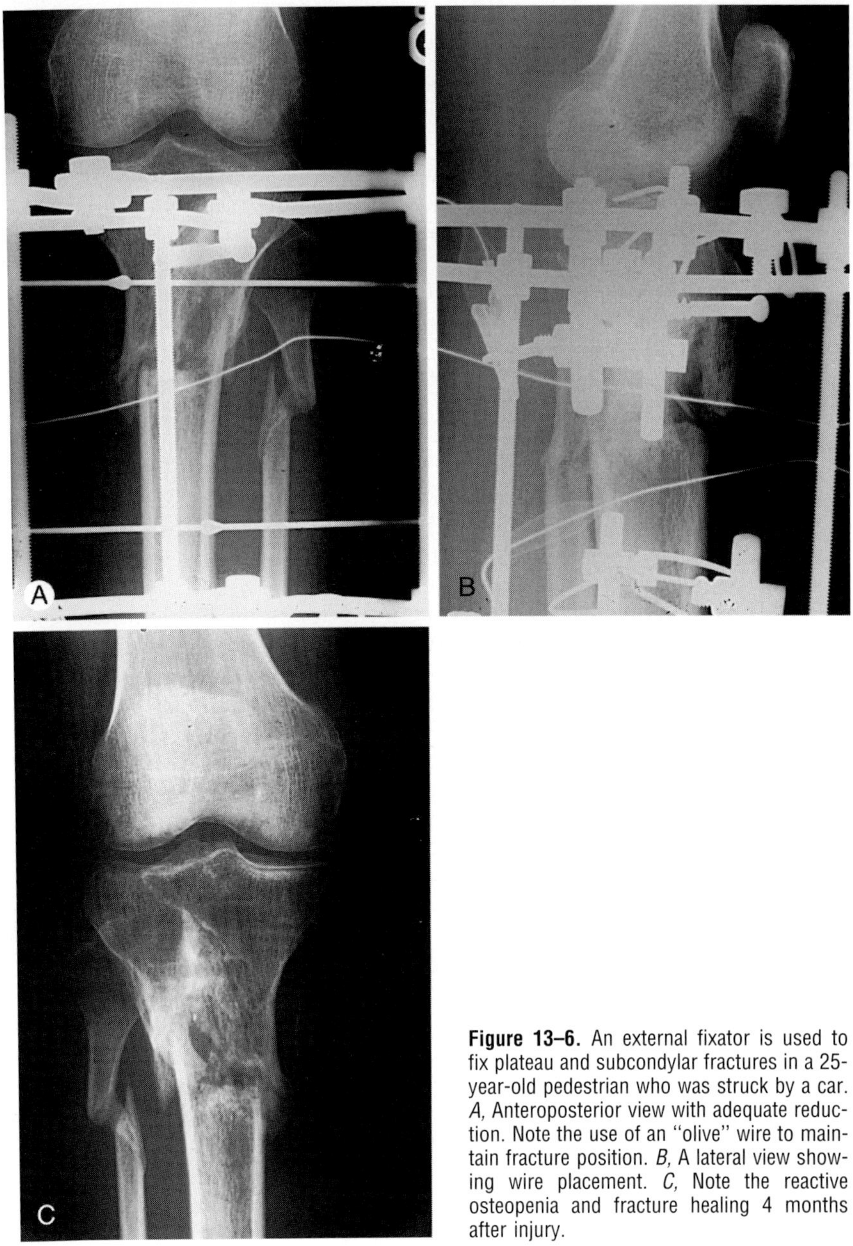

Figure 13–6. An external fixator is used to fix plateau and subcondylar fractures in a 25-year-old pedestrian who was struck by a car. *A*, Anteroposterior view with adequate reduction. Note the use of an "olive" wire to maintain fracture position. *B*, A lateral view showing wire placement. *C*, Note the reactive osteopenia and fracture healing 4 months after injury.

is confirmed by intraoperative x-ray. When reduction is satisfactory, internal fixation devices are inserted. If a buttress plate is to be used, it is contoured to the proximal tibia to provide firm pressure against the condyle to aid in fracture fixation (see Fig. 13–2). After internal fixation has been completed, the stability of the knee is tested. If the knee remains unstable despite reduction and fixation, the status of the collateral ligaments should be determined and torn ligaments should be repaired. The menisci are always preserved unless irreparably damaged. If surgical detachment of menisci through the meniscotibial ligaments is required for visualization of the fractures, then these menisci are reattached with multiple sutures as the first step in wound closure.

POST TREATMENT CARE

The aftercare required following cast, traction, closed reduction, and percutaneous methods has previously been mentioned. Special aftercare is vital to success following complex open reduction procedures. If the desired goal of rigid fracture fixation has been achieved, continuous passive motion decreases postoperative pain and encourages return of knee motion. It is important to ensure that moving the knee does not adversely affect wound healing. Once the wound is healed, recovery of knee motion becomes the priority.

X-rays are taken periodically to carefully compare the current view with the earlier views to ascertain whether the fracture position is changing. Healing of complex bicondylar fractures takes between 10 and 16 weeks, during which time the knee should be moving with appropriate protection. Weight-bearing is deferred until fracture healing is assured. Assumption of full weight-bearing is usually possible by 3 to 4 months after the injury.

COMPLICATIONS

After bicondylar fractures many diverse complications occur that relate both to the nature of the fracture and its treatment. The reported incidence of complications has been highest in bicondylar fractures, and the incidence was 48% in my series. The complication rate in surgically treated patients was 71% and was 32% with closed treatment (Table 13–4).

The incidence of wound infection after open reduction of bicondylar fractures is reported in the literature to be between 7% and 30% and was 13% in my series. A febrile course, swollen, and hot joint or unusual pain should alert the surgeon to the possibility of infection. Aspiration of the wound and also the knee joint for smear and culture should be done early when the possibility of infection is considered. If the smear is positive, the wound should be opened, débrided, irrigated and left open. If the knee joint is infected, either arthroscopic irrigation and débridement or open irrigation and débridement is necessary.

Wound sloughs and wound breakdown usually resulted in wound infection, and bacterial contamination caused sepsis, often involving the knee joint. Every attempt should be made to prevent the spread of infection into the knee or the bone. Repeated débridement at intervals of 2 to 3 days usually brings the infection under control. Keeping the knee in a resting position fosters better wound healing than does knee motion.

In my series loss of fracture reduction of greater than 2 mm occurred in 34 of 163 patients (20%) and had almost the same incidence whether closed or open treatment was used. The development of rigid fixation materials and their use in these challenging fractures has changed the incidence of loss of reduction from 45% before 1970 to 17% since that time.

Table 13–4. COMPLICATIONS IN BICONDYLAR FRACTURES (No. = 163)

COMPLICATION	CLOSED TREATMENT (N = 96)	OPEN TREATMENT (N = 67)	TOTAL (N = 163)
Phlebitis	0	7%	3%
Arterial injury	1%	5%	2%
Compartment syndrome	1%	8%	4%
Peroneal nerve injury	4%	0	4%
Wound infection	1%	13%	6%
Fracture position loss	19%	21%	20%
Avascular necrosis	0	0	0
Open fracture	3%	9%	6%
Other	3%	8%	3%
Total	32%	71%	48%

Table 13–5. FOLLOW-UP RESULTS OF 25 ISOLATED BICONDYLAR FRACTURES

	AVERAGE	RANGE
Point rating	74	(34–99)
Pain	Moderate	0 to severe
Flex deformity	3 degrees	0 to 10 degrees
Knee motion	115 degrees	75 to 135 degrees
Deformity	5 degrees	0 to 15 degrees
Instability	5 degrees	0 to 10 degrees
Arthritis	Mild	0 to severe

Mean follow-up 5 years (2–17 years).

RESULTS

Results after treatment of bicondylar fractures in the author's series were less favorable than after treatment of other plateau fractures. Patients with isolated bicondylar fractures who were followed for more than 2 years (mean 5 years) had an average result of 74 points (Table 13–5). Patients treated by closed methods averaged 77 points, while those treated by open methods averaged 69 points. Those patients with less displaced fractures treated by casting and followed for a year had a point rating of 73. More displaced fractures were usually treated by operative means. Comparison of treatment results between patients in the last 20 years and those before indicated no significant difference in point rating.

If an associated collateral or cruciate ligament injury was present, the results averaged 36 points. If there was an ipsilateral fracture, the results averaged 66 points (Table 13–6).

The 29% of patients who experienced long-term sequelae after closed treatment had rather similar problems than did those noted after open management. Open reduction in bicondylar fractures did, however, lessen the incidence of deformity and instability.

Many anatomically reduced fractures did well, but a few underwent a painful, "chondrolysis-like" joint narrowing. Traumatic arthritis occurred more frequently after this type of fracture because of extensive articular damage and more permanent varus deformity than noted in other fracture types. In large series, 16% were noted to have developed moderate or severe degenerative joint disease within 5 years.[106, 176, 871, 967, 1087]

The prognosis for normal or near-normal function (point rating of 81 to 100) after a bicondylar fracture is not good. Only 31% in my series obtained such results. This group of patients had a 50% incidence of associated fracture and two thirds had been treated by closed methods. Those obtaining poorer results

Table 13–6. RESULTS OF 43 BICONDYLAR FRACTURES WITH IPSILATERAL FRACTURE

	AVERAGE	RANGE
Point rating	66	(32–96)
Pain	Mild–moderate	None to severe
Flex deformity	6 degrees	0 to 15 degrees
Knee motion	105 degrees	60 to 135 degrees
Deformity	8 degrees	0 to 25 degrees
Instability	5 degrees	0 to 10 degrees
Arthritis	Mild–moderate	None to severe

Mean follow-up 6 years (2–20 years).

(less than 80 point rating) had greater initial fracture displacement; two thirds had associated fractures; and 60% were treated by open reduction. Thirty-five percent of bicondylar fractures required later surgical procedures. The most frequent reason for surgery was removal of hardware. The next reason for surgery was subcondylar osteotomy to correct angular deformity or malunion, which was observed more frequently after a bicondylar fracture than after other fracture types.

SUMMARY

Bicondylar fractures have proved to be a major therapeutic challenge throughout the history of plateau fracture treatment. There is some basis for cautious optimism when well-designed internal fixation materials are applied correctly. Nonetheless, these fractures have much associated bone and soft tissue damage that tends to limit the potential for a good result.

Although it is difficult to obtain consistently good results in the treatment of bicondylar fractures, the important factors are the severity of the fracture and the accuracy and rigidity of internal fixation that can be obtained. The high incidence of complications indicates the need for constant vigilance in caring for patients with this difficult injury.

CHAPTER 14

Associated Ipsilateral Fractures

Fractures in the same extremity as a tibial plateau fracture make treatment more complex and results less predictable.[4] The generally accepted principle of treatment is rigid fixation of all fractures in order that rehabilitation of the entire limb may be started early.[947] Treatment compromises, such as cast immobilization or prolonged traction, will tend to limit recovery of knee function.

The problem of ipsilateral fractures is a major one. In the author's series of 1533 patients, 758 (49%) had tibial spine, subcondylar, or other ipsilateral fractures (Table 14–1).

The most frequently associated fracture was the subcondylar fracture, which was present in 21%, whereas tibial spine fractures were noted in 15%. Multiple fractures in the same extremity were much more likely to affect the final result than was a single associated fracture.

The management of plateau fractures with ipsilateral fractures has improved since 1974 because of a more aggressive attitude toward obtaining rigid fracture fixation and promoting early rehabilitation. The average point rating result in the author's series was three points higher than it was during the previous 20 years. The same improvement in average point ratings occurred when there was no associated fracture (Table 14–2).

Operative treatment and nonoperative treatment in 167 patients with ipsilateral fractures resulted in long-term ratings of 76 and 73 points, respectively. In the absence of ipsilateral fractures, operative ratings averaged 78 points and

Table 14–1. IPSILATERAL FRACTURES AND FRACTURE TYPES (N = 1533)

IPSILATERAL FRACTURES	MD	LC	SC	TO	SP	RIM	BIC	TOTAL
Subcondylar	86	49	39	33	10	1	98	316
Tibial spine	46	26	27	42	10	12	64	227
Patella	2	3	1	3	0	0	0	9
Femoral condyle	3	0	2	2	2	1	0	10
Supracondylar	3	0	0	3	0	0	0	6
Femoral shaft	13	2	0	2	0	1	2	20
Hip	4	2	0	2	2	2	4	16
Tibial shaft	23	16	12	10	5	3	9	78
Ankle or foot	2	4	7	4	0	1	2	20
Multiple	15	15	5	11	1	4	5	56
Total	197	117	93	112	39	25	184	758
FIBULAR FRACTURES	106	96	152	46	17	13	113	543

MD = Minimally displaced; LC = Local compression; SC = Split compression; TO = Total depression; SP = Split fracture; RIM = Rim fracture; BIC = Bicondylar fracture.

Table 14–2. RESULTS OF EARLIER AND MORE CURRENT TREATMENT

PLATEAU FRACTURES WITH ASSOCIATED INJURIES	POINT RATING RESULTS BEFORE 1975	AFTER 1974
No associated injury	79 (194)	82 (81)
Associated injury	73 (101)	76 (67)

nonoperative treatment 77 points. Often operative treatment was selected in the more displaced and difficult fractures. Minimally displaced fractures without ipsilateral fractures rated 91 points but with associated fractures the average declined to 83 points (Table 14–3).

TREATMENT CONSIDERATIONS

Based on the aforementioned results and personal experience, it is clear that plateau fractures with associated ipsilateral fractures carry a poorer long-term prognosis. When treating multiple fractures in an extremity, aggressive management of each fracture is suggested to hasten and maximize rehabilitation.

Fixation of a *hip fracture* or inserting a hemireplacement restores stability in the limb so that optimal treatment can be used for the plateau fracture. Rigid internal fixation for the plateau fracture should be carried out, because the use of fracture bracing, cast, or traction may be undesirable for the hip. Early mobilization of the entire limb, concentrating on restoration of knee movement and quadriceps strength, should not compromise healing of the hip fracture and help to maintain necessary strength for later weight-bearing.

Femoral shaft fractures are managed by medullary rod fixation. Comminuted and segmental fractures require an interlocking nail. Once the femur has been fixed, open reduction and fixation of the plateau fracture should be accomplished. When rigid fracture fixation has been achieved, the limb can be free of external support or at the most be encased in a hinged knee support. If it is not possible to internally fix the fractures, skeletal traction using a pin through the distal tibia will often produce a well-moving and probably stable knee but may delay healing of the femoral shaft fracture.

Intercondylar eminence fractures are classified as types I, II, and III by fracture displacement. Type I and some type IIs have insufficient displacement to require open reduction. Indeed, if the plateau fracture has been reduced and the knee can be fully extended, the chances are very good that the intercondylar eminence will heal in a satisfactory position with immobilization and the knee will function satisfactorily. Some type II fractures block knee extension and require operative reduction. Type III fractures are derotated, reduced, and fixed in a normal position. Screw fixation of the fragment is occasionally possible, or the fragment may be locked in as plateau fragments are reduced and fixed (Fig. 14–1). The best method of fixation is most often a wire loop passed around the fragment, through a drill hole in the anterior tibia. With the knee in a few degrees of flexion, the wire is tightened and the fragment is pushed into position. When

Table 14–3. POINT RATING AFTER CLOSED OR OPEN TREATMENT (SINCE 1974) OF PLATEAU FRACTURES WITH COEXISTING IPSILATERAL FRACTURES

TREATMENT	NUMBER	NO. OF POINTS	AVERAGE DEPRESSION (mm)
Closed	15	79	6
Open	50	76	11

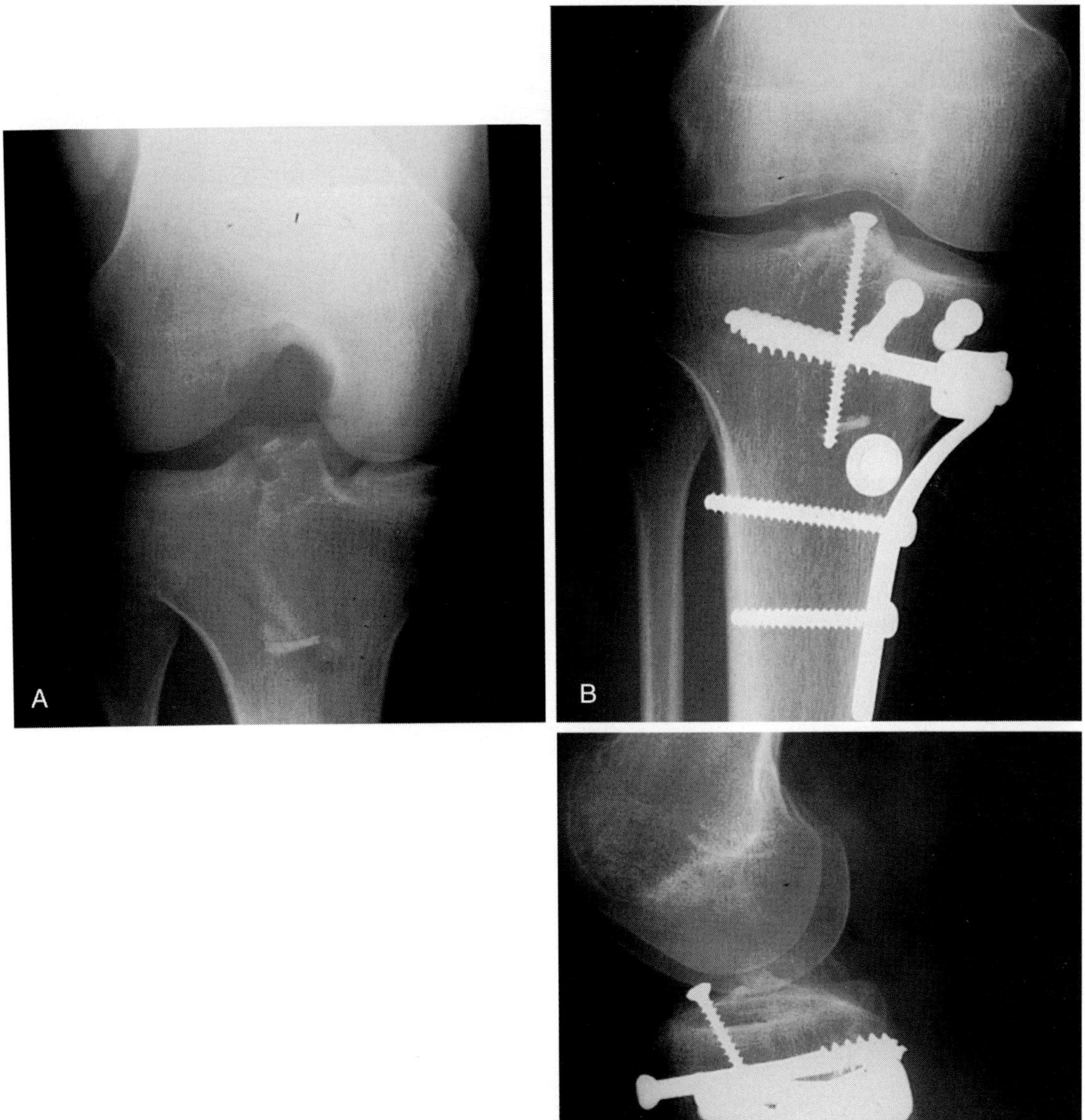

Figure 14–1. Lateral plateau and intercondylar eminence fractures treated by open reduction. *A*, Original tunnel view x-ray. *B*, Anteroposterior view 2 months after reduction. A single screw is used to fix the intercondylar eminence fracture. *C*, Lateral view 2 months after reduction. An accurate fracture reduction has been accomplished.

the wire is secured, the fragment is fixed, but not sufficiently to allow movement of the knee until there is evidence of healing by x-ray.

Tibial tubercle fractures are fortunately seldom seen in association with fractures of the tibial plateau. When present, such fractures accompany comminuted bicondylar fractures, making fixation of the tubercle fragment often difficult and tenuous. Since the function of the quadriceps mechanism depends on the integrity of the patellar tendon and its tubercle attachment, rigid fixation of the turbercle must be provided. It is sometimes possible to nearly reduce the condyles, thus fixing them temporarily with Kirschner wires as a buttress plate is bent to fit and cancellous screws are drilled and partially inserted. Before the condyles are compressed by the lag effect of the screws, the tubercle is replaced and held by a Kirschner wire as the screws are tightened. This often provides tentative fixation, compressing the tubercle region. A screw is then inserted through the tubercle into the posterior tibial cortex. Such internal fixation seldom allows immediate movement of the knee without risk of detachment of the tubercle. A few degrees of movement in a cast-brace or the use of a cast for 3 or 4 weeks after reduction will normally protect the fixation of the tubercle.

Subcondylar fractures occur with great regularity in association with proximal tibial articular fractures, so much so that Schatzker and associates called them type VI.[950] In the author's series, 21% of fractures had a subcondylar extension that effectively detached the shaft of the tibia from the articular condyles. The subcondylar fracture is often undisplaced, but may be angulated or displaced in any direction. Closed reduction is not easy because of the very short proximal lever arm; thus open reduction becomes a more attractive option. When the combination of plateau and subcondylar fractures is treated, there is a tendency for the leg to angulate into varus as the medial cortex of the tibia collapses (Fig. 14–2). This is especially true where there is a bicondylar fracture with the fibula intact.[940] Open reduction requires preoperative planning of what type of internal or external fixation is to be used (often a plate) and also on which side of the tibia it should be applied. When the medial cortex shows comminution or the fibula is intact in a comminuted bicondylar fracture, the medial surface of the tibia is generally the best location for a plate. Even with a single medial plate, a lateral plate may, at times, also be required to achieve rigid fracture fixation (Fig. 14–3). Two buttress plates often occupy so much volume in the leg that wound closure is under tension. In this situation, a smaller medial plate or a medial external fixator is used. Smaller plates with appropriate contouring to the shape of the proximal tibia provide fixation and some buttress effect. The ideal fixation

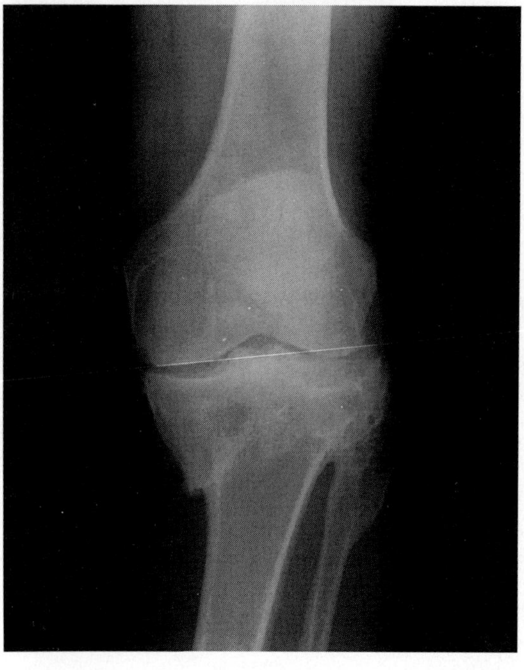

Figure 14–2. Lateral plateau and subcondylar fracture that healed predictably in the varus position after treatment in a plaster cast.

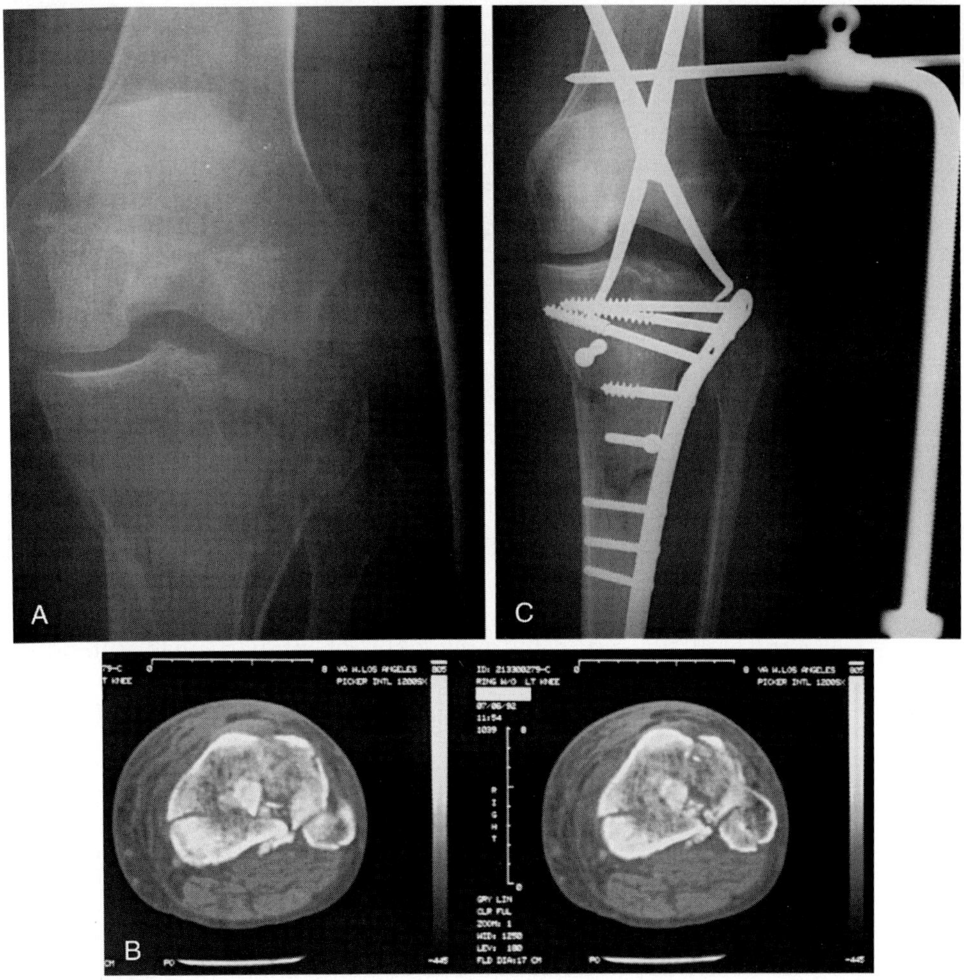

Figure 14–3. Severe split compression fracture with an associated subcondylar fracture. *A*, Initial anteroposterior view. *B*, Axial computed tomography scan showing comminution of the articular surface. *C*, Intraoperative view of a fracture reduction aided by use of a femoral distractor and a tibial plateau plate and screws.

is rigid, after which a cast or brace is not required, and, as Rombold pointed out, early movement of the knee will provide a good result.[910]

External fixation with small pin fixators is being used increasingly in the management of closed or open plateau fractures associated with subcondylar fractures (Fig. 14–4). With these newer techniques, the fractures can be reduced and knee movement encouraged.[214, 729, 971, 1063]

Patellar fractures are rarely associated with plateau fractures; however, when they occur, they should be rigidly fixed along with the plateau fracture to get the knee moving. Knee immobilization sufficiently long to allow healing of the patellar fracture produces dense intra-articular adhesions that make restoration of near-normal knee motion impossible. Thus both the patellar fracture and the plateau fracture need to be fixed rigidly by some means. Fixation methods for the patellar fracture include Kirschner wires or screws, neither sufficient to permit active knee movement. A tension band across the patellar fracture with either of the aforementioned fixation methods will usually be sufficient to permit early passive and probably active knee movement. If a cast-brace is required for the plateau fracture, it will not create additional problems for the patella. If a patellectomy is required, either partial or complete, postoperative hinged knee bracing to partially limit knee flexion temporarily will provide optimal support

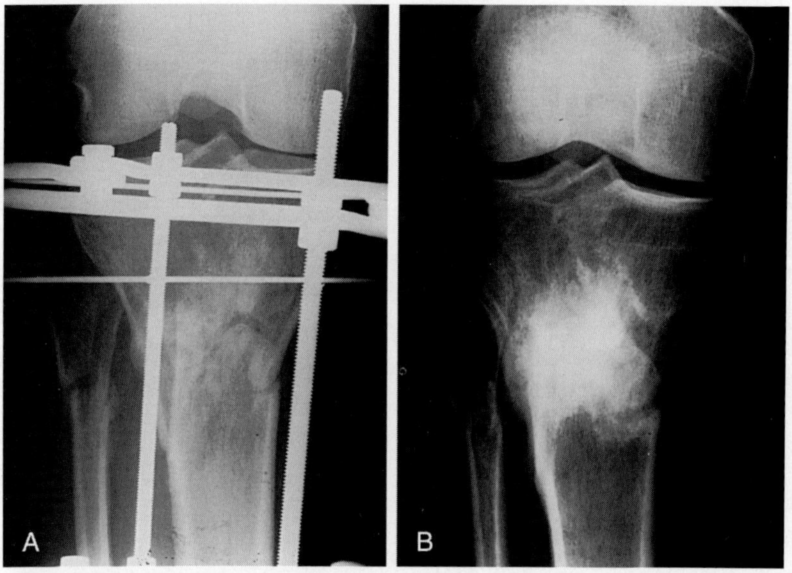

Figure 14–4. Total depression fracture with an associated subcondylar fracture. *A*, Small wires are in place with an external fixator frame. *B*, Fracture well healed 5 months after the injury.

and will still aid in the prevention of intra-articular adhesions. The prognosis with this combination of injuries is some permanent loss of motion and knee extension strength, perhaps with extension lag. A long period of post-healing muscle and joint conditioning is required.

Femoral condylar fracture is infrequently associated with plateau fracture. Open reduction and rigid internal fixation of both femoral condyle and plateau fracture is the best management technique. As a rule, an anterolateral or midline approach will expose both areas of fracture sufficiently to permit accurate articular reduction and insertion of fixation materials. Two or three cancellous screws are usually sufficient to stabilize the femoral condyle, but rarely a condylar plate will serve better. Postoperative external support with a cast-brace or fracture-brace is helpful in hastening rehabilitation.

A *supracondylar femoral fracture* with a plateau fracture is an extremely serious injury combination, rendering the knee very unstable.[4] The objective of treatment is to stabilize both fractures and restore knee movement as rapidly as wound healing will allow. Surgical exposure of the supracondylar fracture depends on its extent and location. If intercondylar extension is present, either a wide anterolateral or midline exposure of the distal femur and proximal tibia is required. Such an approach often reflects the osteotomized tibial tubercle proximalward with the fat pad.[327] The distal femur and both femoral and tibial condyles are exposed to permit accurate reduction and fixation of each fracture. Rigid fixation provides the best possible result.[4] If rigid internal fixation is obtained and the tibial tubercle is rigidly reattached, passive motion and then gentle active motion can be used at an early stage. Traction treatment of this injury combination rarely leads to an acceptable result.

Tibial shaft fractures were associated with 5% of the tibial plateau fractures in the author's series. Some of these tibial shaft fractures were open fractures, which greatly increased the problems of managing the plateau fractures. Since internal fixation of tibial fractures was done infrequently in the series, cast immobilization was often used for 6 to 8 months or more. This caused permanent limitation of knee movement. The challenge of this combination injury is to treat both fractures while preserving knee function. Internal fixation of both fractures is the best choice. Medullary nailing of the tibial fracture is rarely advisable because of the proximity of the plateau fracture. The other options are plate or external fixation. Fixation of the plateau fracture and cast-bracing is not wise because of the inability to begin weight-bearing as a stimulus to tibial shaft healing. External fixators are being used for proximal tibial shaft fractures. Each fracture is a challenge that demands a careful assessment of the advantages and disadvantages of each method of treatment.

Ankle and foot fractures pose little concern and need not alter treatment for the tibial plateau fracture. Techniques for internal fixation of ankle fractures are now standard and are recommended, even if below-knee cast support is needed for a few weeks after the open reduction. Foot fractures are usually treated in plaster casts, which do affect the need for early knee movement.

SUMMARY

The presence of ipsilateral fractures in the same limb poses significant treatment and postoperative care challenges to prevent limitation of knee function. Treatments of the past are not sufficient today, and a much more aggressive approach to the ipsilateral fracture, usually involving rigid internal or external fixation and early knee movement, is more likely to produce better results. Studies are not yet available to assess fully the long-term effects of aggressive treatment.[4]

CHAPTER 15

Early Complications

Treatment of articular fractures of the proximal tibia is beset by a multitude of complications that result from the nature of the fracture, the treatment employed, and also the patient (Table 15–1).

Some complications are normally associated with any injured patient who undergoes either closed or open fracture treatment. Most complications, however, result from the often difficult and capricious behavior of plateau fractures. This chapter deals with complications that occur during the period of active fracture treatment and involves the vascular system, nervous system, internal fixation materials, and the bones themselves. Late fracture sequelae, such as pain, limited motion, knee deformity, instability, and traumatic arthritis, are discussed in the chapter on sequelae (see Chapter 16).

In the author's series, loss of fracture position was the most frequently encountered complication. The overall complication rate in this series of 1267 fractures was 25%, with 16% after closed treatment and 33% after open treatment (Tables 15–2 and 15–3).

In a large series using a narrower definition of complications, Moore reported 8% after closed treatment and 19% after open treatment.[728] The rate of complications was notably highest in bicondylar fractures.[454, 1058, 1091, 1146]

THROMBOPHLEBITIS AND EMBOLISM

Immobilization of a leg or injury to the knee may lead to the development of thrombophlebitis in the calf or thigh. If treatment of the fracture is delayed for a few days, thrombophlebitis may be diagnosed and necessitate postponement or cancellation of planned treatment. In the presence of thrombophlebitis, treatment options may be quite limited and results significantly affected. Thrombophlebitis

Table 15–1. COMPLICATIONS BY FRACTURE TYPE (N = 1267)

COMPLICATION	MD	LC	SC	TO	SP	RIM	BIC	TOTAL
Loss of reduction	20	31	25	33	3	1	34	147
Thrombophlebitis	7	2	8	4	1	3	6	31
Arterial injury	0	1	1	2	3	0	7	14
Compartment syndrome	0	1	2	0	2	0	3	8
Peroneal nerve injury	0	3	7	5	1	0	6	22
Wound infection	0	4	5	2	0	1	11	23
Avascular necrosis	0	2	5	0	0	0	2	9
Nonunion	0	0	0	4	0	0	3	7
Causalgia	0	1	0	0	0	0	0	1
Implant problems	0	0	1	1	1	0	4	7
Open fracture	4	3	5	11	1	2	9	35
Other problems	1	2	4	5	0	3	6	21

MD = Minimally displaced; LC = Local compression; SC = Split compression; TO = Total depression; SP = Split fracture; RIM = Rim fracture; BIC = Bicondylar fracture.

Table 15–2. PERCENT COMPLICATIONS AFTER CLOSED TREATMENT (N = 912)

COMPLICATION	MD	LC	SC	TO	SP	RIM	BIC	TOTAL (%)
Loss of reduction	13	9	7	51	0	11	21	22
Thrombophlebitis	7	3	27	5	0	11	2	7
Arterial injury	0	0	0	0	0	0	1	0.5
Compartment syndrome	0	0	7	0	0	0	1	4
Peroneal nerve	0	0	13	3	0	11	4	3
Open fracture	1	1	2	4	6	5	3	2
Other problems	1	0	7	0	0	11	3	4

MD = Minimally displaced; LC = Local compression; SC = Split compression; TO = Total depression; SP = Split fracture; RIM = Rim fracture; BIC = Bicondylar fracture.

has been observed in from 5 to 10% of patients in larger plateau fracture series.[141, 277, 728, 805, 873, 879, 965, 967, 1058] Only 15 patients (1%) had documented thrombophlebitis in the author's series. That so few were noted undoubtedly represents underobservation or underdocumentation.

Pulmonary embolism was noted in another 1% of 1533 patients in the author's series, with no deaths as the direct result. Other large series in the literature report 1 to 2% embolism.

Patients who are being treated in traction should be considered for prophylaxis against thrombophlebitis, taking into account the extent of other injuries and past history. Low-dose heparin and coumadin have proved to be the most effective prophylactic measures to date. Mechanical measures such as pneumatic or compressive stockings, reverse Trendelenburg position, and movement of the extremities are other useful techniques to prevent thrombophlebitis. If this complication is suspected, duplex sonography is the safest objective demonstration of clot location and size. Venography documents the clot, but its use may cause a further complication because of venous irritation.

Pulmonary embolism sometimes occurs silently but usually causes pleuritic pain, an episode of bloody sputum, or shortness of breath. The diagnosis is reliably established by available tests. The problem then becomes the prevention of additional embolism during the subsequent treatment period. Medical management by heparin and coumadin is indicated.

FAT EMBOLISM

Fat embolism is one of the earliest recorded complications in the history of plateau fracture treatment; the embolism was believed to have caused the

Table 15–3. PERCENT COMPLICATIONS AFTER OPEN TREATMENT (N = 355)

COMPLICATION	MD	LC	SC	TO	SP	RIM	BIC	TOTAL (%)
Loss of reduction	0	18	17	23	0	10	22	18
Thrombophlebitis	11	1	5	5	10	0	9	5
Arterial injury	0	1	1	2	0	0	8	3
Compartment syndrome	0	1	1	0	0	0	0	0.5
Peroneal nerve	0	3	7	9	0	10	3	5
Wound infection	0	1	5	5	0	0	16	6
Avascular necrosis	0	1	0	0	0	0	0	0.3
Nonunion	0	0	1	0	0	0	5	0.3
Implant problems	0	0	1	2	10	0	6	3
Open fracture	2	1	3	7	0	0	6	4
Other problems	0	1	3	5	0	25	5	12

MD = Minimally displaced; LC = Local compression; SC = Split compression; TO = Total depression; SP = Split fracture; RIM = Rim fracture; BIC = Bicondylar fracture.

patient's demise.[331] No patient in the author's series was definitely diagnosed with a fat embolism. The diagnosis is usually established by the presence of petechial hemorrhages, changes in fatty enzymes, and decreased pO_2 in arterial blood. Treatment consists of oxygen to improve respiratory exchange, corticosteroids, and other supportive methods.

COMPARTMENT SYNDROME

Compartment syndrome, in which one or more fascial compartments in the calf develop elevated pressure, is a rarely reported complication of proximal tibial articular fractures. It is manifested clinically by pain, increasing with time, most frequently located over the proximal portion of the anterior compartment, and is tested for by measuring pressures in all leg compartments. Early and complete release of fascia encompassing the affected compartments is the indicated treatment. As a prophylactic measure to avoid compartment syndrome after open reduction of a lateral plateau fracture, the fascia should not be tightly closed.

The possibility of compartment syndrome must be considered when treating any proximal tibial fracture, especially bicondylar fractures or those with an associated subcondylar fracture.[23, 393, 1058] Unusual complaints of pain or numbness signal the need for careful examination of the leg. To accomplish this, all circular bandages and casts must be removed. Compartment pressures are then measured, and if these pressures are increased over normal values or are increasing, early fascial release must be accomplished to avoid muscle necrosis.

Early diagnosis with appropriate and timely management usually preserves the limb and most of the musculature; however, because of open fasciotomy wounds or delayed healing, ideal treatment of the fracture may not be possible. Eight patients with compartment syndrome were observed in the author's series, one of whom, diagnosed late, underwent amputation through the knee. Tscherne reported 20% compartment syndromes in comminuted plateau fractures.[1058]

ARTERIAL INJURY

Bicondylar fractures with sharp spicules of bone or any plateau fracture, especially those with an associated subcondylar component, may injure the popliteal artery. Only 14 arterial injuries (1%) were noted in the author's series. Other series report 1 to 2% arterial injury.[273, 873, 905, 1041] Ottolenghi noted 3.8% vascular injuries in plateau fractures.[801]

A diagnosis of arterial injury is strongly suspected when there is pallor of the foot, absence of foot pulses, and abnormalities of sensation in the leg and foot. An arteriogram can pinpoint the site of an arterial lesion (Fig. 15–1).

Surgical repair of the lacerated or occluded artery is carried out as an emergency, reserving fracture fixation until circulation has been re-established. Internal fixation is accomplished after arterial repair, but closed management techniques may also be used effectively. Prophylactic fasciotomies should be considered, depending on the duration of circulatory interruption. If repair is delayed for 4 to 6 hours, prophylactic fasciotomy should be strongly considered.

Although the prognosis for limb survival after vascular repair is generally good, pulses and compartment pressures should be observed closely for several days.

PERONEAL NERVE PARALYSIS

The anatomic course of the common peroneal nerve around the neck of the fibula makes it vulnerable to injury by direct trauma against the lateral aspect of the knee or by the same type of stretching that may also damage lateral knee

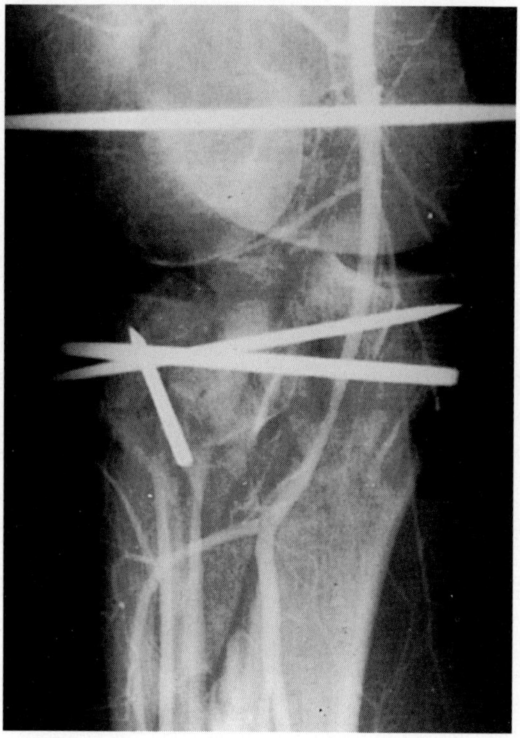

Figure 15–1. Normal arteriogram after manipulation and percutaneous pinning of an open displaced bicondylar fracture.

ligaments. Peroneal nerve damage usually occurs at the time of fracture but can also result from direct pressure against a plaster cast or traction sling, or from retraction in surgery. Most series report peroneal nerve injury in from 1 to 4%.[68, 762, 1115] Tscherne noted 23% in complex knee trauma.[1058] There were 22 peroneal palsies in the author's series (1.5%).

It is important to examine the status of the peroneal nerve initially, prior to definitive treatment, and again at intervals. During routine open reduction of a lateral plateau fracture, the peroneal nerve is not exposed but should be protected against unnecessary dissection or strong retraction. If nerve palsy is noted preoperatively, it is reasonable to ascertain nerve continuity by exploring the nerve at the time of open reduction. The surgical findings are usually of a contused nerve with some hemorrhage in the nerve sheath or stretching of the nerve around a fracture fragment.[762] Late neurolysis of the peroneal nerve is seldom required, and the prognosis for recovery is favorable. Most injured nerves recover the majority of their function within a period of 6 months. The progress of reinnervation can be documented by electromyography.

LOSS OF FRACTURE REDUCTION

Fractures that involve the articular surface of the proximal tibia are affected by strong muscle forces across the knee joint. Because of these forces, fractures tend to displace owing to pressure of the femoral condyle against the tibial plateau. Closed and open methods of treatment vary in their ability to control displacement.

A plaster cast to "immobilize" the leg does not protect against loss of fracture reduction. Studies have shown that flexion-extension and valgus-varus movement occurs even within a cast.[564] The author's clinical experience leads him to treat only stable lateral fractures in a cast, because corrective forces exerted by a cast cannot be relied on to maintain fracture reduction. Leg traction, on the other hand, holds knee joint surfaces apart by exerting its pull on the proximal tibial fracture fragments through capsular and ligamentous attachments and thus holds reduction quite well. Even when a fracture fragment displaces during knee movement or muscle contraction, it returns to its reduced position. Open reduction and internal fixation do not guarantee retention of reduction.[35, 172, 1052, 1134] Rigid internal fixation with plates and screws, however, provides the best protection against loss of reduction.[950, 1058]

In the author's series of 1533 patients, 4% of knees lost more than 4 mm of postreduction position (see Fig. 8–8). Since 1980, loss of more than 2 mm of fracture position occurred after closed treatment in 9% and after open reduction in 18% of patients in that series (Table 15–4).

Fewer fractures lost reduction when a buttress plate rather than bolts or screws was used. Point ratings for openly reduced fractures with no loss of reduction averaged 80 points, whereas those with loss of reduction of more than 2 mm averaged 62 points. The quality of the final result deteriorated with progressive loss of reduction. Bicondylar fractures treated closed lost 2 mm or more position in 19%. When treated by internal fixation, a third of these fractures lost 2 mm of reduction. The average point ratings declined from 73 to 59 points for this difficult fracture if there were 2 mm or more loss of reduction. These data indicate the importance of using methods of treatment most likely to retain fracture position.

Critical evaluation of x-rays taken during the early follow-up period after fracture treatment is important in order to detect subtle position loss in time to prevent loss.[454] A change of treatment from closed to open may solve the problem at times, and after open treatment the use of external support in the form of traction or cast-bracing may be helpful.

WOUND INFECTION

Open reduction of a plateau fracture carries with it the risk of wound infection. Wound healing problems were noted most frequently after operative treatment of bicondylar fractures, probably because of the extensive exposure required, retraction, metallic implants, and operating time.[608, 1091, 1146] The surgical approach used has a bearing on wound healing. Surgeons became aware of wound healing problems after using the Y incision, because skin necrosis often developed at the apex of the Y.[934, 1091] Deep infection ensued in some patients.

Wound infection has been reported in recent larger series, from 5 to 38%, depending on the mix of fractures subjected to open reduction.[1091, 1146] Since 1980 there were 10 infections in 290 open reductions for an incidence of 3.4% in the author's series.

Prophylactic antibiotics and newer techniques have fostered the current favorable attitude toward operative fracture management. Careful attention to skin condition, intraoperative antibiotics, surgical approaches requiring little retraction, and rigid fracture fixation have minimized the risk. Thin skin flaps should not be developed; instead, incisions through skin and subcutaneous tissue should be generous enough to minimize retraction pressure against the skin edges. Wound closure should minimize dead space, and wound suction should be used in some patients to prevent accumulation of hematoma. Tight

Table 15–4. LOSS OF REDUCTION BY FRACTURE TYPE SINCE 1980 (MORE THAN 2 MM)

LOSS OF REDUCTION	MD	LC	SC	TO	SP	RIM	BIC
After closed reduction	12%	2%	4%	19%	6%	3%	19%
After open reduction	0%	26%	15%	19%	6%	7%	18%

MD = Minimally displaced; LC = Local compression; SC = Split compression; TO = Total depression; SP = Split fracture; RIM = Rim fracture; BIC = Bicondylar fracture.

skin closure and strongly compressive bandages, splints, or casts must be avoided. Surgical wounds should be redressed frequently if there is persistence of systemic temperature elevation. A swollen, reddened suture line suggests the need for wound and knee joint aspiration for smear and culture. If there is any question of wound sepsis, the earlier the wound is opened and débrided the better the opportunity for complete eradication of the infection. Appropriate systemic antibiotics are helpful in preventing dissemination of infection. If there is concern over the possibility of infection, the knee should be aspirated and cultured. If the knee joint itself is infected, arthroscopic débridement and irrigation or arthrotomy should be performed promptly and repeated as necessary.

The prognosis after wound infection depends on the extent and spread of the infectious process. If infection is detected early and controlled while only soft tissues are involved, the result is likely to be satisfactory. When the infection results in osteomyelitis or joint infection, the proliferation of scar pannus within the joint and in the capsule usually leads to considerable loss of motion in the knee and an inferior result. In the author's series the average point rating result for knees that became infected was 61; for knees not infected it was 82 points.

AVASCULAR NECROSIS

Exposure of fractured tibial plateaus by their near complete release from soft tissue attachments may produce avascular changes. Necrosis of elevated fragments in local compression or split compression fractures is seen rarely. Bringing these already avascular, impacted bony fragments up to articular level moves them a significant distance from vascularized bone and increases their chance of remaining avascular and undergoing absorption within the knee joint. When this happens, a bony depression in the articular surface and knee deformity result (Fig. 15–2).

Bony fragments need to be exposed to accomplish accurate reduction and rigid fixation. Minimum soft tissue dissection will lessen the risk of avascular changes in the bony fragments. Percutaneous methods of fixation run no risk of producing avascular changes and should be used whenever possible.

Elevation of impacted articular fragments in local or split compression fractures is controversial in many centers, where it is believed that the results are as good with or without reduction. If reduction is accomplished and the fragments undergo avascular necrosis and absorb, the patient is no better off after the procedure. Only 7 of 267 surgically treated patients with local or split compression fractures in the author's series were left with an articular defect that resulted from avascular necrosis. When such operative reduction is performed, additional support must be given to these fragments to allow ingrowth of vessels promptly. Although metallic internal fixation is often not practical, multiple Kirschner wires and occasionally screws have been used. Most often the fragments are held in place by the firm impaction of copious bone grafts underneath. In the absence of excessive pressure of the femoral condyle on the elevated plateau, the fragments will usually remain in position and again become vascularized.

NONUNION

Pseudoarthrosis of a tibial plateau fracture is quite uncommon. Cancellous bone in the tibial plateau region is richly supplied with vascularity, which favors rapid bony union. Nonetheless, failure of fracture union happens in about one of 200 plateau fractures.[544, 951] Muggler and associates mentioned pseudoarthrosis in 1975.[752] The first published case was by Hohl[454] in 1978 with another by Schatzker and Schulak[951] in 1979; both involved the medial plateau. In the author's series of 1533 fractures, there were seven nonunions, all in total depression or bicondylar fractures (see Table 15–1).

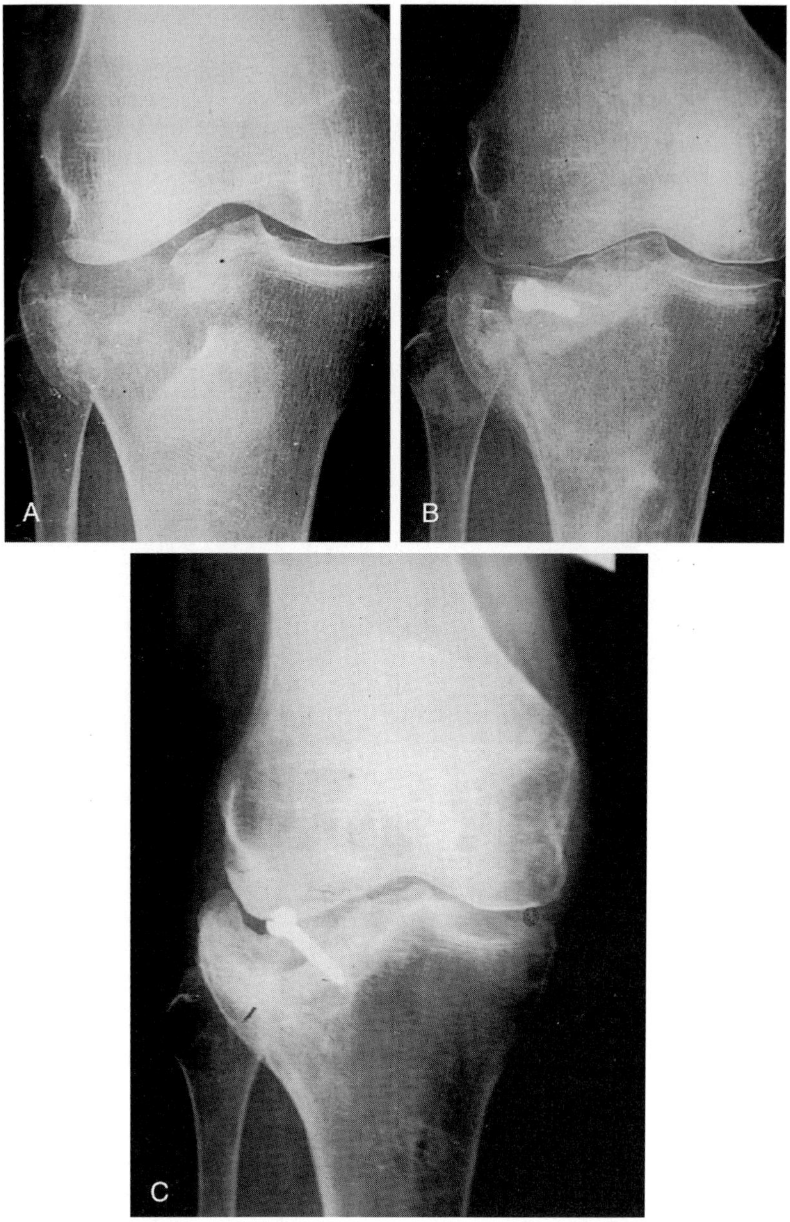

Figure 15–2. Markedly depressed local compression fracture in a 67-year-old woman. *A*, Note the depressed central fragment in metaphysis. *B*, Postoperative view with a fragment that is elevated and fixed. *C*, Absorption of an elevated avascular fragment has occurred.

In most cases nonunion is caused by lack of bony apposition or instability of the fragments. Good apposition of bony fragments and rigid fixation must be the goal of open reduction. Buttress plates or screws rather than Steinman pins, Kirschner wires, or bolts, provide the best assurance of fixation.

The knee does not tolerate nonunion, because it is incompatible with weight-bearing. The diagnosis is suggested by painful weight-bearing and is confirmed either by stress films showing movement of the fragment, by tomogram, or by computed tomography.

Treatment of nonunion must be aggressive. Experience with cast-bracing of two delayed unions convinced the author that prolonged closed treatment does not favor bony union. Surgical exposure and grafting are usually successful when combined with rigid internal fixation.[951] Drilling of the nonunion site and filling several drill holes with cortical peg bone grafts has proved to be successful (Fig. 15–3). Postoperative cast-bracing provides sufficient external support while at the same time preserving knee movement.

The prognosis after nonunion depends on how long it has existed and the amount of articular damage present. The lack of support occasioned by a

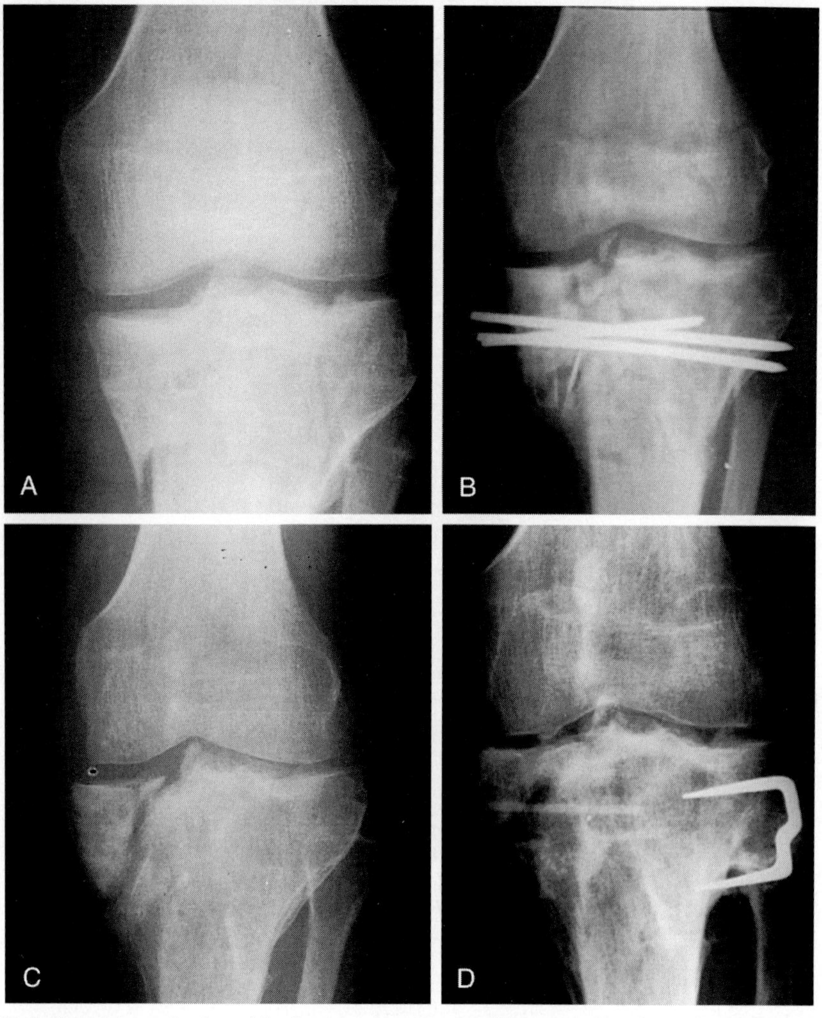

Figure 15–3. Bicondylar and subcondylar fractures in a 40-year-old man. *A*, After 2 months of cast immobilization. *B*, Bone graft and pin fixation 8 months later. *C*, One year later—an ununited medial plateau. *D*, Four years after fixation and peg grafting of nonunion and subsequent subcondylar osteotomy. (From Hohl, M.: Complications of fractures about the knee. *In* Epps, C. H. Jr. (Ed.): Complications in Orthopedic Surgery. Philadelphia, J.B. Lippincott, 1994, p. 546.)

nonunited condyle places greater stress on the remaining intact portion of the condyle and may cause knee deformity and damage to articular cartilage. Several patients with nonunions have recovered serviceable knees after surgical treatment, but their knees went on to develop traumatic arthritis.

IMPLANT COMPLICATIONS

Internal fixation devices can break, slip, or cause irritation. When skeletal traction or external fixation pins were used, infection of pin tracts with osteomyelitis was observed rarely. This complication is minimized by daily skin care and using pins that are under tension or are of such a size that bending and skin pressure are not a problem. Whereas Apley used traction with a pin through the mid-tibia, others favored a pin through the distal tibia, and still others a pin through the heel. The common denominator in the avoidance of pin tract infection seems to be to prevent the pin from rotating or sliding from side to side. One way to avoid these problems is to apply a cast over the portion of the leg into which the pin is inserted. The pin thus remains fixed. Once infection has been diagnosed, the pin should be changed to a different location. Local treatment should be given to the infected site, and systemic antibiotics should be used.

Hardware breakage or displacement occurs more often when wires or bolts are used rather than cancellous screws or buttress plates. In the author's series, there were only seven significant hardware complications. Many other patients had minor hardware-related problems, including the subcutaneous prominence of a bolt or screw that might have to be removed prematurely. Of 347 internal fixations performed, 20% of the fixation devices were later partially or completely removed. Fortunately, the types of fixation devices used currently tend to produce fewer complications than those used when less than rigid fixation was the rule.

CAUSALGIA

Causalgia about the knee is a rare complication; only one was noted in the author's series of 1533 fractures. It usually follows incomplete injury to the infrapatellar branch of the saphenous nerve, such as by stretching at surgery or by local bruising from the initial injury. The symptoms are typical of causalgia with pain, and the findings are of shiny, swollen skin that may be hypersensitive. The treatment is local anesthetic injection of the involved nerve, exploration of the nerve with neurolysis, or paravertebral sympathetic blocks. Over a period of 12 to 18 months the condition usually subsides spontaneously. In the meantime, function has been adversely affected because of chronic knee swelling and fibrosis. Patients with causalgia have difficulty in restoring knee movement because of continuing discomfort and knee stiffness.

OPEN FRACTURE

The incidence of open fracture varies between 6 and 24% in larger series.[1058] There were 3% open tibial plateau fractures in the author's series. Depending on the grade of soft tissue injury, the contamination, and time elapsed since injury, a number of treatment options can be considered. Grade I and II injuries encountered within 4 to 6 hours of injury are débrided and irrigated promptly, after which the fracture is treated by the optimal method, even internal fixation. If the same grade of open injury is treated after 6 hours, the wound is débrided and left open or only deep tissues are closed. Redébridement daily is advised, and the wound is closed when appropriate. Currently small pin external fixators are being used to manage both the bone and soft tissue injuries, and results have been more encouraging than with previous methods.[760] Open treatment should not be used unless conditions of skin and tissue are optimal, so that few grade III open fractures can qualify for open management.

The prognosis after open fracture is for an inferior result. Internal fixation seems to add injury to the tissues, promoting at best additional tissue fibrosis and capsular contracture. On the other hand, the use of traction to maintain reduction and knee motion has produced some satisfactory results. The advantage of external fixation in maintaining reduction while allowing knee movement and wound care is obvious, and it will now be used more frequently.

SUMMARY

Despite best efforts to avoid complications, they will still occur in the treatment of tibial plateau fractures because of their nature. When a complication occurs, prompt treatment will minimize its effect on the result. Awareness of the pitfalls of treatment and potential complications will result in a greater number of good and excellent results.

CHAPTER 16

Long-Term Sequelae

The most significant long-term sequelae that result from tibial plateau fractures are pain, limited knee movement, lack of knee extension, angular deformity, instability, and traumatic arthritis. These problems occur because of the nature of the fracture and, to some extent, the success of treatment and aftercare. By anticipating the possibility that one or more of these sequelae might occur, one can develop appropriate treatment and aftercare strategies (Table 16–1).

In this chapter, the incidence of sequelae and their effects on the knee are analyzed using results from patients in the author's series followed in excess of 2 years (mean of 6.1 years). Only 36% of patients followed in excess of 2 years had no adverse sequelae. The average point rating for fractures without sequelae was 93 but only 74 in those with sequelae. A normal or near-normal knee (average point rating of 90 or more) was achieved in only 29% of fractures with sequelae.

PAIN

Thirty-two percent of patients followed after tibial plateau fractures had sufficient pain to limit use of the knee. The majority of these patients felt pain only in the fractured compartment. Traumatic arthritis with loss of articular cartilage was the primary reason for pain. Eighty percent of patients with traumatic arthritis complained of pain. Of the patients with pain, 38% had some traumatic arthritis. Pain from strain on capsular ligaments can be anticipated when a fracture heals with a valgus or varus deformity. Pain follows more severe fractures, such as bicondylar types, more often than minimally displaced fractures.

LIMITATION OF KNEE MOVEMENT

It is well accepted that the process of healing articular injuries utilizes scar tissue that tends to envelop all articular structures. If the knee is immobilized

Table 16–1. SEQUELAE OF TIBIAL PLATEAU FRACTURES
(444 Fractures Followed from 2 to 20 Years)

Sequelae No. of Patients	MD 54	LC 146	SC 93	TO 65	SP 10	RIM 14	BIC 62	Total 444
Pain	22%	25%	26%	40%	33%	36%	58%	142
Limited range of motion	9%	34%	53%	46%	60%	43%	60%	182
Lack of extension	4%	8%	19%	14%	10%	7%	13%	51
Deformity	11%	36%	24%	35%	20%	14%	31%	126
Instability	15%	31%	36%	28%	30%	43%	47%	137
Arthritis	7%	16%	26%	28%	40%	21%	26%	93

Note: Sequelae represent "significant" symptoms or impairment. Limited motion is less than 110 degrees. Lack of extension is 10 degrees or more. Deformity and instability are greater than 8 degrees. Arthritis is moderate to severe.

MD = Minimally displaced; LC = Local compression; SC = Split compression; TO = Total depression; SP = Split fracture; RIM = Rim fracture; BIC = Bicondylar fracture.

during the period of intense scar formation, dense adhesions arise from the fracture to the synovia, encompassing menisci and fat pad. Experimental studies in a variety of animal models have clearly defined this reaction.[418, 459, 709, 983] Late arthrotomy and arthroscopy have also confirmed the presence of multiple intra-articular adhesions.[814, 1004] Hohl and Luck studied the effect of knee movement versus immobilization on the development of adhesions in rhesus monkeys.[459] Identical defects made in the articular cartilage and cortex of both knees were evaluated at different times after one knee had been placed in a cast and the other had been left free to move. The conclusion of these studies clearly indicated that immobilization fosters adhesions, whereas cage movement limits the extent of adhesions (Fig. 16–1). Salter went a step further by developing the innovative concept of continuous passive motion, which in rabbits was clearly advantageous over cage ambulation or immobilization.[927, 928] A clinical study has also addressed the recovery of motion as a function of various periods of immobilization.[367] It appears from this study that knee immobilization should not be continued longer than 40 days, if the knee is to recover more than 120 degrees of motion.

Historically, immobilization of knee fractures was continued until they

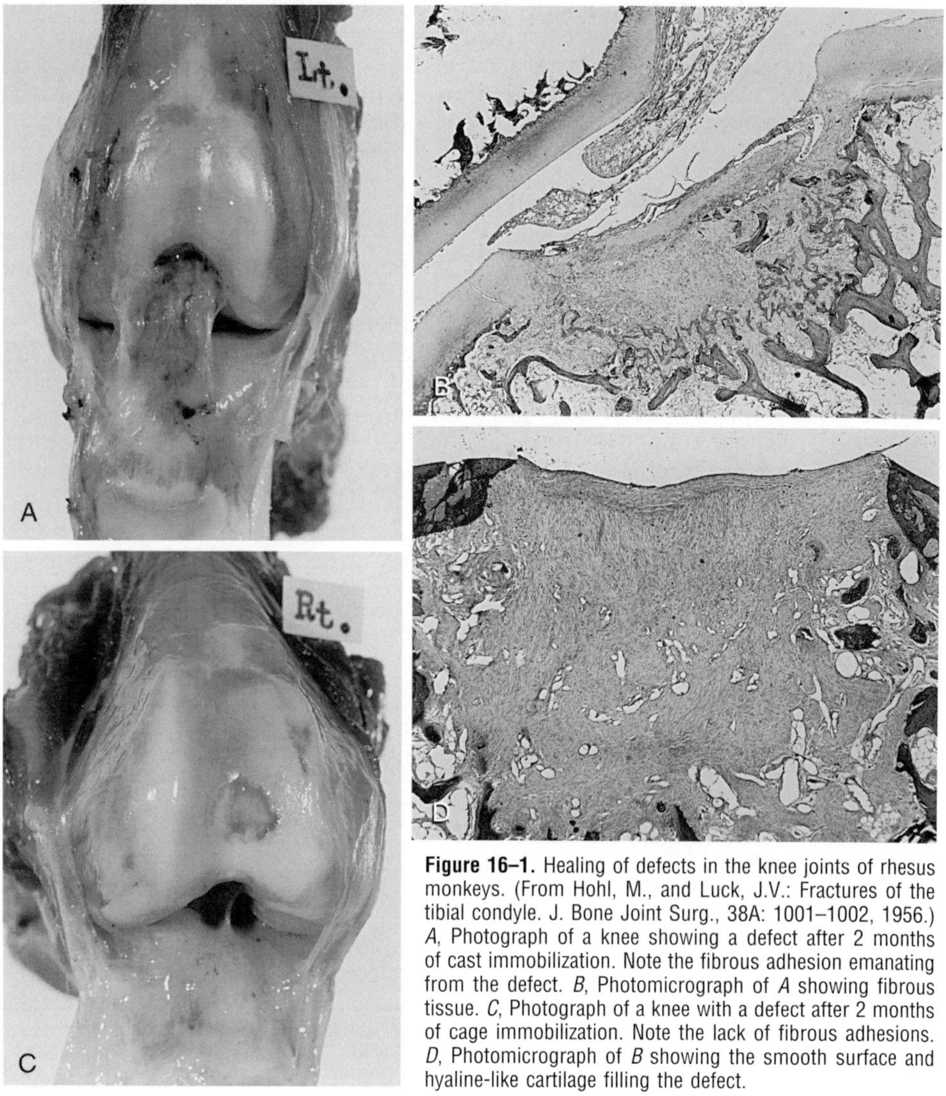

Figure 16–1. Healing of defects in the knee joints of rhesus monkeys. (From Hohl, M., and Luck, J.V.: Fractures of the tibial condyle. J. Bone Joint Surg., 38A: 1001–1002, 1956.) *A*, Photograph of a knee showing a defect after 2 months of cast immobilization. Note the fibrous adhesion emanating from the defect. *B*, Photomicrograph of *A* showing fibrous tissue. *C*, Photograph of a knee with a defect after 2 months of cage immobilization. Note the lack of fibrous adhesions. *D*, Photomicrograph of *B* showing the smooth surface and hyaline-like cartilage filling the defect.

Table 16–2. PERCENT KNEE MOTION AFTER CLOSED TREATMENT (N = 235)*

FRACTURE TYPES	DEGREES >135	120–134	91–119	<90	TOTAL NO. OF CASES
Minimally displaced	50	22	18	10	50
Local compression	38	31	14	17	82
Split compression	23	27	23	27	30
Total depression	25	31	13	31	32
Split fracture	0	100	0	0	1
Rim fracture	0	50	0	50	10
Bicondylar fracture	16	30	7	47	30
Total	32	30	14	24	235

*38% had less than 120 degrees.

healed. Then a program of rehabilitation was begun that often continued for many months until maximum recovery was obtained. Despite this rehabilitation effort, eventual recovery of knee movement was often short of normal or near-normal knee function. Because of this problem, a variety of strategies to move knees earlier and earlier have been attempted over the years.

Traction has been used successfully for many years. It was recognized early that fractures change position with knee movement and that traction restores the original position. Because traction tends to straighten the normal knee valgus position, Badgley modified it to ensure knee alignment.[39] Traction mobilization remains a standard treatment in many areas of the world.[165, 482]

Early methods of internal fixation rarely fixed tibial plateau fractures rigidly enough that the surgeon felt confident in leaving the leg unprotected. A plaster cast was used to "protect the operation." All too often, stiff knees resulted and this led many surgeons to abandon open reduction in favor of closed methods of treatment. The development of modern internal fixation materials and techniques has permitted an ever larger number of plateau fractures to be rigidly fixed, so as not to require postoperative cast immobilization. These new techniques are the major reason for the surge of interest in internal fixation in the last 20 years.

The best way to ensure a functional range of knee movement after a plateau fracture is to use a method of treatment that allows early knee motion (Tables 16–2 and 16–3).

Many factors are important in determining when to begin knee movement, including healing of a surgical wound and other soft tissue structures. If rigid fixation has been obtained, early motion should be encouraged. Continuous

Table 16–3. PERCENT KNEE MOTION AFTER OPEN TREATMENT (N = 204)*

FRACTURE TYPES	DEGREES >135	120–135	91–119	<90	TOTAL NO. OF CASES
Minimally displaced	0	100	0	0	1
Local compression	28	61	6	5	64
Split compression	25	38	25	12	63
Total	27	52	18	3	33
Split fracture	13	25	25	37	8
Rim fracture	33	67	0	0	3
Bicondylar fracture	9	47	16	28	32
Totals	24	49	16	11	204

*27% had less than 120 degrees.

passive motion machines help to mobilize knees rapidly during the first few days after surgery. If less than rigid fixation has been obtained at surgery, a cast-brace or a fracture-brace can often be used to supplement internal fixation and permit early movement of the knee in most patients. Another possibility is the use of traction for 2 or 3 weeks after surgery to allow recovery of at least 90 degrees of movement prior to using some form of external knee support. Knee immobilization should be discontinued as soon as practicable and should certainly not exceed 40 days if at all possible.[367]

In the author's series of 444 fractures followed in excess of 2 years (average of 6 years), the mean knee movement was 114 degrees. After cast immobilization of less than 6 weeks, 71% of patients had a range of motion that exceeded 120 degrees, and after traction, and in 56%, the range of motion exceeded 120 degrees. After open reduction prior to 1970, only 46% exceeded 120 degrees; however, after 1970, 67% had over 120 degrees. After rigid fixation had been obtained, 69% exceeded 120 degrees.

LACK OF KNEE EXTENSION

If the knee cannot be extended fully, the gait is altered and walking becomes more difficult. Even a few degrees of flexion contracture causes some gait impairment. Loss of knee extension is an often avoidable sequel after tibial plateau fractures. Ten degrees or more lack of knee extension was found in 12% of followed patients in the author's series (Table 16–4).

In the author's experience the most frequent cause of contracture is prolonged immobilization in a flexed position. When cast immobilization or traction is used, the knee should be kept fully extended. The resting position in traction must be with the knee fully extended.

When an associated subcondylar fracture heals with anterior angulation flexion contracture occasionally results. Careful assessment of the position of the fracture during the healing process enables the surgeon to anticipate whether such a malunion might affect the final result. If healing in malposition occurs, a late subcondylar osteotomy is used to correct the deformity.

Failure to reduce and maintain articular fragments in their anatomic position can also cause flexion contracture. Careful attention to the accuracy of articular reduction can alert the surgeon to this possibility, permitting early correction.

During rehabilitation of the knee, emphasis should be placed on regaining extension and quadriceps strength first and flexion second.

ANGULAR DEFORMITY

A frequent and distressing outcome observed after a tibial plateau fracture is an angular knee deformity, most frequently a valgus deformity. One reason for the predominance of valgus deformity is the almost 4:1 ratio of lateral to medial plateau fractures.

Table 16–4. PERCENT FLEXION CONTRACTURE AND FRACTURE TYPES (N = 443)

	PERCENTAGE				
FRACTURE TYPES	NONE	5 DEGREES	10 DEGREES	15 + DEGREES	TOTAL NO. OF CASES
Minimally displaced	83	13	4	0	53
Local compression	76	15	6	3	146
Split compression	67	14	9	16	93
Total depression	63	24	6	7	65
Split fracture	50	40	0	10	10
Rim fracture	64	29	0	7	14
Bicondylar fracture	61	26	8	5	62
Totals	70	19	6	5	443

There are two reasons for angular deformity: (1) healing of a plateau below its normal level, and (2) traumatic arthritis with loss of articular cartilage and erosion of the articular bony surface. If the articular surface has not been maintained at its normal level and has instead healed in a depressed position, an angular deformity is the result. Prevention of deformity is usually easier than cure. It is prevented by accurate reduction of the plateaus to normal position and maintenance of that reduction. During the weeks following a fracture, it is important to check the position of the fracture by x-ray. If a fracture has lost reduction, another form of treatment (e.g., open reduction) should be considered immediately. The result of unreduced tibial plateaus is angular deformity as well as instability (Table 16–5).

An angular deformity can also result from the loss of articular cartilage as traumatic arthritis occurs. After the cartilage has been eroded, there is progressive bony erosion that leads to an angular deformity. Rarely, avascular necrosis of elevated articular fragments occurs and leaves a variable-sized joint surface defect (see Fig. 15–2).

Treatment of an angular deformity depends on the patient's age and future requirements. If one tibial plateau is depressed but the articular surface is relatively smooth, a single plateau osteotomy can be considered. The line of osteotomy extends from the tibial cortex to the intercondylar area. After the plateau has been levered into proper position, a bone graft is sandwiched in the resulting defect, and a buttress plate is used for rigid internal fixation. This type of osteotomy is indicated primarily for younger patients. A subcondylar osteotomy is frequently used and does correct knee alignment (Fig. 16–2).[217] Unicondylar or total knee replacement may be a better choice than osteotomy for patients in poor health or older than 70 years of age.[99, 352, 592]

INSTABILITY

Three reasons for late instability after tibial plateau fractures are recognized. The first is failure to reduce and maintain reduction of the plateau surface. The second is ligament laxity secondary to an unrepaired collateral or cruciate ligament injury. The third is traumatic arthritis with loss of articular cartilage and erosion of the articular cortex.

In the chapter on soft tissue injuries, many problems associated with ligament injury are discussed (see Chapter 4). Late instability was noted in 10 to 45% of patients reported in long-term follow-up.[450, 727, 901] Instability of greater than 5 degrees was found in 36% of patients in the author's series treated with closed reduction and 26% of those treated with open reduction (Table 16–6).

Knee instability is often responsible for late knee pain and the development of traumatic arthritis. In the author's series, 60% of patients with arthritis had knee instability. If knee instability can be recognized early in treatment and stability restored, this will help to minimize pain later on and possibly the degree

Table 16–5. DEFORMITY AND INSTABILITY (N = 434)

	INSTABILITY					
DEFORMITY	NONE	5 DEGREES	10 DEGREES	15 DEGREES	20 DEGREES	TOTAL NO. OF CASES
None	110	34	17	3	2	166
5 Degrees	53	55	26	3	2	139
10 Degrees	20	36	23	19	7	105
15 Degrees	4	2	14	5	3	28
20 Degrees	2	0	2	1	1	6
Totals	189	127	82	31	15	434

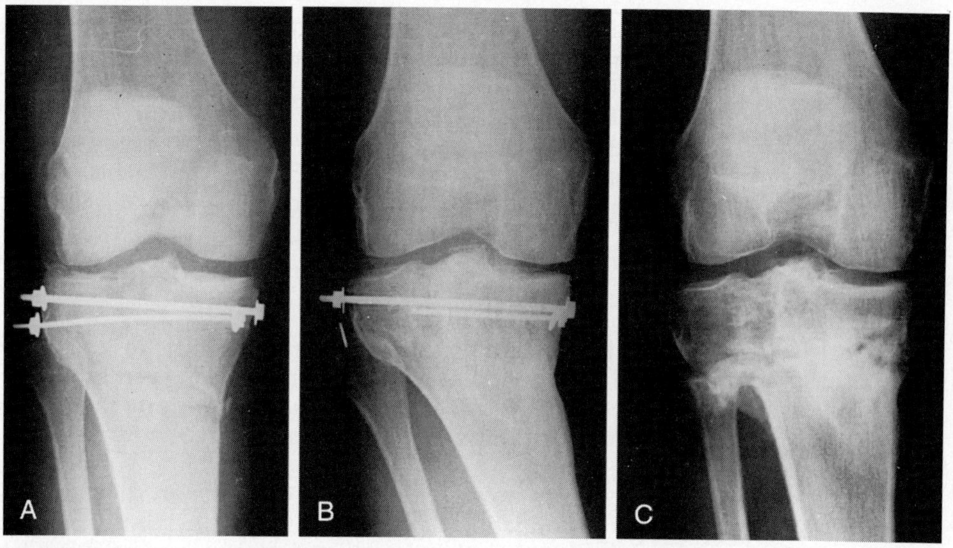

Figure 16–2. Total depression fracture in a 40-year-old man treated inadequately with two tibial bolts. (Reprinted with permission from Southern Medical Journal 68: 990, 1975; and from Epps, C.H., Jr. (Ed.): Complications in Orthopedic Surgery. Epps, Philadelphia, J.B. Lippincott, 1994, p. 548.) *A*, Postoperative view appears to be satisfactory. *B*, Fracture redisplaced into a marked varus. *C*, Knee alignment improved by subcondylar osteotomy.

of traumatic arthritis (Table 16–7). In many patients with articular depression, the pain is felt on the side opposite the fracture because of collateral ligament and capsular strain.

Moore used an apparatus to document stability in both knees and concluded that only 10% had an instability of 10 degrees or more.[727] For this reason he doubted the long-term significance of torn ligaments. In patients of the age group in which so many plateau fractures occur, many collateral ligament injuries are actually avulsions from the femoral condyles that tend to heal well with a cast or brace. Nonetheless, an analysis of the results of fractures in which operative ligament repair was carried out demonstrated better stability and a significantly increased average point rating compared with those fractures without ligament repair.[244]

The exceptions were fractures with associated cruciate ligament insubstance tears that rated the same, with or without ligament repair. Only cruciate injuries with an avulsion fracture were more stable after being internally fixed. Late ligament reconstruction can help to increase knee stability.

Table 16–6. KNEE INSTABILITY AT FOLLOW-UP (N = 439)

	INSTABILITY					
TYPE	NONE	5 DEGREES	10 DEGREES	15 DEGREES	20 DEGREES	TOTAL
Minimally displaced	33	11	5	2	2	53
Local compression	45	55	36	9	1	146
Split compression	38	26	21	7	0	92
Total depression	26	21	14	3	1	65
Split fracture	2	5	3	0	0	10
Rim fracture	2	6	4	2	0	14
Bicondylar	18	12	22	5	2	59
Totals	164	136	105	28	6	439

Table 16–7. KNEE INSTABILITY AT FOLLOW-UP

	% WITH INSTABILITY							
	MD	LC	SC	TO	SP	RIM	BIC	TOTAL
All follow-ups	15%	31%	30%	28%	33%	43%	47%	32%
No ligament injury	12%	30%	24%	24%	22%	33%	49%	29%

MD = Minimally displaced; LC = Local compression; SC = Split compression; TO = Total depression; SP = Split fracture; RIM = Rim fracture; BIC = Bicondylar fracture.

The degree of instability is related to final articular depression below normal anatomic level (Table 16–8).

Avascular necrosis of elevated fragments in compression fractures results in a cup-shaped depressed plateau in which the femoral condyle dips upon weight-bearing. Lessening of deformity and instability can be effected by an osteotomy or by using a composite frozen allograft to replace the damaged condyle by the method of Gross.[399, 658]

If traumatic arthritis in one compartment is the cause of instability, one might consider a subcondylar osteotomy or knee replacement, depending on the patient's age. Although the knee may be improved, it will be far from normal.

Operative treatment deserves full consideration when a patient with a plateau fracture presents with clinical instability.[873] Like so many of the other long-term sequelae, the problem of instability is best anticipated and controlled at the time of the initial fracture treatment rather than dealt with later when only partial solutions are available.

TRAUMATIC ARTHRITIS

There is no universal agreement as to what constitutes traumatic arthritis in the knee, and thus the reported incidence following plateau fracture varies greatly, from about 10 to 78%.[106, 176, 871, 967, 1087] The criteria that are used most often are those of Fairbank or Albeck.[317, 871] Squaring of the femoral and tibial condyles is the earliest change seen on x-ray. Then other changes occur, including spurring on the tibial spines and joint margins, sclerosis of the subchondral bone, joint space narrowing, and finally cyst formation in the articular subcortex. Squaring and spurring at joint margins suggest a mild arthritic change, whereas joint narrowing and articular sclerosis make the diagnosis of moderate or severe arthritis, depending on the extent of changes.

One variable to be considered in a study of traumatic arthritis is elapsed time since the injury (any study should start at 5 years), comparing the result with the opposite knee. Moore noted 19% arthritic changes in the injured knee and 9% in the uninjured in a 3.7-year average follow-up, for a net incidence of

Table 16–8. ARTICULAR DEPRESSION AND INSTABILITY (N = 443)

	% WITH INSTABILITY							
FINAL DEPRESSION	MD	LC	SC	TO	SP	RIM	BIC	TOTAL
2 mm or less	17	17	17	15	33	71	32	19
3 mm or more	0	42	21	42	29	14	58	44
5 mm or more	0	52	47	53	99	20	68	53
7 mm or more	0	53	54	63	0	33	77	59

MD = Minimally displaced; LC = Local compression; SC = Split compression; TO = Total depression; SP = Split fracture; RIM = Rim fracture; BIC = Bicondylar fracture.

10%.[724] Rasmussen,[871] in a follow-up averaging 7.3 years, noted 21% arthritic changes in the injured knee and 2% in the uninjured knee. Dustmann compared the length of follow-up with the incidence of arthritis and noted a 56% incidence at 5 years and 78% at 20 years.[287] Chow, using Kaplan-Meier analyses of the author's series, noted 16% arthritis at 5 years, 32% at 10 years, and 49% at 15 years.[176]

Most observers, including the author, did not routinely document osteoarthritis in the other knee and thus report a gross incidence of arthritic change. Patients in the author's series had a 21% overall incidence of any arthritis with a follow-up time of 6.1 years. Severe arthritis was noted in 8% of patients at 15 years and 24% at 20 years (Table 16–9).

For at least 50 years traumatic arthritis has been recognized to be a frequent sequel to tibial plateau fractures. Several articles have described the problem well, citing articular damage and residual incongruities as the causes.[106, 871, 967, 1087] Other articles stress the importance of malalignment in the development of arthritis[873] (Fig. 16–3). Varus is generally conceded to promote more rapid development of arthritic change.

Those devoted to accurate operative reduction and rigid fixation believe that by achieving these goals the incidence of traumatic arthritis will be minimized. In 1973, Muggler reported on 150 operatively treated patients and noted that 53% developed arthritic changes.[752] Boszotta found arthritis in 71% of knees after open reduction of plateau fractures.[106] Some authors believe that early passive and active movement of the knee keeps arthritis away, but there is no scientific evidence to support this concept.

Moore observed that neither final plateau reduction position, nor the choice of treatment affected the incidence of arthritic change.[724] Postoperative infection, however, always resulted in arthritic changes.

There is thus far little scientific evidence to indicate why arthritis develops after injury to the tibial plateau. It is assumed that direct surface damage destroys cartilage cells, and the pannus healing reaction after a plateau fracture tends to digest and partially destroy some of the articular cartilage.[634] Bicondylar fractures immobilized for more than 6 weeks were compared with others that were allowed free mobility after open reduction or treatment in traction. The incidence of arthritis was 34% in both groups.

Fracture types differ considerably in their propensity to induce knee arthritis. The highest incidence of any arthritic change (mild to severe) was 67% in bicondylar fractures. The lowest incidence (10%) was in fractures that healed without angular deformity (Fig. 16–4). Local compression fractures had a 17% incidence, and fractures that healed with varus deformity had 33% incidence of arthritis at 5 years. Traumatic arthritis developed in 48% of patients whose fracture healed with varus deformity and 32% whose fracture healed with valgus deformity (Table 16–10).

Table 16–9. ARTHRITIS AND FOLLOW-UP INTERVAL (N = 279)

	% WITH ARTHRITIS			
ARTHRITIS	5 Yr	10 Yr	15 Yr	20 Yr
None	45	31	36	17
Mild	38	42	36	24
Moderate	11	23	20	35
Severe	6	4	8	24
Patients	126	55	39	29

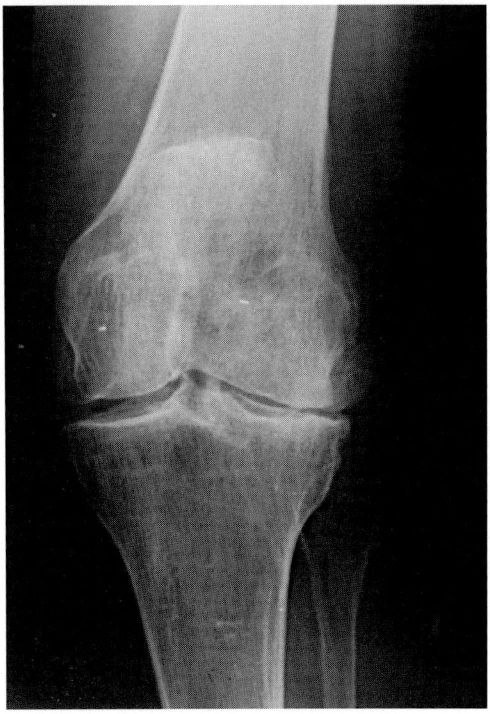

Figure 16–3. Seven years after a lateral plateau fracture. Note the moderate traumatic arthritic change, especially in the lateral compartment, that is associated with a valgus deformity.

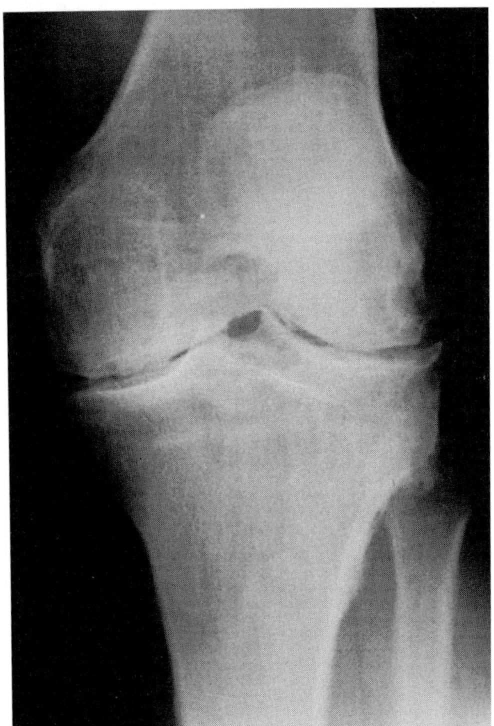

Figure 16–4. Twenty years after a tibial plateau fracture. Note the loss of cartilage space and arthritic spurring.

Table 16–10. TRAUMATIC ARTHRITIS AND DEFORMITY (N = 121)

	VARUS DEFORMITY	VALGUS DEFORMITY	TOTAL (%)
Arthritic change	12	34	38
No arthritis	11	64	62
Total patients	23	98	100

SUMMARY

The surgeon treating fractures of the tibial plateau should be aware of long-term sequelae that could occur. Such awareness during treatment may help one to avoid or minimize some sequelae. The results of treatment in the 36% of patients without sequelae indicated mostly near-normal or normal knees with a mean point rating of 93 points. The 64% with sequelae had a mean point rating of 74.

REFERENCES

1. Abdalla, F. H., Tehranzadeh, J., and Horton, J. A.: Avulsion of the lateral tibial condyle in skiing. Am. J. Sports Med., 10:368–370, 1982.
Four cases of nonarticular avulsions from the lateral tibial condyle in skiing are reported. The injuries were not appreciated on x-ray, and the leg was splinted. Late instability was the rule. Early diagnosis and surgical treatment were advocated.
2. Abdollahi, K., Lee, J., and Vangsness, C. T.: Nonoperative tibial plateau fractures: Prevalence of associated soft tissue injuries as determined by MRI. (To be published.)
Nineteen acute plateau fractures had magnetic resonance imaging knee studies. Of those fractures, 74% were found to have meniscal tears and 47% had torn ligaments. There were five medial collateral, three lateral collateral, three anterior cruciate, and three posterior cruciate ligament injuries.
3. Acker, P. van: (Follow-up study of 75 patients with fractures of the tibial plateau.) Ned. Tijdschr. Geneeskd, 105:2181–2184, 1961.
4. Adamson, G. J., Wiss, D. A., Lowery, G. L., and Peters, C. L.: Type II floating knee: Ipsilateral femoral and tibial fractures with intra-articular extension into the knee joint. J. Orthop. Trauma, 6:333–339, 1992.
Treatment was given to 34 patients with ipsilateral femoral and tibial fractures extending into the knee joint. Of those, 68% of tibial fractures extended into the joint and 62% were open fractures. Ninety percent were treated surgically, and only 24% had good or excellent results. All lost significant extension and flexion. Ten of 34 were plateau fractures. Although excellent or good results were obtained in less than 30%, open reduction was advised.
5. Aglietti, P., and Chambat, P.: Tibial plateau fractures. *In* Insall, J. (Ed.): Surgery of the Knee. New York, Churchill Livingstone, 1984.
6. Agrifoglio, E., Rettagliata, F., and De Miglio, G.: Le fratture del piatto tibiale. Osp. d'Italia Chir., 10:317, 1964.
7. Ahern, G. S., and Lipscomb, P. R.: Fracture of the tibial plateau: Report of a case. Proc. Staff Mayo Clin., 23:288–290, 1948.
This case report involves a split compression fracture associated with an upper third tibial fracture, which was treated by screw fixation with a satisfactory result.
8. Aichner, H., and Due, G.: Contributo allo studio delle fratture monocondiloidee del piatto tibiale. Arch. Ortop., 69:297–315, 1956.
9. Akeson, W., Woo, S., Amiel, D., and Frank, C.: The chemical basis of tissue repair: The biology of ligaments. *In* Hunter, L., and Funk, F. (Eds.): Rehabilitation of the Injured Knee. St. Louis, C.V. Mosby, 1984.
10. Albers, E.: Beitrag zur kenntnis des compressionsfrakturen des oberen endes der tibia. Berl. Klin. Wchnschr., 31:1153–1157, 1894.
Four patients sustained compression-type plateau fractures as the result of an elevator accident. All were treated with closed reduction.
11. Alglave, P.: Fracture du condyle tibial externe abordé par voie transrotulienne transversale. Bull. Mem. Soc. Chir. Paris, 47:1968, 1921.
12. Allaben, C. M.: Fractures into and around the knee joint. N. Y. J. Med., 40:1279–1282, 1940.
After treating 80 plateau fractures, the author concluded that open reduction and internal fixation were rarely needed, and conservative care with traction was preferred.
13. Allaria, A., and Bertini, S.: Fratture del piatto tibiale da invernali trattate con vite percutanea. Atti S.E.R.T.O.T. 5:491, 1960.
14. Allegreni, R., and Dell'Orto, R.: Indicazioni e limiti al trattamento incruento delle fratture del piatto tibiale. Minerva Ortop., 18:377–381, 1967.
Thirty-one plateau fractures were treated by closed means with generally fair to good results.
15. Allgower, M.: Die behandlung der tibiakopffraktur im wandel der zeit. Hefte Unfallheilk., 158:417–421, 1982.
The history of plateau fracture treatment and the development of treatment principles are reviewed.
16. Alling: Fracture de l'extrémité supérieure du tibia. Bull. Soc. Anat. Paris, 46:347–348, 1871.
The author describes a plateau fracture found at the autopsy of a fatally injured person.
17. Alonzo, F., and Magrini, G.: La nostra esperienza sui trattamento delle fratture del piatto tibiale. Minerva Ortop., 18:415–418, 1967.
The authors report on the treatment of 220 plateau fractures treated both with closed and open reduction.
18. Anderson, P. W., Harley, J. D., and Maslin, P. U.: Arthrographic evaluation of problems with united tibial plateau fractures. Radiology, 119:75–78, 1976.
Arthrography delineated the articular surface better than did any other method in older fractures. It can be useful in making late treatment decisions.
19. Anderson, R., and Loughlen, I.: Fractures of the tibial plateau: Treatment by the assured fixation technique. Clin. Orthop. 4:10–23, 1954.
The method of closed reduction on the fracture table is discussed. Pins are placed above and below the knee and incorporated in a cast. Knee movement is started after healing is complete.
20. Andreesen, R.: Zur operativen behandlung der schienbeinkopfbruche. Zentralbl. Chir., 65:2759–2760, 1938.
A type of tibial bolt was used to fix a split compression fracture.
21. Andreesen, R.: Die behandlung der schienbeinkopfbruche. Chir. Praxis, 1:49–60, 1959.
Ninety-seven fractures were treated, mostly nonoperatively, using traction or plaster. When fractures were opened, bolt fixation was used.
22. Andreini, G., and Cabras, G.: Contributo clinico alla terapia chirurgica delle fratture intra-articolari del ginocchio. Ort. Traum. App. Mot., 3:747–764, 1957.
23. Andrews, J. R., Tedder, J. L., and Godbout, B. P.: Bicondylar tibial plateau fracture complicated by compartment syndrome. Orthop. Rev., 21:317–319, 1992.
A case report is given of a 54-year-old woman with a Schatzker type VI fracture who developed compartment syndrome within hours of the fracture. The fracture was treated by fasciotomy and open reduction.
24. Anger, R., Naett, R., Wolff, F., et al: Étude critique du traitement des fractures articulaires de l'extrémité superior du tibia. Rev. Chir. Orthop., 54:259–274, 1968.
The authors reviewed 175 plateau fractures and made the finding that early knee mobilization and accurate reduction were important.
25. Angerer, W.: Traitement des fractures graves du genou et du coude dans la prâtique campagnarde. Zentralbl. Chir., 63:1581–1585, 1936.
26. Anglen, J. O., and Healy, W. L.: Tibial plateau fractures. Orthopedics, 11:1527–1534, 1988.
The results of 128 plateau fractures were analysed in relation to their treatment. The authors proposed guidelines for closed or open treatment.
27. Anzoletti, A.: La frattura indiretta dei condili tibiali ed il suo meccanismo. Arch. Int. de Chir. Gand., 3:267–304, 1906.

28. Apley, A. G.: Fractures of the lateral tibial condyle treated by skeletal traction and early mobilisation. J. Bone Joint Surg., 38B:699–708, 1956.
The author reports 60 bumper fractures with 48 fractures treated in traction. After a follow-up of 27 patients for more than 5 years, the author suggested that these fractures should be treated nonoperatively and without plaster.
29. Apley, A. G.: Fractures of the tibial plateau. Orthop. Clin. North Am., 10:61–74, 1979.
The author observed that plateau fractures are treated by plaster, metal, or traction. Plaster immobilizes the knee; metal immobilizes the fracture but allows the knee to move. Traction keeps the knee comfortable so that it can be moved. He favors the use of traction.
30. Apoil, A., Langlais, F., and Vivier, J.: Les fractures de la marge tibiale dans les entorses graves du genu. J. Chir. (Paris), 107:611–616, 1974.
31. Arnold, M. H.: Fractures of the tibial plateau as a cause of immobility. Aust. N Z J. Med., 25:178, 1995.
32. Armani, L.: La frattura parcellare della epifisi superiore esterna della tibia. Arch. Ortop., 53:241, 1935.
33. Arnaud, M.: (Late results of surgical reposition and osseous graft of fractures of the external plateau. 2 cases.) Bull. Mem. Soc. Chir., 59:1479–1484, 1933.
34. Arriula, F., and Elosegui, J.: (Compression fractures of the lateral tibial plateau.) Acta Ortop. Traumatol. Iber., 1:491–494, 1953.
35. Aufranc, O. E.: Fracture of the lateral tibial plateau. J.A.M.A., 176:676–679, 1961.
This case report involves a 58-year-old person with a moderately depressed local compression fracture treated by open reduction, Barr bolt, and early knee motion. The result was satisfactory despite some loss of reduction.
36. Aufranc, O.: Depressed fracture of the lateral tibial plateau. J.A.M.A., 177:564–567, 1961.
This case report concerns a missed local compression fracture associated with a medial ligament injury. The author believed that oblique x-ray views may be beneficial. Twenty months after open reduction and internal fixation without ligament repair, the knee was stable.
37. Aufranc, O. E., Jones, W. N., and Harris, W. H.: Depressed lateral tibial plateau fracture. J.A.M.A., 178:835–837, 1961.
This case report concerns a 75-year-old woman with a slightly depressed local compression fracture who was treated by early splinting then movement of the knee. A good result was attained at 18 months with no further depression.
38. Baar: Z. Org. Ges. Chir., 104:551, 1942.
39. Badgley, C. E., and O'Connor, S. J.: Conservative treatment of fractures of the tibial plateau. Arch. Surg., 64:506–515, 1952.
This report concerns 17 plateau fractures treated in skeletal traction with early knee mobilization. Traction was used for 8 to 12 weeks, with emphasis on active muscle strengthening and movement.
40. Bajardi, A., and Fantato, S.: Il trattamento delle fratture intraarticolari dell'arto inferiore, nell'eta senile. Minerva Ortop., 12:488–489, 1961.
41. Bakalim, G., and Wilppula, E.: Fractures of the tibial condyles. Acta Orthop. Scand., 44:311–322, 1973.
The authors studied 197 plateau fractures in which 53% were treated conservatively. Of the "dislocated" cases, 79% were operated on. Operative treatment and repair of torn collateral ligaments are suggested. Functional results were better when anatomic reduction was obtained.
42. Balgramo, M., Roncalli-Benedetti, L., and Soave, G.: Le fratture del piatto tibiale. Minerva Ortop. 18:331–346, 1967.
43. Ballerait, G.: Contribution au Diagnostic Tomographique des Fractures du Plateau Tibial. Paris, Thesis No. 1072, 1957.
44. Ballerio, A.: Sulle fratture del piatto tibiale. Arch. Ortop. Milano, 2:101–121, 1952.
45. Baltensweiler, J.: Konservativ therapie der frischen tibiakopffrakturen. Hefte Unfallheilk., 126:236–241, 1976.
The author discusses indications for conservative treatment of plateau fractures. He believed that because of late arthritic changes, some fractures should be treated by open reduction.
46. Baltensweiler, J.: Die abstutzung der tibiaplateaufraktur mit gabelplatte. Z. Unfallchir. Versicherungsmed Berufskr., 78:237–247, 1985.
This author designed a three-pronged plate to provide wide support under a tibial plateau. Some cases were illustrated.
47. Barbarin: Paris Chirurgie, 16:306, 1923.
48. Barbieri, E., Tognolo, P., and Rienzo, C.: On physiokinesitherapy in sequelae of fractures of the tibial plateau. Minerva Ortop., 21:57–64, 1970.
49. Barbilian, N.: Les fractures du plateau tibial. J. Chir. (Paris), 6:663, 1926.
50. Barlassine, G., Bracale, M., and Doldi, M.: Fractures of the tibial plateau. Arch. Ital. Chir., 92:777–797, 1966.
51. Barr, J. S.: The treatment of fracture of the external tibial condyle (bumper fracture). J.A.M.A., 115:1683–1687, 1940.
This is a general discussion of lateral plateau fractures, including treatment and results based on 30 cases.
52. Barrington, T. W., and Dewar, F. P.: Tibial plateau fractures. Can. J. Surg., 8:146–152, 1965.
This article concerns 147 patients on workers' compensation who were treated in Canada. The plea is made for early mobilization and more conservative treatment.
53. Basom, W. C.: Threaded pins for tibial plateau fractures. Southwest. Med., 45:216–217, 1964.
54. Basset, A.: Sur la necessité de l'arthrotomie dans les opérations pour articulaires de l'extrémité supérieure du tibia. Mem. Acad. Chir., 62:427–428, 1936.
This discussion advocates an arthrotomy to reduce fractures accurately and to remove torn menisci.
55. Battisti, B.: (Fractures of the upper end of the tibia. 2 cases.) Gazz. Osped. e Clin., 54:1340–1344, 1933.
56. Baumann, C., and Ziegler, A.: Nachkontrolle von 44 operativ und konservativ behandelten tibiakopffrakturen. Helv. Chir. Acta, 43:443–445, 1976.
The authors briefly report on the operative treatment of 44 plateau fractures with 70% satisfactory results.
57. Baumgartner, J.: Z. Org. Chir., 84:733, 1936.
58. Baumgartner, J.: Fracture du plateau tibial externe. Lyon Chir. 34:179–182, 1937.
This case report concerns a split compression fracture treated by two wood screws with a good result.
59. Bec, and Hadengue: Un cas de fracture cuneiform de l'extrémité supérieure du tibia. Paris Med., 27:301, 1918.
60. Becker, F.: Tibiakopffrakturen. Dtsch. Z. Chir., 243:189–208, 1934.
The author used 52 plateau fractures to describe various types encountered. Some were treated operatively, but most were treated by closed means. The sequelae of instability, deformity, and arthritis were noted.
61. Becker, T.: Die bruche des schienbeinkopfes un ihre versorgung. Zentralbl. Chir., 74:1040–1046, 1949.
The author reviewed 21 plateau fractures and found satisfactory results with conservative treatment. He reserved surgery for those showing meniscal incarceration.
62. Belenger, M.: À propos d'une fracture de l'extrémité supérieure du tibia. Acta Orthop. Belg., 23:305–310, 1957.
63. Belgrano, M., Roncalli-Benedetti, L., and Soave, G.: Le fratture del piatto tibiale. Minerva Ortop., 18:331–346, 1967.
The authors treated 184 plateau fractures and followed 84 fractures. Closed treatment was satisfactory in 40 of 52 cases. Open treatment was satisfactory in 24 of 32 cases.
64. Belluomini, P.: Contributo clinico-statistico al trattamento delle fratture del piatto tibiale. Minerva Ortop., 21:177–179, 1970.
65. Benirschke, S. K., Agnew, S. G., Mayo, K. A., et al: Immediate internal fixation of open, complex tibial plateau fractures: Treatment by a standard protocol. J. Orthop. Trauma, 6:78–86, 1992.
The authors reported on patients with 46 complex Schatzker V or VI fractures and 14 grade II or III open fractures who were given antibiotics in the emergency room, and taken to surgery where internal fixation was performed and often with delayed primary wound closure. There were no deep infections and the average Hospital for Special Surgery score was 81.5.
66. Bennett: Comminuted fracture of the head of the tibia. Dublin J. Med. Sc., 68:162–164, 1879.
The author describes a knee specimen of a comminuted proximal tibial fracture and describes it in relation to Heydenreich's 1877 classification.
67. Bennett, G. A., and Bauer, W.: Further studies concerning the repair of articular cartilage in dog joints. J. Bone Joint Surg., 17:141–150, 1935.

The authors created cartilaginous defects in the patellar groove of seven puppies. There was generally incomplete healing of cartilage despite the age of the dog.

68. Bennett, W. F., and Browner, B.: Tibial plateau fractures: A study of associated soft tissue injuries. J. Orthop. Trauma, 8:183–188, 1994.
A prospective evaluation was made of 30 patients by x-ray and stress testing before and after fixation. Fifty-six percent had soft tissue injury. Collateral ligament injuries were noted in 23%, meniscal injuries in 20%, cruciate injury in 10%, and peroneal nerve injury in 3%. Pre- and postfixation stress testing were recommended.
69. Berard: Fracture grave du plateau tibial par traumatisme léger. Lyon Chir., 1925.
70. Bergemann, S. A.: Uber ide mit kalkablagerung einhergehende entzundung der schulterschleimbeutel. Munch. Med. Wochenschr., 55:2699, 1908.
71. Berger, P. E.: MRI demonstration of radiographically occult fractures: What have we been missing? Radiographics, 9:407–436, 1989.
72. Beris, A. E., Glisson, R. R., Seaber, A. V., and Urbaniak, J. R.: Load tolerance of tibial plateau depressions reinforced with a cluster of K-wires (Abstract). Trans. Orthop. Res. Soc., 13:301, 1988.
Six fresh cadaveric tibias were mounted, and local compression fractures were created. The depression was elevated, bone grafts packed underneath, and one of seven patterns of K-wire fixation were used. A load was applied. Thirty percent of normal strength was obtained when K-wires were used with grafts.
73. Bertin-Sans, H., and Jeanbrau, E.: Fracture du condyle interne du tibia avec fissures epiphyseo-diaphysaire et subluxation du genou endelhors. Arch. d'Eléctricité Med. Bordeaux, 8:461–465, 1900.
74. Betz: Tibial head fractures. Chirurgie, 60:732–738, 1989.
75. Bezouglis, C. P., and Eliopoulos, C. S.: Perkutane osteosynthese der tibiakopffrakturen und sofortige mobilisierung des knies. Z. Orthop., 110:983–985, 1972.
The authors treated 41 plateau fractures by percutaneous pins or bolts with traction and early mobilization.
76. Bianchi-Maiocchi, A., and Fantato, S.: L'osteosintesi metallica nelle fratture recenti del piatto tibiale e dei condili femorali con speciale riferimento alla vite di Barr. Arch. Ortop., 67:512–545, 1954.
77. Bick, E. M.: Fractures of the tibial condyles. J Bone Joint Surg., 23:102–108, 1941.
The authors divided 61 fractures into undisplaced or displaced groups and reviewed the results. They advocated a plaster cast for 6 to 7 weeks and believed that open reduction and internal fixation were seldom indicated. Lateral instability was a temporary phenomenon.
78. Bielski, T., and Ciecko, R.: Zachowawcze leczenie zlaman klykcia bocznego piszczeli. Chir. Narz. Ruchu Ortop. Pol., 34:651–655, 1969.
The authors applied traction and angular force to use collateral ligament tension to reduce lateral plateau fractures. Forty-three of 45 patients treated in this manner achieved satisfactory results; only two bad results were noted.
79. Biencke: Munch. Med. Wochenschr., 73:87, 1926.
80. Bimler, R.: Band-, knorpel- und spongiosaheilung unter fruhfunktioneller behandlung auf der bewegungsschiene am beispiel der tibiakopftrummerfrakturen. Hefte. Unfallheilk., 81:568–576, 1978.
The authors treated 48 plateau fractures in traction with movement of the knee. A follow-up for 10 years indicated that good function was preserved.
81. Bistolfi, S.: Contributo allo studio delle ossificazion traumatische paracondiloidee e paraepicondiloidee del Ginocchio. Arch. Ital. Chir., 30:233–313, 1931.
82. Bistolfi, S.: Contributo allo studio del meccanismo delle fratture monocondiloide dello tibia da causa inderetta. Chir. Organi Mov., 16:451–498, 1931.
This discussion of plateau fracture injury mechanisms involves body weight, varus or valgus forces, the role of ligamentous structures, and the femoral condyles.
83. Bistolfi, S.: Z. Org. Chir., 56:767, 1932.
84. Biyani, A., Reddy, N. S., Chaudhury, J., et al: The results of surgical management of displaced tibial plateau fractures in the elderly. Injury, 26:291–297, 1995.
The authors treated and reviewed 32 patients older than 80 years of age with displaced tibial plateau fractures. There were two cases of deep vein thrombosis. The results were: 9—excellent; 14—good; 5—fair; and 4—poor. The best results were those treated by continuous passive motion postoperatively and a cast-brace.
85. Black, R. B., Morandi, M., Watson, J. T., et al: Treatment of complex tibial plateau fractures with circular external fixators (Abstract). J. Orthop. Trauma, 17:167–168, 1993.
Thirty Schatzker VI fractures were treated using the thin wire circular fixator. Twenty-seven fractures had associated severe soft tissue injuries. Motion was started immediately, and all united with a mean range of motion of 106 degrees. One amputation and two subcondylar nonunions were recorded. The authors use this method when open reduction and internal fixation are not practical.
86. Blackburn, J. E.: Maintenance of reduction of tibial plateau fractures with Charnley compression device. Clin. Orthop., 123:112–113, 1977.
This general discussion is about the use of the Charnley device to distract the knee to prevent redepression after closed or open treatment. No case reports are given.
87. Blake, J.: Diagnosis and treatment of fractures involving the knee joint. Ann. Surg., 58:27–38, 1913.
The author noted that knee joint fractures were easily misdiagnosed, and this resulted in liability actions. He noted that the prognosis after treatment was guarded and that open reduction with plate or wire was sometimes necessary.
88. Blanchard, J., and Samuel, P.: Les fractures articulaires de l'extrémité supérieure du tibia. Encyclop. Med. Chir., 44805:1–8, 1966.
89. Bloch, J. C.: Affaissement de la tuberosité tibiale externe après fracture traitée par visage: Operation plastique secondaire. Mem. Soc. Nationale Chir., 62:401–409, 1936.
90. Block, W.: (Discussion.) Zentralbl. Chir., 65:614, 1938.
The author discussed using bayonet wires and pulling them to right angles to effect and hold reduction.
91. Blokker, C. P., Rorabeck, C. H., and Bourne, R. B.: Tibial plateau fractures: An analysis of the results of treatment in 60 patients. Clin. Orthop., 182:193–199, 1984.
The authors studied 60 plateau fractures, of which 39% were bicondylar. Thirty-eight of 60 fractures were treated with open reduction, and the others were treated by closed methods. The overall results were 75% satisfactory. Unsatisfactory results were associated with more than 5 mm of articular offset.
92. Blumenfeld, I., and Pressmann, A. A.: Fractures des plateaux du tibia. Prensa Med. Argent., 27:2114–2118, 1957.
93. Boeckel, M.: Fracture du condyle externe du tibia. Union Med., 7:387–390, 1869.
This case report involves a man injured in a fall. There was effusion, crepitus, and valgus deformity. After bandaging, healing occurred in a good position.
94. Boero, G., and Bignardi, A.: (Treatment of tibial plateau fractures.) Minerva Ortop., 18:383–388, 1967.
95. Bohler, J.: Frakturen im kniegelenk. Langenbecks Arch. Chir., 313:502–509, 1965.
The author discusses the value of open reduction in the treatment of plateau fractures.
96. Bohler, J.: Intraartikulare frakturen des kniegelenks. Langenbecks Arch. Chir., 325:789–794, 1969.
The author advocates accurate reduction, rigid fixation, and early knee motion. The author thought that percutaneous fixation might be acceptable.
97. Boll, K. L.: (Fractures of the lateral tibial plateau. Results of surgical treatment.) Ugeskr. Laeger, 150:224–226, 1988.
98. Bombelli, R.: Le fratture del piatto tibiale. Arch. d'Ortop., 69:88–112, 1956.
99. Bomler, J., and Arnoldi, C. C.: Resurfacing of depression fractures of the lateral tibial condyle. Acta Orthop. Scand., 52:231–232, 1981.
Five patients with old depressed lateral plateau fractures were treated by a Marmor modular knee replacement. The authors believed that cartilage tolerated polyethelene well, but they have no follow-up information.
100. Bone, L. B.: Indirect fracture reduction: A technique for minimizing surgical trauma. J. Orthop. Trauma, 2:247–254, 1994.
Internal fixation has been evolving away from rigid internal fixation towards stable, biologically benign internal fixation. A femoral distractor is used while percutaneous fixation or open reduction is performed.
101. Bonnet: 1847.

102. Borch-Madsen, P.: (Symmetric bilateral fracture of the tibial tuberosities.) Arch. Orthop. Scand., 24:44–48, 1954.
103. Borghi, M.: Contributo allo studio degli esiti delle fratture intrarticolari dell'estremita superiore della tibia. Arch. Ortop., 43:178, 1926.
104. Borghi, M.: Il Trattamento delle fratture articolari dell'estremo superiore della tibia, Considerato in base allo studio anatomo-patologico ed alla constatazione dei loro esiti lontani e definitivi. Arch. Ortop., 34:407–535, 1927.
105. Bossi, L.: Intervento chirurgico secondario in un caso di frattura obliqua della tuberosita esterna della tibia. J. Chir., 39:133, 1923.
106. Boszotta, H., Helperstorfer, W., Kolndorfer, G., and Prunner, K.: Langzeitergebnisse nach operativer versorgung von tibiakopffrakturen. Aktuel Traumatol., 23:178–182, 1993.
107. Bottger, G.: Patellatransplantation bei tibiakopfbruch. Mschr. Unfallheilk., 71:77–81, 1968.
This case report concerns a 53-year-old man who fell and sustained a markedly comminuted lateral plateau fracture. The lateral third of the patella was used to replace the articular surface.
108. Bouger, D.: Fractures des Plateaux Tibiaux: Osteosynthèse par plaque en T. Paris, Medical Thesis, 1972.
109. Bowes, D. N., and Hohl, M.: Tibial plateau fractures: Evaluation of treatment and outlook. Clin. Orthop., 171:104–108, 1982.
The authors analysed 110 plateau fractures retrospectively with 52 seen more than 1 year after injury. The results were acceptable in 84%. Twenty-eight percent of patients were operated on.
110. Boyer: 1819. (Quoted in Thiele.)
Thiele indicated that Boyer and Richter described the first tibial plateau fracture.
111. Braciforti, S., and Zappoli, S.: Contributo alla therapia delle fratture del piatto tibiale. Chir. Organi Mov., 37:275, 1952.
112. Bradford, C. H., Kilfoyle, R. M., Kelleher, J. J., and Magill, H. K.: Fractures of the lateral tibial condyle. J. Bone Joint Surg., 32A:39–47, 1950.
The authors reviewed treatment principles and proposed a therapeutic classification: Crush, split, and shatter. The shatter fracture carried the worst prognosis.
113. Branciforti, S., and Zappoli, S.: Contributo alla terapia delle fratture del piatto tibiale. Chir. Organi Mov., 37:275–294, 1952.
114. Brandesky, G., and Salem, G.: Die fraktur der tuberositas tibiae. Der Chirurg., 32:517–519, 1961.
115. Brandt, G.: Ergebn. Chir. Orthop., 33:1, 1940.
116. Brechot, A., and Girard: Fractures fissuraires du plateau tibial. Prog. Med., 53:2151–2152, 1935.
117. Brehm, O.: Ein Fall von seltener fraktur im kniegelenk. Petersbrg. Med. Ztschr., 38:189–191, 1913.
118. Bressan, G., Fusco, A., and Pappalardo, G.: Le fratture del piatto tibiale. Minerva Ortop., 8:11, 1957.
119. Breyer, H., and Rahmanzadeh, R.: (The pros and cons of postponed primary osteosynthesis.) Aktuel Traumatol., 10:327–331, 1980.
120. Briese: Ein seltener fall von fraktur der tibia. Zentralbl. Chir., 24:633–634, 1887.
This case report concerns a 36-year-old person who was struck by a wagon and died. The autopsy showed a comminuted fracture involving the proximal tibia.
121. Brocq, P., and Panis, G.: Technique de l'entervention sanglante dans les fractures condyliennes du tibia. J. Chir., 25:417–437, 1925.
122. Brown, G. A., and Sprague, B. L.: Cast brace treatment of plateau and bicondylar fractures of the proximal tibia. Clin. Orthop., 119:184–193, 1976.
The authors used cast-bracing in 30 plateau fractures. It was possible to unload the fractured condyle. Five fractures were placed in the brace postoperatively. None lost fracture position in the cast-brace. The majority of fractures in this series were minimally displaced. Weight-bearing was allowed in the cast.
123. Brown, T., Anderson, D., Nepola, J., et al: Contact stress aberrations following imprecise reduction of simple tibial plateau fractures. J. Orthop. Res., 6:851–862, 1988.
The authors created sagittal fractures in seven cadaver knees; then, using pressure testing with pressure film and digitization of results, they noted that 1.5 to 2 mm of displacement created very little increased pressure, but more than 2 mm of displacement did.
124. Brunner, W.: Les fractures du plateau tibial. Z. Unfallmed. V. Berufs Krk., 32:146, 1938.
125. Brunner, W.: Z. Org. Chir. 92:638, 1939.
126. Buchanan, W., Lenihan, M., and Dossick, P.: Percutaneous reduction and stabilization of tibial plateau fractures: A new method of articular fracture management. Orthop. Trans., 14:601, 1990.
The authors treated 35 plateau fractures by miniarthrotomy to see the reduction obtained by percutaneous fixation. Eighteen were augmented by an external fixator that was attached to pins and could manipulate and impact articular fragments. Some had hinged fracture braces postoperatively. Motion averaged 90% of normal.
127. Bucholz, R. W., Carlton, A., and Holmes, R.: Interporous hydroxyapatite as a bone graft substitute in tibial plateau fractures. Clin. Orthop., 240:53–62, 1989.
Coralline porous hydroxyapatite was used as a substitute for iliac bone in 28 plateau fractures. No difference was noted in healing patterns or complication rates, and there was no loss of reduction. Biopsies taken at the time of hardware removal demonstrated bone regeneration.
128. Buckle, R., Blake, R., Watson, J. T., et al: Treatment of complex tibial plateau fractures with the Ilizarov external fixator (Abstract). J. Orthop. Trauma, 7:167–168, 1993.
129. Buckner, H. T.: Bumper fractures of the tibia. Northwest. Med., 37:102–105, 1938.
Open reduction with fixation are achieved by wires tightened over buttons. Accurate reduction and early motion were advised.
130. Buckner, H. T.: Fractures of the upper end of the tibia with lateral displacements. Am. J. Surg., 51:707–721, 1941.
The authors describe a technique of compression wiring that would allow accurate reduction and early motion.
131. Buechel, F.: A simplified evaluation system for the rating of knee function. Orthop. Rev., 11:97–101, 1982.
The author proposed a 100-point knee rating system that allows 30 points for pain, 25 points for function, 15 points for motion, 12 points for deformity, 10 points for stability, and 8 points for strength.
132. Bulloch, B., Stills, M., Lyman, J., et al: Cast bracing for severe tibial plateau fractures. Orthop. Trans., 18:944, 1994.
The authors used cast-braces on 49 patients with severe plateau fractures after internal or external fixation. They believe that cast-braces provide good supplementary fixation.
133. Burghele, N., and Ciocilan, S.: (Indications for Zanoli's method in treating fractures of the tibial plateau.) Rev. Chir. Oncol. Radiol., 33:435–438, 1984.
134. Burkhart, S. S., and Peterson, H. A.: Fractures of the proximal tibial epiphysis. J. Bone Joint Surg., 61A:996–1002, 1979.
These authors discuss the various types of proximal tibial epiphyseal fractures.
135. Burkle de la Camp, H.: Chirurgie, 7:582, 1935.
136. Burkle de la Camp, H.: Die behandlung der scheinbeinkopfbruche. Zentralbl. Chir. 67:367–368, 1940.
This article gives a very brief description of the author's operative technique.
137. Burnham, A.: Compression fractures of the upper extremity of the tibia. Med. Record, 86:1004–1006, 1914.
This case report concerns a split compression fracture treated by manipulation under anesthesia and cast. The result was restriction of knee movement that prompted the author to believe that the prognosis for these fractures was poor.
138. Burri, C.: Die aussasekraft des roentsenbildes bei der operativen versorgung von tibiakopffrakturen im hinblick auf das entstehen posttraumatische gonarthrosen. Hefte Unfallheilk., 110:176, 1971.
139. Burri, C.: Fractures of the Tibial Plateau. Philadelphia, J.B. Lippincott, 1975 (?).
140. Burri, C.: Die frischen verletzungen des kniegelenks. Langenbecks Arch. Chir., 345:459–460, 1977.
This is a short round-table type of discussion about plateau fractures.
141. Burri, C., Bartzke, G., Coldewey, J., and Muggler, E.: Fractures of the tibial plateau. Clin. Orthop., 138:84–93, 1979.
The authors treated 342 plateau fractures, mainly by anterior oblique technique. Of these fractures, 278 were followed more than 1 year (average of 32 months). Two groups were set up: The first group was treated by very experienced surgeons and the other group by less experienced surgeons. Better reductions and results were noted from experienced surgeons. Arthritis was noted in about 50% at follow-up.
142. Burrows, H. J.: Fractures of the lateral condyle of the tibia (Editorial). J. Bone Joint Surg., 38B:612–613, 1956.

This editorial comment compares Apley's article with Slee's article, both of which showed good results after traction treatment.

143. Buttermann, F.: Klinik der tibiakondylenbruche. Arch. Klin. Chir., 190:580–603, 1937.
Of 17 plateau fractures reported, 10 were treated with closed reduction and 7 were operated on. Bone grafts were used under elevated surfaces, and wires were used for internal fixation.
144. Cabanie: Fractures de l'extrémité supérieure du tibia. Maroc Med., 75:87, 1928.
145. Cadore, V.: Le fratture dell'estremita superiore della tibia. Rass. Prev. Soc., 9:25–59, 1933.
146. Caldwell, E. H.: Fractures of the condyles of the tibia. Surg. Gynecol. Obstet., 63:518–522, 1936.
The author studied 58 plateau fractures and reviewed 48, 1 to 5 years after injury. Closed treatment and nonrepair of torn ligaments were recommended.
147. Camargo, B.: Fractura rara da extremidade superior da tibia. Gaz. Clin. S. Paulo, 22:240–242, 1926.
148. Campbell, O. J.: Bumper fractures of the tibia. Minn. Med. 19:593–603, 1936.
After using closed reduction, the author became convinced that open techniques might give better results.
149. Canteri, L., and Cereser, C.: (Our experience in the treatment of closed fractures of the tibial plateau.) Chir. Organi Mov., 66:371–379, 1980.
The authors followed 182 of 341 plateau fractures and concluded that most fractures do well after closed treatment, except those with cavities, which are best operated on.
150. Carling, E.: A note on two cases of vertical or cuneiform fracture of the tibia. Westminst. Hosp. Rep., 14:133–136, 1905.
Two case reports are given—one with x-rays showing a sagittal split fracture, and the other with a bicondylar fracture. Rest and massage were used for the split fracture, and plaster was used for the bicondylar fracture.
151. Carlson, D. H.: CT evaluation of intra-articular fractures. South. Med. J., 73:820–821, 1980.
This case report concerns a bicondylar fracture shown axially on a computed tomography scan.
152. Carlson, H.: Reaction of rabbit patellar cartilage following operative defects: A morphological and autoradiographic study. Acta Orthop. Scand., 28 (Suppl.), 1957.
153. Carr, D. E.: Arthroscopically assisted stabilization of tibial plateau fractures. Techniques Orthop., 6:55–57, 1991.
154. Cary, N.: 1932.
155. Caspari, R. B., Hutton, P. M., Whipple, T. L., and Meyers, J. F.: The role of arthroscopy in the management of tibial plateau fractures. Arthroscopy, 1:76–82, 1984.
The authors concluded that arthroscopy can be valuable in the treatment of plateau fractures. The advantages were accurate diagnosis of soft tissue and the ability to reduce and fix percutaneously 14 of 30 fractures. Seven soft tissue injuries were diagnosed as well as one medial collateral, one lateral collateral, and one posterior cruciate ligament injury.
156. Catalano, V.: L'osteosintesi metallica con vite nel trattamento delle fratture del piatto tibiale. Bol. Mem. Soc. Tosco-Umbra Chir., 6:610–629, 1950.
157. Cauchoix, J., and Deburge, A.: Fractures de l'extrémité supérieure du tibia. Appl. Locomoteur, 2:1–10, 1966.
158. Cavazza, F.: Trattamento cruento delle fratture del piatto tibiale. Taranto Med., 3:10, 1957.
159. Cave, E. F.: Fractures of the tibial condyles involving the knee joint. Surg. Gynecol. Obstet., 86:289–294, 1948.
The author recommends surgical treatment for moderately displaced fractures and closed treatment for lesser displacements. The author treated 98 plateau fractures with 24 opened and internally fixed.
160. Cazeneuve, A.: Des Fractures de l'Extrémité Supérieure du Tibia par Arrachement et de la Lenteur de Leur Consolidation. Paris, Thesis, 1875.
161. Cecil, M. L., McGee, J. P., Ebraheim, N. A., and Jackson, W. T.: Response of the lateral meniscus of the dog to wide incision and repair of the meniscotibial ligament. J. Orthop. Trauma, 9:141–144, 1995.
The lateral meniscus was detached through the meniscotibial ligament and repaired in nine dogs. At 6 weeks, vascularity had recovered and there were no observed degenerative meniscal changes. Healing occurred by fibrovascular scar.
162. Celestin Dallas, J.: Des Fractures de l'Extrémité Supérieure du Tibia. Paris, Thesis, 1854.
163. Cericola, G., and Manetta, F.: Sul trattamento delle fratture del piatto tibiale con metodo mobilizzante in trazione continua. Arch. C.T.O. dell'INAIL, 4:387, 1964.
164. Cerrini, L.: Trattamento delle fratture dell'estremo superiore articolare della tibia. Chir. Organi Mov., 48:279–292, 1960.
165. Chaix, B.: La méthode de traction-mobilisation immédiate dans le traitement des fractures articulaires de l'extrémité supérieure du tibia. Lyon Med., 210:145–146, 1963.
The authors have briefly analysed plateau fractures treated by the traction-mobilization method with 72% satisfactory results. In lateral plateau fractures the results were satisfactory in 77% of cases but were only 65% satisfactory in bicondylar fractures.
166. Chaix, B.: La Méthode de Traction-Mobilisation Immédiate dans le Traitement des Fractures Articulaires de l'Extrémité Supérieure du Tibia. Lyons, Thesis, 1962.
Satisfactory results were reported in 82% of plateau fractures that were treated by the traction-mobilization method.
167. Chaix, O., Herman, S., Cohen, P., et al: Osteosynthèse par plaque epiphysaire dans les fractures des plateaux tibiaux: A propos de 111 cas. Rev. Chir. Orthop., 68:189–197, 1982.
The authors treated 100 plateau fractures by open reduction and AO fixation with a plate and graft. The results were satisfactory in 86%. Patients in poor condition were advised to avoid surgery.
168. Chalnot, P., Michon, J., and Vichard, P.: La place de l'intervention chirurgicale et de l'arthrotomie dans le traitement des fractures récentes des plateaux tibiaux (à propos de 81 observations). Ann. Med. Nancy, 3:848–861, 1964.
169. Chalochet, P.: Sur le Traitement des Fractures Unituberositaires du Tibia. Paris, Thesis, 1942.
170. Chambry, C.: Su un caso di frattura da schiacciamento del piatto tibiale. Acta Orthop. Ital., 5:1, 1959.
171. Chandeclerc, M.: Les Fractures Articulaires Récentes de l'Extrémité Supérieure du Tibia. Toulouse, Thesis, 1971.
172. Charles-Bloch, J.: Affaissement de la tuberosité tibiale esterne après fracture traitée par visage. Operation plastique secondaire: Restituto ad integrum. Mem. Acad. Chir., 62:401–409, 1936.
This case report concerns a 34 year old with a split compression fracture treated by open reduction and screw fixation. The fracture lost reduction and 3 months later reoperation and grafting were performed.
173. Chen, H. T.: Fractures of the tibial plateaus. J. Formosa Med. Assoc., 60:138–147, 1961.
174. Chevassu: Fracture de la tuberositie externe du tibia. Bull. Mem. Soc. de Chir. de Paris, 32:270–272, 1906.
This case report concerns a 30-year-old person who fell onto the knee. After aspiration of hemarthrosis, healing occurred. Good movement was obtained with some tibial widening.
175. Chevrier, L.: Enclouage d'une fracture unicondylienne du tibia. Rev. d'Orthop., 1:351–356, 1910.
176. Chow, G. H., and Hohl, M.: Osteoarthritis of the knee following tibial plateau fracture: A survivorship analysis. Orthop. Trans., 16:631, 1993.
Kaplan-Meier analyses were applied to 693 plateau fractures that were followed for 1 to 42 years. Moderate or severe arthritic changes in the knee were determined as the endpoint of survival. Arthritis was 16% at 5 years, 32% at 10 years, and 49% at 15 years. The accuracy of final reduction and subcondylar fracture were the most likely predictors of arthritis.
177. Christel, P., Herman, S., Benoit, S., et al: Percutaneous arthrolysis under arthroscopic control and manipulation under anesthesia in the treatment of postoperative stiffness of the knee. Rev. Chir. Orthop., 74:517–525, 1988.
The authors discuss 40 stiff knees after ligament injury. Half of the knees were manipulated under anesthesia and the other half had arthroscopic lysis of adhesions followed by manipulation. Those patients who had arthroscopic lysis recovered motion twice as fast as those treated by manipulation alone. Manipulation was most effective when done within 3 months of injury.
178. Christensen, K. P., Powell, J. N., Bucholz, R. W., and Stills, M.: Early results of combined internal-external fixation for the treatment of high grade tibial plateau fractures. J. Orthop. Trauma, 4:226, 1990.
179. Chuinard, E. G.: Fractures of the condyles of the tibia. Clin. Orthop., 37:115–129, 1964.
This author classified plateau fractures into those needing manipulation and those not requiring manipulation. Traction was used without early motion, and operative treatment was rarely used.

180. Claeys, C.: Les fractures uni-condyliennes du tibia. Arch. Prov. Chir., 20:223–233, 1911.
181. Clarke, H. J., Robertson, J. A., and Schearer, J. R.: Tibial plateau fractures: A comparison of autograft and organic solvent treated allograft bone for reconstruction. Orthop. Proc. Suppl. 1, 1993.
Human allografts were prepared with solvents and used in 37 of 73 patients operated on for plateau fractures. After a mean of 3.4 years, there was no difference noted between an autograft and an allograft. Recurrent depression occurred in both the allograft and autograft cases (four of each). All grafts incorporated well.
182. Clarke, H. O.: Discussion on fracture of the tibia involving the knee joint. Proc. R. Soc. Med., 28:1035–1043, 1935.
The author analysed 19 plateau fractures in detail and presented suggestions for treatment of various fracture types.
183. Clarke, R.: Arthroscopic assisted management of tibial plateau fractures. Orthop. Trans., 14:715, 1990.
The author treated 14 plateau fractures by arthroscopic-assisted reduction and concluded that it is a useful method.
184. Claussen, T.: Intra-articular fractures in the upper end of the tibia and lower end of the femur. Acta Chir. Scand., 94:407–428, 1946.
185. Clymer, D., and Reckling, F. W.: Roentgenographic and clinical assessment of patients with tibial plateau fractures. Orthop. Trans., 9:482, 1985.
186. Cobey, M. C.: Lag-screw fixation in fractures of the tibial tuberosity. J. Bone Joint Surg., 28:273–276, 1946.
This author reports four plateau fractures that were treated by lag screw, lock washer, and spur.
187. Coblentz: Étude des Lesions Ligamentaires dans les Fractures du Plateau Tibial. Strasbourg, Thesis, 1961.
188. Coche, A.: De Quelques Phénomènes Consécutifs aux Fracture de l'Extrémité Supérieure du Tibia. Paris, Thesis, 1879.
189. Collert, S.: Tibiakondylfrakturer-operation och omedelbar mobilisering. Nord. Med., 79:263–264, 1968.
Fifty-four plateau fractures were operated on, and early mobilization was promoted. Forty-one fractures were followed with 16 excellent results, 15 good results, and 10 fair results.
190. Collins, A.: Tibial fractures into the knee joint. Minn. Med., 13:285–292, 1930.
The author reports 20 plateau fractures treated by cast, traction, or rarely manipulative reduction. The open treatment was considered to be too complicated. Early motion, within 2 to 3 weeks, was recommended.
191. Colton, C. L.: Telling the bones. J. Bone Joint Surg., 73B:362–363, 1991.
In this editorial the AO fracture classification is promoted as a step forward.
192. Constantz, B. R., Ison, I. C., Fulmer, M. T., et al: Science, 267:1796–1799, 1995.
These authors describe a calcium paste that can be injected into fractures and that sets hard after an interval providing stability and resisting compression only to be integrated into real bone. This calcium paste is used in Colles fractures.
193. Contiades, X. J., and Politis, A. M.: À propos du traitement chirurgical des fractures sous articulaires récentes d'un plateau tibial par enfoncement. Presse Med., 43:44–46, 1935.
Two local compression fractures of the lateral plateau were treated by elevation and grafting with local bone.
194. Convery, F. R., Akeson, W. H., and Keown, G. H.: The repair of large osteochondral defects. Clin. Orthop., 82:253–262, 1972.
Full-thickness osteochondral defects were made (9 to 15 mm) in the femoral condyle of nine mature Shetland ponies. A 3-mm defect was also made in a non–weight-bearing part of the same condyle. The small defects all healed and could hardly be identified after 3 months. None of the defects 9 mm or more completely repaired even after 9 months. Microscopic studies were made.
195. Cooper, A.: A Treatise on Dislocations and on Fractures of the Joints. Boston, Wells & Lilly, 1825.
This is a textbook description of the tibial plateau fracture and its reduction by manipulative methods. The author points out that ankylosis occurs with immobilization.
196. Cornacchia, M., Marre, F., and Raffelini, R.: Rilievi comparativi trattamento cruento e incruento delle fratture del piatto tibiale. Minerva Ortop., 18:346–351, 1967.
These authors treated 63 plateau fractures, some operatively, and discussed the indications for various forms of treatment.
197. Cornell, C. M., and Hardy, R. C.: Plateau fractures of the tibia. Surgery, 28:735–743, 1950.
These authors studied 111 plateau fractures that were treated mainly by closed methods and did some early follow-up studies.
198. Correa do Lago: (Posterior marginal fractures of the tibial plateau.) Rev. Bras. Orthop. Traumatol., 1:375–384, 1940.
199. Corvisy: Fractures de l'Extrémité Supérieure du Tibia. Bordeaux, Thesis, 1912.
200. Costa, P., and Dall'Aglio, S.: (Considerations on the surgical treatment of fractures of the tibial plateau.) Chir. Organi Mov., 69:247–255, 1984.
201. Costa, V., et al: (The use of Barr's bolt in treatment of proximal tibial epiphyseal fractures.) Atti Acad. Med. Lombard, 20:24–30, 1965.
202. Cotte: Deux cas de fracture avec éclatement du plateau tibial. Lyon Chir., 718, 1929.
203. Cotton, F. J.: Fender fractures. Surg. Gynecol. Obstet., 62:442–443, 1936.
A fender fracture is defined as a crush fracture of the lateral plateau. Closed reduction under anesthesia is advocated because of the results noted after open surgery.
204. Cotton, F. J., and Berg, R.: Fender fracture of the tibia at the knee. N. Engl. J. Med., 201:989–995, 1929.
A fender fracture is defined as a crush fracture of the lateral plateau. Closed reduction under anesthesia is advocated because of the poor results noted after open surgery.
205. Coulomb: Arch. Med. Pharm. Nav., 108:139, 1919.
206. Couloum, P.: Architecture du Plateau Tibial. Toulouse, Thesis, 1928.
207. Courvoisier, E.: Les fractures intraarticulaires de l'extrémité supérieure du tibia. Helv. Chir. Acta, 32:257–263, 1965.
The author classified plateau fractures and illustrated methods of internal fixation using plates and screws.
208. Courvoisier, E.: Traitement des fractures des plateaux tibiaux. Med. Hyg., 27:750, 1969.
209. Courvoisier, E.: Les fractures des plateaux tibiaux; Étude clinique. Traitement: Résultats de 129 cas. Bull. A.O., Nov., 1973.
This detailed thesis is based on 186 fractures with 129 cases followed.
210. Courvoisier, E.: Fractures des plateaux tibiaux: Comparaison du traitement opératoire et du traitement conservateur. Helv. Chir. Acta, 41:283–286, 1974.
This author describes results after closed and open treatment of plateau fractures and concludes that although stability is better after open reduction, motion of the knee is the same. This was considered to be a complex problem.
211. Courvoisier, E.: (Fractures of the tibial plateau: Surgical or conservative treatment?) Rev. Chir. Orthop., 61 (Suppl.): 280–285, 1975.
This author treated 129 plateau fractures, 62 closed and 67 open. The conclusion was that each method has advantages and can produce satisfactory results when properly applied.
212. Courvoisier, E.: Die behandlung der tibiakopffrakturen. Hefte Unfallheilk., 120:137–144, 1975.
This author followed 129 plateau fractures, 62 treated closed and 67 open, and compared the results of closed versus open treatment methods. The author noted that operative results were better.
213. Courvoisier, E.: Fractures des plateaux tibiaux: Traitement opératoire ou traitement conservateur? SO. F.C.O.T. Ann. Reunion, 49:280–285, 1975.
This author used immediate motion in undisplaced fractures and traction and open reduction and internal fixation in others. Of 186 plateau fractures that were treated, these selected treatments provided satisfactory results.
214. Covall, D. J., Fowbie, C. D., Foster, T. E., and Whitelaw, G. P.: Bicondylar tibial plateau fractures: Principles of treatment. Contemp. Orthop., 28:115–122, 1994.
These authors treated 23 bicondylar fractures either by open reduction and internal fixation (in seven cases), arthroscopic reduction and fixation in six cases, or Monticelli-Spinelli external fixation (in 10 cases). Infection was a major problem after open reduction and internal fixation, but pin tract infections occurred after fixators were used. The arthroscope was considered to be a very valuable method for assessing reduction.
215. Crellin, R.: Macintosh prosthesis for tibial-plateau fractures (Abstract). J. Bone Joint Surg., 47B:196, 1965.
This author reports on three plateau fractures that were treated

primarily by use of a Macintosh prosthesis. The results were generally good.

216. Creyssel, J., Berard, M., and Dargent, M.: Le boulonnage transcutane dans le traitement des fractures cuneiformes de l'extrémité supérieure du tibia. J. Chir., 53:758–767, 1939.
217. Creyssel, J., and Chaix, D.: L'osteotomie tibiale haute complementaire dans le traitement secondaire des fractures de l'extrémité supérieure du tibia. Lyon Chir., 60:760–767, 1964.
The authors analysed the results of an osteotomy for deformity after a plateau fracture and concluded that an early osteotomy produced better results than did a late osteotomy.
218. Crillovich, R.: Uber geschlossense frakturen und traumatische luxationen des kniegelenkes. Arch. Orthop., 35:94–124, 1927.
219. Cubbins, W. R., Conley, A. H., Callahan, B. S., and Scuderi, C. S.: Fractures of the lateral condyle of the tibia: Classification, pathology, and treatment. Surg. Gynecol. Obstet., 59:461–468, 1934.
These authors studied 125 lateral plateau fractures. Half were treated by open surgery. A classification was developed with a treatment plan for each type.
220. Cubbins, W. R., Conley, A. H., and Seiffert, G. S.: Fractures of the lateral tuberosity of the tibia with displacements of the lateral meniscus between the fragments. Surg. Gynecol. Obstet., 48:106–108, 1929.
The authors noted in several cases that the meniscus prevented reduction by wedging into the fracture. After a meniscectomy, reduction was possible.
221. Dambrin, C.: Sur trois cas de fractures condyliennes du tibia. Arch. Med. Toulouse, 11:531–541, 1905.
This author reported three plateau fractures prior to x-rays. The physical findings and the diagnosis were discussed. Pseudoarthrosis was mentioned as a possibility, but one had not been seen.
222. Damholt, V.: (Conservative treatment of fractures of the tibial condyles.) Rev. Chir. Orthop., 74 (Suppl.)2:281–282, 1988.
223. Damiot, G.: Contribution à l'Étude des Fractures de l'Extrémité Supérieure du Tibia. Paris, Thesis, 1906.
224. Daniel, D., and Rice, T.: Valgus-varus stability in the hinged cast used for controlled mobilization of the knee. J. Bone Joint Surg., 61A:135–136, 1979.
These authors found that the thigh portion of a cast-brace must be molded onto the femoral condyles for optimum control of valgus and varus. They used six cadaver knees in 20 degrees of flexion and a medial opening documented after stress, with the medial collateral ligament intact and cut, in a long-leg cast and in a cast-brace.
225. D'Aubigne, R. M.: De l'emploi de boulons légers pour le traitement des fractures avec diastasis. Rev. Orthop., 26:51, 1933.
226. D'Aubigne, R. M.: À propos du traitement des fractures par enfoncement du plateau tibial. Mem. Acad. Chir., 68:249–250, 1942.
227. D'Aubigne, R. M.: À propos du traitement des fractures unituberositaires du tibia. Rev. Orthop., 33:107–108, 1947.
This author divided plateau fractures into those above or below the insertion of the medial collateral ligament. Those fractures below reduce by manipulation, those above do not. Six osteotomies were done to correct malalignments.
228. D'Aubigne, R. M., and Mazas, F.: (The anatomic types and treatment of fractures of the upper end of the tibia.) Rev. Chir. Orthop., 46:289–318, 1960.
Seventy-six plateau fractures were studied, and 60 followed for more than 3 years. A simple classification was suggested. The results indicate that certain treatments are better for selected types of fractures.
229. D'Aubigne, R. M., and Mazas, F.: Formes anatomiques et traitement des fractures de l'extrémité supérieure du tibia. Rev. Orthop., 46:289–318, 1961.
230. Daubenspeck, K.: Z. Orthop., 86:237, 1955.
231. David, J.: Étude du traitement Orthopédique et des Résultats des Fractures des Plateau Tibiaux. Bordeaux, Medical Thesis, 1979.
232. Davidson, R. L., Russell, T. A., Kuester, D. J., and Klinar, D. F.: Fibular head autograft for severely comminuted lateral plateau fractures of the tibia. Orthop. Trans., 14:601–602, 1990.
These authors treated five severely comminuted lateral plateau fractures with the fibular head as an articular surface replacement. With cadaver dissection, it was noted that there was 3.2 cm of articular surface on the fibular head. Using Hospital for Special Surgery rating at 1 year, there were three excellent and one good (one lost).
233. DeBoeck, H., and Opdecam, P.: Posteromedial tibial plateau fractures: Operative treatment by posterior approach. Clin. Orthop., 320:125–128, 1995.
These authors used a posteromedial approach across the popliteal fossa, partially dividing the medial gastrocnemius head and the popliteus to expose the fracture. A T plate fixes the fracture. Seven patients had good results, except for a mean extensor lag of 7 degrees.
234. De Jure, T., and Ghisellini, F.: Il trattamento cruento delle fratture del piatto tibiale. Atti S. E. R. T. O. T., 9:801, 1964.
235. De Racker, C.: Un cas de fracture du plateau tibial externe. Acta Orthop. Belg., 23:467–469, 1957.
236. De Marneffe, R. de: Fracture de l'extrémité supérieure du tibia. Acta Orthop. Belg., 23:247–251, 1957.
237. DeCoster, T. A., Nepola, J. V., and El-Khoury, G. Y.: Cast brace treatment of proximal tibial fractures: A ten year follow-up study. Clin. Orthop., 231:196–204, 1988.
The Brown-Sprague cast-brace treated series was followed again more than 10 years after the initial treatment. Of the 29 survivors, 27 showed 61% good results, but 32% had developed moderate or severe arthritic changes.
238. Decoulx, J., and Capron, J. C.: Traitement chirurgical à foyer fermé de certaines fractures de l'extrémité supérieure du tibia. Rev. Chir. Orthop., 60 (Suppl.):324–330, 1974.
The author describes techniques of reduction and application of external fixators or with percutaneous internal fixation. Case reports are illustrated.
239. Decoulx, P., and Razemon, J. P.: Fractures de l'extrémité supérieure du tibia (à propos de 50 observations). Lille Chirurg., 13:149–163, 1958.
These authors classified 50 fractures to determine if surgical treatment would produce a satisfactory result. They recommended surgical treatment for unicondylar fractures but cautioned about bicondylar fractures.
240. Dehelly, M.: Écrasement du plateau tibial: Reconstitution de ce plateau par greffons osteoperiostiques. Bull. Soc. Nat. Chir., 53:1296–1299, 1927.
This case report concerns a lateral plateau fracture treated by closed reduction with a persistent deformity. On the 8th day, an osteoperiosteal graft was used to restore the plateau, and grafts were placed underneath.
241. Dehne, E., and Torp, R. P.: Treatment of joint injuries by immediate mobilization. Clin. Orthop., 77:218–231, 1977.
These authors reported 11 plateau fractures that were treated by functional methods with 10 of 11 achieving a good range of motion.
242. Dejour, H., Chambat, P., Caton, J., and Melere, G.: Les fractures des plateaux tibiaux avec lésion ligamentaire. Rev. Chir. Orthop., 67:593–598, 1981.
These authors found ligament injuries by bone fragments, stress x-rays, or tomograms. Twenty-five ligament injuries were identified. They included tibial spine fractures as evidence of ligament injury. They suggested operative repair of the ligament followed by 1 month in a cast.
243. Delamarter, R. B., and Hohl, M.: The cast brace and tibial plateau fractures. Clin. Orthop., 242:26–31, 1989.
A cast-brace was used as part of the treatment in 141 of 306 plateau fractures. One year follow-up was possible in 99 patients. Fifteen percent lost between 4 and 8 mm of reduction, and this was noted more in medial plateau and bicondylar fracture types. Cast-bracing can be used in all types of plateau fractures but should be used cautiously if the medial plateau is involved.
244. Delamarter, R. B., Hohl, M., and Hopp, E.: Ligament injuries associated with tibial plateau fractures. Clin. Orthop., 250:226–233, 1990.
Thirty-nine tibial plateau fractures with concomitant ligament injuries were evaluated 1 to 15 years after an injury (mean of 3.9 years). Two groups were analysed: Group 1 had no ligament repair (20 cases of which 13 had open reduction of the fracture). Group 2 had ligament repair (19 cases all with open reduction of the fracture). Results in group 1 were an average of 6.1 degrees of instability and a point rating of 73. Group 2 had 4.5 degrees of instability and a point rating of 80.
245. Delchef, J.: Le traitement des condyles du tibia avec déplacement. Le Scalpel, 21, 1935.

246. Dell'Orto, R., and Allegreni, R.: Sul trattamento cruento delle fratture del piatto tibiale. Minerva Ortop., 18:374–377, 1967.
These authors used operative treatment in 43 plateau fractures with tibial bolts. Although functional results were mainly good, the anatomic results were not good.
247. Del Torto, U., and Mangiaricina, A.: Considerazioni sulle fratture del piatto tibiale da incidenti stradali. Atti S.I.O.T., 44:143, 1959.
248. Del Vecchio, E., and Antongiovanni, G.: Fratture del piatto tibiale. Minerva Ortop., 28:657–678, 1977.
249. Demoulin: Bull. Mem. Soc. Chir. Paris., 44:2628, 1916.
250. Demoulin: Arch. Gen. Med., 2:737, 1894.
This case report concerns a 29 year old who sustained a medial plateau fracture that was thought to be incomplete and that healed satisfactorily.
251. Denks, H.: Zentralbl. Chir., 65:613, 1938.
252. Denny, L., Keating, E., Englehardt, J., and Saha, S.: A comparison of fixation techniques in tibial plateau fractures (Abstract). Trans. Orthop. Res. Soc., 1986.
The authors studied the biomechanics of fixation of cadaveric plateau fractures using screws or buttress plates. Judging by deformation resistance, the plates were clearly superior to screws.
253. Depalma, L., and Serra, F.: (Surgical treatment of fractures of the tibial plateau.) Chir. Patol. Sper., 23:325–343, 1975.
254. Desgouttes, D., and Ricard, A.: À propos du traitement des fractures de l'extrémité supérieure du tibia. J. Chir., 26:481–485, 1925.
These authors reported three plateau fractures that were treated by closed reduction and casting. There were more problems with irregularity medially than laterally.
255. Desgouttes, D., and Ricard, A.: À propos des fractures de l'extrémité supérieure du tibia: Résultat du traitement non sanglant. Lyon Chir., 26:749–753, 1929.
This author makes a plea for closed reduction and cast treatment based on treatment of six plateau fractures.
256. Desguin, M.: De la fracture unicondylienne du tibia à trait vertical. Presse Med., 17:703, 1909.
This author reports on five plateau fractures, two of which were treated before and three after x-rays. The fractures split off the lateral plateau and were associated with fibular fractures.
257. Desguin, M.: De la fracture unicondylienne du tibia à trait vertical. Bull. Acad. R. Med. de Belge, 1909.
258. Deubner: Eine neue schraubenzwinge fur knockenbruche (kompressarium). Munch. Med. Wochenschr., 83:1094–1095, 1936.
259. Deuticke, H. J.: Zentralbl. Chir., 62:708–709, 1935.
Two brief reports are made of plateau fractures—one open and both treated by traction and reduction.
260. Dezzani, D., and De Lucio, O.: Sulle fratture dell'estremita superiore della tibia. Arch. Ortop., 69:333–359, 1956.
261. Di Natale, L.: Le fratture dell'estremita superiore della tibia (Escluse le fratture delle eminenze intercondiloidee). Arch. Ortop., 62:77–121, 1949.
262. Diamond, B.: Tibial plateau fractures. Med. Trial Tech. Q., 11:1–13, 1965.
This is a general discussion for lawyers regarding plateau fractures.
263. Dias, J. J., Stirling, A. J., Finlay, D. B., and Gregg, P.: Computerised axial tomography for tibial plateau fractures. J. Bone Joint Surg., 69B:84–88, 1987.
These authors studied 16 plateau fractures by x-ray, tomography in two planes, and computed tomography (CT) scans. They concluded that CT scans allowed better classification and assessment of displacement compared with standard views.
264. Dickson, J. A.: Fractures of the tibia involving the knee joint: Bumper or fender fractures. Am J. Surg., 38:700–705, 1937.
A technique of closed reduction using traction and varus casting was employed initially. If reduction was not satisfactory by x-ray, the cast was windowed and open reduction was carried out with no fear of redisplacement.
265. Didier: Les Fractures en Tiroir de l'Extrémité Supérieure du Tibia. Bordeaux, Thesis, 1959.
266. Dietz, G. W., Wilcox, D. M., and Montgomery, J. B.: Segond tibial condyle fracture: Lateral capsular ligament avulsion. Radiology, 159:467–469, 1986.
These authors reported 20 Segond fractures (lateral capsular ligament avulsion) from the lateral plateau.
267. Dobelle, M.: A new method of closed reduction of fractures of the lateral condyle of the tibia. Am. J. Surg., 53:460–462, 1941.
A method of closed reduction is proposed in terms of a hinged cast with the hinges placed anteriorly and posteriorly to control valgus-varus alignment.
268. Doizon, R.: Fractures du plateau tibial externe (anatomie Pathologique et Traitement.) Paris, Thesis, 1955.
269. Dondoglio, M. A.: (Arthrosis of the knee as a sequel of fractures of the lateral tibial plateau.) Diabet. Med., 35:1032–1033, 1963.
270. Dondoglio, M. A.: (Lesions associated with fractures of the tibial plateaus.) Dia. Med., 35:2156–2157, 1963.
271. Dorrance, F. S.: An unusual fracture of the upper end of the tibia. Can. Med. Assoc. J., 31:184–185, 1934.
This case report concerns a 36-year-old football player who sustained fracture of the upper tibia and intercondylar eminence after kicking. The treatment was rest followed by early motion and a 1-year follow-up.
272. Dovey, H., and Heerfordt, J.: Tibial condylar fractures. Nord. Med., 83:830–831, 1970.
These authors operated on 62 plateau fractures and used Kiel bone as graft material. Early mobility gave the best results, and good results were observed even when the reduction was not good and the articular surfaces were displaced.
273. Dovey, H., and Heerfordt, J.: Tibial condyle fractures: A follow-up of 200 cases. Acta Chir. Scand., 137:521–531, 1971.
These authors reviewed 200 plateau fractures for 1 to 10 years after injury. Sixty-two were operated on, most of which were depressed fractures that were supported by Kiel bone, often with tibial bolt fixation. Early mobilization was the key to good function, and function was also improved when the meniscus was not removed.
274. Dragonetti, L., and Ottaviani, C.: Considerazioni sulle lesione meniscali e ligamentore associate a fratture del piatto tibiale. Minerva Ortop., 18:394–398, 1967.
These authors operated on 43 plateau fractures and found 13 meniscal tears, peripheral tears, and radial tears.
275. Drennan, D. B., Locher, F. G., and Maylahn, D. J.: Fractures of the tibial plateau: Treatment by closed reduction and spica cast. J. Bone Joint Surg., 61A:989–995, 1979.
Sixty-one of 187 plateau fractures were treated by heavy traction on a fracture table, manipulating the fracture using varus or valgus straps and a single spica cast applied for 6 weeks. Only 15% of results were unsatisfactory.
276. Dujarier: Bull. Mem. Soc. Chir. Paris, 46:1103, 1920.
277. Duparc, J., and Cavagna, R.: Résultats du traitement operatoire des fractures des plateaux tibiaux (À propos de 110 cas). Int. Orthop., 11:205–213, 1987.
A complete review is given concerning plateau fractures, especially complications and sequelae. The advantages and disadvantages of the available treatment methods are cited. The study is based on 172 personal plateau fractures.
278. DuParc, J., and Ficat, P.: Fractures articulaires de l'extrémité supérieure du tibia. Rev. Chir. Orthop., 46:399–486, 1960.
These authors describe plateau fractures from anatomy and mechanism to classification and treatment. Ligament injuries and meniscal injuries are illustrated. Each type of fracture is described in one and both condyles.
279. Duparc, J., and Filipe, G.: Fractures spino-tuberositaires ou fractures avec subluxation de l'extrémité supérieure du tibia. Rev. Chir. Orthop., 61:705–716, 1975.
The "entire" fracture type is described and illustrated in detail with drawings of probable mechanisms of injury. Ligament and meniscal lesions were often noted to be present.
280. Duplay, M., and Marot, E.: Sur une variété de fracture de l'extrémité supérieure du tibia. Prog. Med., 4:325–327, 1876.
This case report concerns a 60 year old whose knee was injured by a falling stone. Chloroform was given, and the knee was examined. A fracture reduction was noted in flexion. Gangrene developed because of politeal artery laceration. An autopsy was performed.
281. Dupuis, P. V.: Traitement des fractures par enfoncement du plateau externe. Rev. d'Orthop., 41:268, 1945.
282. Dupuis, P. V.: Artifice de technique facilitant la reduction sanglante des fractures recentes par enfoncement central du plateau tibial externe. Presse Med., 62:135–136, 1954.
This author reported six split compression plateau fractures that

were treated operatively by elevating the depressed fragment and by nailing the split fragment with good results.
283. Dupuis, P. V.: Étude de diverses variétés de fractures du plateau tibial externe et leur traitement. Acta Orthop. Belg., 21:113–121, 1955.
284. Dupuis, P. V.: Traitement des fractures par enfoncement du plateau tibial externe. Rev. Chir. Orthop., 41:268–270, 1955.
285. Durochas, M.: Des Fractures de l'Extrémité Supérieure du tibia; de Leur Prognostic, des Causes de la Lenteur de Leur Consolidation. Paris, Thesis, 1867.
286. Dustmann, H. O., and Schulitz, K. D.: Konservativ oder operative behandlung von scheinbeinkopfbruchen. Z. Orthop., 111:160–168, 1973.
287. Dustmann, H. O., and Schulitz, K. D.: Das problem der arthrose nach schienbeinkopffrakturen. Chirurg., 46:358–362, 1975.
This long-term study of 180 plateau fractures was followed up to 20 years. Arthritis was noted in 56% of patients at 5 years and 78% at 20 years. (The criteria for arthritis and a comparison with the other knee was not mentioned.)
288. Dustmann, H. O., Schulitz, K., and Puhl, W.: Der schienbeinkopfbruch als praarthrose. Z. Orthop., 112:637–640, 1974.
These authors describe microscopic synovial changes occurring after a plateau fracture. These changes were similar to villonodular synovitis.
289. Duwelius, P. J., and Connelly, J. F.: Closed reduction of tibial plateau fractures: A comparison of functional and roentgenographic end results. Clin. Orthop., 230:116–126, 1988.
In this multicenter study of 100 plateau fractures, the end results were graded by functional and radiographic criteria. The 73 fractures that were treated by closed reduction and cast-bracing got 89% satisfactory results, whereas the fractures treated by open reduction and internal fixation were less good but were not comparable.
290. Dyas, F. G., and Goren, M. L.: Bumper and fender fractures. Surg. Gynecol. Obstet., 65:690–694, 1937.
This discussion article contributes the idea of taking a cortical graft removed from the uninjured leg to use under an elevated plateau.
291. Ebner, E.: Zur behandlung schwerer oberschenkel-und scheinbeinkopf-bruche (pelottenapparat). Zentralbl. Chir., 60:2665–2668, 1933.
This author used a device like a Braun frame fitted with shoes to maintain leg alignment. No case reports are given.
292. Edeland, H. G.: Open reduction of central compression fractures of the tibial plateau: Preliminary report of a new method and device arrangement. Acta Orthop. Scand., 47:686–689, 1976.
A curved probe was used to aid in the elevation of compression fractures. Five cases were cited.
293. Edeland, H. G.: A method for treatment of rim fractures of the tibial condyle: Description of a new surgical technique and a new fracture fixation device. Acta Orthop. Belg., 44:393–396, 1978.
This author describes an osteotomy that was used in two patients, in which a block of bone is elevated, including the tibial rim, and fixed with a staple-like device.
294. Ehalt, W.: Trummerbruche am oberen schienbeinende mit gleichzeitiger zerreissung des ligamentum patellae proprium als typische motorradverletzung (traversenverletzung). Unfallheilk., 44:417–427, 1937.
Three motorcyclists sustained plateau fractures associated with tearing of the patellar tendon. It was determined that soft tissue injuries into the knee require careful débridement and repair in order to get good results.
295. Ehalt, W.: Sitzungsberichte aus chirurgischen gesellshaften. Zentralbl. Chir., 64:1298–1301, 1937.
This author describes three compression fractures of the articular surface that were incurred in motorcycle accidents.
296. Ehalt, W.: Frische kniegelenks frakturen. Behandlung der frakturen im bereich des kniegelenks. Z. Orthop., 96(Suppl.), 1962.
297. Ehlert, H.: (Fractures of the tibial head.) Med. Monatsschr., 5:169–172, 1951.
298. Eisenbach, J.: Spatergebnisse und erfahrungen bei der konservativen und operativen behandlung frischer frakturen des tibiakopfes. Bruns. Beitr. Klin. Chir., 215:148–154, 1967.
This author followed 150 plateau fractures, 94 of which were treated closed and 56 were treated open. Functional results in both groups were the same. The author thought that more fractures should be operated on.
299. El Sobky, A., and Fisk, G.: Fractures of the upper end of the tibia, treated by early mobilization on Fisk's traction: Assessment of long term results. Ain-Shams Med. J., 32:15–24, 1981.
These authors treated 17 plateau fractures in England using Fisk's traction. After 2 years of follow-up, results were quite good in 13 of 15 patients.
300. Eliason, E. L., and Eberling, W. W.: Non-operative treatment of fractures of the tibia and femur involving the knee joint. Surg. Gynecol. Obstet., 57:658–667, 1933.
These authors treated 40 plateau fractures of the tibial head and femoral condyles by closed reduction and a cast. Of those followed, 80% had satisfactory results.
301. Ellacheff, A.: Z. Org. Chir., 91:237, 1939.
302. Elstrom, J., Pankovich, A. M., Sassoon, H., and Rodriguez, J.: The use of tomography in the assessment of fractures of the tibial plateau. J. Bone Joint Surg., 58A:551–555, 1976.
Tomography proved useful in the accurate diagnosis and classification of 21 plateau fractures.
303. Elyashev, A. I.: Die bruche des scheinbeinkopfes. Ortop. Traumat., 12:78–86, 1938.
304. Ender, J.: Bruche des schienbeinkopfes. Zentralbl. Chir., 78:253–256, 1953.
The author briefly reviewed 130 follow-up plateau fractures after 8 years. The bicondylar fractures did less well. Arthrosis was noted frequently after 7 years of follow-up.
305. Ender, J.: Bruche des schienbeinkopfes (Abstract). Zentralbl. Chir., 78:731, 1953.
306. Ender, J.: (Therapeutic results of fractures of the tibial head.) Arch. Orthop. Unfallchir., 47:287–306, 1955.
307. Ender, J.: B. H. Z. Orthop., 86:207, 1955.
308. Ender, J.: Zur behandlung schwerer scheinbeinkopfbruche. Arch. Orthop. Unfallchir., 57:16–25, 1965.
309. Enneking, W. F., and Horowitz, M.: The intra-articular effects of immobilization on the human knee. J. Bone Joint Surg., 54A:973–985, 1972.
The authors studied the effects of immobilization on 10 knees in legs amputated for various problems during which the knee remained partially or completely limited in movement for a prolonged period. Gross and histologic changes found in these knees were similar to observations made experimentally in animal studies.
310. Erfurth, F.: Uber einen fall von kompressionsfraktur der tibia. Mschr. Unfallheilk., 19:19–21, 1912.
This case report involves a 36 year old with a bicondylar fracture that was treated by therapy and early motion, leaving some permanent impairment of knee function.
311. Esteve, E.: Les Fractures de l'Extrémité Supérieure du Tibia avec Subluxation et Accrochage Condylien. Toulouse, Medical Thesis, 1971.
In this thesis 10 entire type plateau fractures were studied. The author concluded that open reduction and plate fixation should be used.
312. Eucher, L.: Deux cas de fracture des plateaux tibiaux traités par greffe de rotule. Acta Chir. Belg., 60:804–816, 1961.
Two plateau fractures are reported in which the lateral facet of the patella was used as a graft to replace the articular surface with good results 1 to 3 years after fracture.
313. Eulert, J., Apoil, A., and Baux, S.: Les fractures récentes des plateaux tibiaux. Ann. Chir., 25:285–304, 1971.
These authors treated 133 plateau fractures and followed 86 to the end result. The authors stressed the need for anatomic reduction and early motion.
314. Exner, G.: Zu operativen behandlung veralteter kniegelenks frakturen. Z. Orthop., 96 (suppl.), 1962.
315. Exner, O.: Uber bruche der tibia an ihren oberen ende. Berlin, Inaugural Dissertation, 1888.
316. Fagerberg, S.: Tomographic analysis of depressed fractures within the knee joint and of injuries to the cruciate ligaments. Acta Orthop. Scand., 27:219–227, 1958.
The author used tomography, sometimes with added contrast, in 200 cases. This demonstrated the absolute superiority of tomography over other available diagnostic methods.
317. Fairbank, T. J.: Knee joint changes after meniscectomy. J. Bone Joint Surg., 30B:664–670, 1948.
The author compared premeniscectomy and follow-up x-rays,

noting late spurring, squaring, or narrowing of cartilage spaces. The author concluded that the meniscus is important to knee function and that its absence leads to degenerative changes.

318. Fairbank, T. J.: Condylar fractures of the knee-joint. Proc. R. Soc. Med., 48:95–96, 1954.
The author makes a plea for treatment with traction and immediate movement of the knee.
319. Fairbank, T. J.: Fractures des plateaux du tibia. Acta Orthop. Belg., 21:456–468, 1955.
320. Faldini, A.: Indicazioni alla meniscectomia nelle fratture del piatto tibiale. Atti. 1 Congr. Soc. Ort. Traum., 133–139, 1965.
321. Fallus, J.: Sur le traitement des Fractures Unituberositaires du Tibia. Paris, Thesis, 1949.
322. Fama, G., Turra, S., and Bonaga, S.: (Plate osteosynthesis in complex fractures of the tibial plateau.) Arch. Putti Chir. Organi Mov., 39:181–188, 1991.
The authors report their experience with a Kerboull plate and autografts in complex fractures of the plateau. They believe that the plate is important to allow early knee movement, and they emphasize early treatment of soft tissue injuries with meniscal preservation. No data are given.
323. Fargeaud, F.: Des Fractures de l'Extrémité Supérieure du Tibia. Paris, Thesis, 1866.
324. Fassbender, A.: Ein fall von compressionsfraktur des oberen tibiaendes mit subluxation der tibia nach aussen. Kiel, Inaugural Dissertation, 1901.
Riedl's article cites Fassbender as being the first surgeon to operate on a tibial plateau fracture.
325. Felsenreich, F.: (On the therapy of fissure fracture of the tibial head.) Wien Med. Wochenschr., 100:88–89, 1951.
326. Fenoglio, V., and Pisani, P.: Studies on fractures of the tibial plateau. Minerva Ortop., 18:346–351, 1967.
327. Fernandez, D. L.: Anterior approach to the knee with osteotomy of the tibial tubercle for bicondylar tibial fractures. J. Bone Joint Surg., 70A:208–219, 1988.
The author described a midline approach to the knee in which a long tongue of tibial tubercle and an anterior shaft is osteotomized and reflected proximally, with the patellar mechanism allowing simultaneous visualization of both plateaus and secure tubercle replantation.
328. Ferre, R. L., Comolli, E. P., Valenghi, L. A., and Esteban, H. V.: Fracturas de platillo tibial externo. Rev. Ortop. Traumatol., 22:16–18, 1952.
329. Ficat, P., and Duparc, J.: Rapport: les fractures articulaires de l'extrémité supérieure du tibia. J. Chir. (Paris), 81:388–392, 1961.
330. Ficatier: Contribution à l'Étude des Traumatismes du Genou. Paris, Thesis, 1878.
331. Finotti, E.: Tod durch fettembolie der lungen nach compressions-fracturen der unteren extremitaten. Z. Chir., 508–515, 1894.
This case report concerns an 18 year old who fell and sustained a compression fracture of the plateau. Death was due to a fat embolism. An autopsy showed a bicondylar fracture with comminution.
332. Fisk, G.: Lancet, May:654–661, 1944.
333. Flamand, C.: Les fractures du plateau tibial. Le Scalpel, 38:90, 1937.
334. Flamand, C.: Les fractures du plateau tibial. Ann. Soc. Chir. de Belge, 36:235–258, 1937.
335. Flamand, J., and Danis, A.: Réflexions à propos de 60 cas de fractures des plateaux tibiaux. Acta Chir. Belg., 66:673–691, 1967.
The authors treated 60 plateau fractures, half open and half closed. Fifty-three fractures had good results, and seven had fair results. They concluded that open reduction should be used in certain fractures and that a cast should be avoided.
336. Foged, J.: (Surgical therapy of condylar fractures.) Ugeskr. Laeger, 105:1301, 1943.
337. Foged, J.: Osteosynthesis of the tibial condyle. Acta Chir. Scand., 91:143–160, 1944.
This author treated 41 plateau fractures over a period of 6 years. Closed versus open methods are discussed. The author used a bolt to permit early knee motion.
338. Follin: Paris, Thesis, 1967.
This case report concerns a 40 year old run over by a wagon. Banding and massage were used for 5 weeks, resulting in proximal tibial fracture healing.
339. Foltin, E.: Bone loss and forms of tibial condylar fracture. Arch. Orthop. Trauma Surg., 106:341–348, 1987.
The author assessed bone quality in 358 plateau fractures, grading porosis into five categories and fractures into cleavage, split compression, local compression, and entire types. Osteoporotic bone tended to have compression fractures, whereas stronger bone tended to have cleavage fractures.
340. Foltin, E.: Osteoporosis and fracture patterns: A study of split-compression fractures of the lateral tibial condyle. Int. Orthop., 12:229–303, 1988.
This author studied the pattern and size of the split fragment in relation to the degree of osteoporosis present. The size of the fragment decreased with increasing osteoporosis.
341. Fontan: Fracture du tibia dans les condyles; Desarticulation du genou; Guerison. Arch. Med. Nav. (Paris), 33:388–393, 1880.
342. Fontanesi, G.: Lesioni meniscali e recupero funzionale nelle fratture del piatto tibiale. Atti S.E.R.T.O.T., 9:1949, 1964.
343. Forrester, C. R. G.: Fractures of the head of the tibia involving the knee joint: A new method of reducing. Am. J. Surg., 21:230–234, 1933.
The author developed a redresser (compressor) like a C clamp with buttons of wood that he used to compress and impact plateau fractures.
344. Forster, E., Mole, L., and Coblentz, J.: Étude des lesions ligamentomes dans les fractures du plateau tibial. Ned. Tijdschr. Geneeskd., 105:2173–2181, 1961.
These authors studied 90 consecutive plateau fractures in which stress x-rays in valgus and varus were taken under anesthesia. They found 22 collateral ligament injuries in this group and recommended routine stress x-rays.
345. Fowler: External dislocation of the knee. J.A.M.A., 62:2124, 1911.
This case report concerns a severely injured knee with a fracture of the lateral plateau and knee dislocation.
346. Fowbie, C. D., Zimmer, J. W., and Schepsis, A. A.: The role of arthroscopy in the assessment and treatment of tibial plateau fractures. Arthroscopy, 9:584–590, 1993.
These authors compared open and arthroscopic reduction in 23 local and split compression fractures. All 12 arthoscopic reduction and internal fixations were anatomically reduced; only 6 of 11 open reduction and internal fixation (ORIF) were reduced; and one later lost reduction. Complications were greater and more severe in cases of ORIF cases. The authors used guide, grafts, and later continuous passive movement.
347. Franke, C.: Langenbecks Arch. Klin. Chir., 270:473, 1951.
348. Freehafer, A. A., Goldman, S., and Chapman, K.: Stubbins arthroplasty for fractures of the tibial condyle. Clin. Orthop., 90:140–145, 1973.
These authors used a full-thickness ilium as a replacement for a severely damaged articular surface in severe tibial plateau fractures. They report on five cases, four of which had a good result.
349. Fregnani, I., and Pirazzini, R.: La riduzione cruenta con vite nelle fratture del piatto tibiale. Clin. Ortop., 15:473, 1963.
350. Frey, M.: Beitrag zur behandlung der tibiakopffrakturen. Helv. Chir. Acta, 29:317–334, 1962.
This author studied 25 plateau fractures, nine operated and the remainder treated as closed. He concluded that the results were not so good when a cast was used. Results in nondisplaced fractures varied considerably.
351. Freyer, S., and Connell, J.: Three unusual fracture cases from Fresham Hill Military Hospital. Practitioner. 96:259–260, 1916.
This case report concerns a 51 year old with a split compression fracture.
352. Friedebold, G.: Die arthroplastik nach schienbeinkopfbruchen. Hefte Unfallheilk., 126:275–281, 1976.
This author describes specific indications for the use of a prosthetic replacement after a plateau fracture. A Macintosh or a McKeever may be used, but total replacement should be used with arthritic involvement.
353. Friedl, W., Ruf, W., and Krebs, H.: (Study of the correlation between early and late changes in the x-ray and functional status after conservative or surgical treatment of plateau fractures.) Unfallchirurgie, 13:192–206, 1987.
354. Fries, L., and Willenegger, H.: Spatresultate nach gebolzten tibiakopfbruchen. Z. Unfallmed. Berufskr., 51:242–251, 1958.
355. Fripp, A. T.: Fracture into the knee joint. Proc. R. Soc. Med., 28:1043–1047, 1935.

The author discusses the philosophy of treating single condyle fractures and bicondylar fractures by conservative means. A cast is advocated.

356. Fripp, A. T.: (Fractures of the tibia involving the knee joint.) Clin. J., 65:20–23, 1936.
This general discussion of knee fractures concluded that early knee movement was important and that the knee improves for 18 to 24 months.
357. Fryjordet, A. Jr.: Operative treatment of tibial condyle fractures. Acta Chir. Scand., 133:17–24, 1967.
This follow-up study of 101 plateau fractures is treated by open reduction and fixation by a wire loop with early knee movement. The author believes that anatomic reduction, firm fixation, and early motion would give good results.
358. Fuhrmann, F.: Leipzig, Dissertation, 34, 1935.
359. Fyshe, T. G.: Fractures of the condyles of the tibia immobilized by the stader splint. Can. Med. Assoc. J., 67:103–107, 1952.
Eight plateau fractures were reduced openly and then supported in a Stader splint. The results included well-functioning knees "which do not call attention to themselves."
360. Gaenslen, E. S., Schaefer, R. S., and Lambert, K. L.: Arthroscopic assisted reduction and internal fixation of tibial plateau fractures. Orthop. Trans., 16:316, 1993.
The authors treated 21 plateau fractures of all types by arthroscopic assisted reduction and followed eight fractures. The results were excellent in four cases, good in two cases, and poor in two cases. One poor result lost reduction.
361. Gahr, Von R., Thierack, C., and Kramer, G.: Die percutane aufrichtung und fixierung bei geschlossenen scheinbeinkopfbruchen. Zentralbl. Chir., 111:1241–1247, 1986.
One hundred and five closed plateau fractures were treated by percutaneous elevation and fixation. A follow-up of patients for more than 2 years after fractures indicated results that were equal to those found after open reduction and internal fixation. Low risk and trauma with minimum fixation were advocated. The best results were found after early intensive active exercises.
362. Gaiser, M.: Arch. Orthop. Unfallchir., 51:201, 1959.
363. Gallinaro, P., and Crova, M.: Eziopatogenesi e classificazione delle fratture del ginocchio. G.I.O.T., 23–34, 1977.
364. Gandolfi, M., and Prignacchi, V.: Le fratture del condilo tibiale esterno. Atti S.E.R.T.O.T., 1:829, 1956.
365. Garrison, L. E., and Garrison, M.: The use of periosteal sutures in open fixation of fractures of the tibial condyle. J. Bone Joint Surg., 20:498–500, 1938.
This case report concerns a 15 year old with avulsion of the tibial tubercle and an anterior plateau treated by open reduction with anatomic reduction.
366. Gaudinez, R., Mallik, A. R., and Szporn, M.: Hybrid external fixation of comminuted tibial plateau fractures. Clin. Orthop. 328:203–210, 1996.
These authors treated 16 Schatzker type V or VI fractures by small pin external fixation. They also graded soft tissue injuries. External fixation was used for about 15 weeks, and all fractures healed. Varus malunion occurred in three cases, and early traumatic arthritis occurred in 15 of 16 cases. A follow-up was done for 4 to 19 months.
367. Gausewitz, S. H., and Hohl, M.: The significance of early motion in the treatment of tibial plateau fractures. Clin. Orthop., 202:135–138, 1985.
The authors studied 112 plateau fractures and divided them into undisplaced, displaced treated nonoperatively, and displaced treated operatively. Fractures that were treated operatively tended to develop knee stiffness after only 2 weeks. Undisplaced and displaced fractures that were treated nonoperatively recovered motion well.
368. Gebhardt, K.: Der bandschaden des kniegelenkes. 1933.
369. Geel, C., Leutenegger, A., and Ruedi, T.: (Cortico-spongiosa chips in tibial head impression fractures.) Z. Unfallchir. Versicherungsmed. Berufskr., 81:66–67, 1988.
370. Georgescu, N., Iancu, C., and Carafil, R.: (The therapeutic options in tibial plateau fractures.) Rev. Med. Chir. Soc. Med. Nat. Iasi, 94:113–116, 1990.
371. Georgiadis, G. M.: Combined anterior and posterior approaches for complex tibial plateau fractures. J. Bone Joint Surg., 76B:285, 1994.
The author treated four severe closed bicondylar fractures with a posteromedial fragment using both anterior and posterior approaches. The patient was placed on the back, and a midline anterior approach and then a posteromedial approach was made, retracting the medial gastrocnemius. A plate is used after reducing the posterior fragment.
372. Gerard-Marchant, P.: Fractures des plateaux tibiaux. Rev. Orthop., 26:499–546, 1939.
This lengthy article reviews issues of classification, treatment, and postoperative care.
373. Gerard-Marchant, P.: Fractures des plateaux tibiaux. Presse Med., 26 Oct.: 709, 1946.
374. Gherlinzoni, G.: Trattamiento chirurgico delle fratture del piatto tibiale. *In* XI Simposio Instituto Ortopedico Rizzoli. Chir. Organi Mov., 61:638–643, 1972.
375. Girardi, V. C., and Plaghos, A. H.: (Therapy of fractures of the tibial plateau.) Prensa Med. Argent., 39:1659–1661, 1952.
376. Girshin, S. G., Dubrow, V. E., and Komarov, A. A.: (Surgical treatment of fractures of the tibial condyle.) Khirurgiia (Mosk.), 12:30–36, 1991.
These authors studied the choice of treatment in 23 patients. They recommend a computed tomography scan for an accurate diagnosis. Surgery is recommended for all displaced fractures and for undisplaced fractures with associated ligament injuries or associated ipsilateral fractures. The authors prefer to avoid postoperative immobilization for best results.
377. Gjessing, M. H.: Uber die anwendung des elastichen schraubendrucks in der knochenbruchbehandlung. Acta Chir. Scand., 76:472–484, 1935.
This author used a screw device percutaneously to push and hold displaced proximal tibial fractures.
378. Glauser, T., Abdel Baki, G. R., and Noesburger, B.: Langzeitresultate operativ behandelter tibiaplateaufrakturen. Helv. Chir. Acta, 54:477–481, 1987.
This author followed 32 patients who had undergone open reduction and internal fixation using an AO technique from 6 to 15 years. Subjective results were excellent in 31% and satisfactory in 84%. Functional results were excellent in 53% and satisfactory in 91%. Radiologic appearances at follow-up correlated well with the functional results. Severe arthritis was noted in three patients.
379. Goddi, N.: Terapia delle fratture del piatto tibiale, Chir. Organi Mov., 62:235–267, 1975.
380. Godinot, C., and Gignoux, M.: Considerations anatomo-cliniques et therapeutiques: À propos de 39 observationes et fractures des plateaux tibiaux. Lyon Chir., 59:842–852, 1963.
The authors studied 39 plateau fractures, eight of which were operated on, and concluded that early motion was necessary to achieve a good result.
381. Godlee, R. J.: A case of longitudinal fracture of the tibia. Lancet, 1:504–505, 1904.
This case report involves an injury caused by a direct blow to the knee. There was genu valgum and instability with widening of the tibia. After closed reduction and casting, the knee healed with limited movement.
382. Godoli, N., Guerra, A., Lanfranchi, R., et al: Limiti del trattamento incruento nelle fratture del piatto tibiale. Chir. Organi Mov., 62:237–267, 1973.
The authors analysed 258 plateau fractures. They advocated closed treatment for fractures without much displacement or for open fractures. Many unicondylar and bicondylar fractures were opened. A curved plate was used for bicondylar fractures.
383. Gomar-Sancho, F., and Gastaldi Orquin, E.: Repair of osteochondral defects in articular weight-bearing areas in the rabbit's knee: The use of autologous osteochondral and meniscal grafts. Int. Orthop., 11:65–69, 1987.
384. Goodman, S. B.: Iliac autograft for reconstruction of severely depressed fracture of the lateral tibial plateau: A brief note. J. Bone Joint Surg., 68:475, 1986.
385. Goodwyn, T. P.: Fractures of the upper end of tibia involving the articular surfaces. South. Surgeon, 1:209–215, 1932.
The author believed that late disability was due to uneven joint surfaces, which led to arthritis. He thought that stable fractures could be treated with closed reduction but that certain fractures needed open reduction.
386. Gosset, J.: Anatomie pathologique et traitement des fractures du plateau tibial externe. Mem. Acad. Chir., 73:670–679, 1947.
Eight open reductions were done, seven of which were for split compression fractures. The results were good. The author believes that pure split fractures are rare and that mixed fractures are the rule.

387. Gosset, J.: Fractures de l'extrémité supérieure du tibia. Encycl. Med. Chir., 10:1–6, 1955.
388. Gossling, H. R., and Peterson, C. A.: A new surgical approach in the treatment of depressed lateral condylar fractures of the tibia. Clin. Orthop., 140:96–102, 1979.
The authors resected the fibular head to expose the lateral plateau. The meniscus was preserved. Grafts were internally fixed.
389. Gottfries, A., Hagert, C. G., and Sorensen, S. E.: T- and Y-fractures of the tibial condyles: A follow-up study of cases treated with closed reduction and surgical fixation with a wire loop. Injury, 3:56–73, 1971.
The authors treated 14 bicondylar fractures with traction, closed reduction, and fixation by wire loop. Ten fractures were followed for 6 to 12 years after treatment. There were no excellent results, six good results, three fair results, and three poor results. Moderate to severe arthritic changes followed in 50%.
390. Gordan, F.: (Experience with the surgical management of fractures of the tibial head.) Magy Traumatol. Orthop. Kezseh. Plaszlikai Seh., 36:305–311, 1993.
391. Gould, N.: Early mobilization of the joint in intraarticular fractures with special attention to the elbow joint. Surg. Gynecol. Obstet., 115:575–584, 1962.
The author reports treating a plateau fracture by open reduction and internal fixation and a cast for 4 weeks followed by knee movement. He suggests early movement of the knee based on his work on moving elbow joint fractures early.
392. Goyo, G. C., and Zanuso, G.: Use of the Putti screw in fractures of the tibial plateau. Can. Med. Assoc. J., 68:160–162, 1953.
393. Graham, B., and Loomer, R. L.: Anterior compartment syndrome in a patient with fracture of the tibial plateau treated by continuous passive motion and anticoagulants (Case report). Clin. Orthop., 195:197–199, 1985.
This case report involves a 30-year-old woman with a bicondylar fracture treated by open reduction and internal fixation, taking down the tibial tubercle. She developed phlebitis and was given anticoagulants. The patient then bled, causing compartment syndrome. An immediate anterior fasciotomy was done.
394. Grauer, D., Kabo, J., Dorey, F., and Meals, R.: The effects of intermittent passive exercise on joint stiffness following periarticular fractures in rabbits. Clin. Orthop., 220:259–265, 1987.
These authors did experimental joint movement and noted that ankle joints with periarticular fractures were more swollen and stiffer, suggesting that passive motion caused additional trauma to healing joint tissues.
395. Greco, A.: (Meniscal lesions in fractures of the tibial plateau.) A. Reforma Med., 79:845–848, 1965.
396. Greinemann, H.: Scheinbeinkopfbruche aus scheinbarer gelegenheitsursache. Arch. Orthop. Unfallchir., 68:79–87, 1970.
This biomechanical study indicated that a 70-kg male places a 541-kg load on the condyles of the flexed knee. The author reported seven compression plateau fractures caused by pressure in flexion.
397. Groh, H., and Weinmann, E. L.: Uber die am kniegelenk auftretenden krafte. Z. Orthop., 96:527–530, 1962.
The authors discuss the forces and angles that occur on a knee that is very flexed.
398. Grosglik, F.: Étude des traitements des Fractures des Plateaux Tibiaux. Toulouse, Thesis, 1947.
399. Gross, A., McKee, N., Pritzker, K., and Langer, F.: Reconstruction of skeletal deficits at the knee: A comprehensive osteochondral transplant program. Clin. Orthop., 174:96–106, 1983.
The authors performed osteochondral grafts in tibial defects. Some grafts for old plateau fractures had very encouraging results.
400. Gross, G., and Sencert: Fracture unicondylienne du plateau du tibia. Rev. Med. de l'Est, Nancy, 37:310–313, 1905.
401. Groth: Ueber unicondylare frakturen des kniegelenks usw. Leipzig, Inaugural Dissertation, 1902.
Three case reports are made of plateau fractures treated with plaster casts.
402. Grugni, C.: Sul trattamento delle fratture del plateau tibiale. Rass. Internaz. Clin. Ter., 34:177–189, 1954.
403. Gualtieri, G., Hendriks, M., Gualtieri, I., and Prosperi, P.: (Fracture of the tibial plateau: Results of surgical treatment.) Chir. Organi Mov., 74:13–20, 1989.
The authors reviewed 93 plateau fractures for 7 to 13 years after surgical treatment. The fractures that had poor results showed instability or arthritis.
404. Guanche, C. A., and Markham, A. W.: Arthroscopic management of tibial plateau fractures. Arthroscopy, 9:467–471, 1993.
The authors treated five plateau fractures of Schatzker types I, II, and III by arthroscopic reduction and fixation using guide and two screws with a postoperative brace. The technique is described in detail, and the results are good.
405. Guarda, E.: Sulle fratture del piatto tibiale. Clin. Ortop., 17:193, 1965.
406. Gui, L.: Le fratture dell'estremo superiore della tibia. Chir. Organi Mov., 27:133–161, 1942.
407. Gui, L.: Indicaziono e resultati della cura chirurgica delle fratture monocondelade e del femora e del piatto tibiale. Chir. Organi Mov., 31:308–331, 1947.
408. Gui, L.: Le fratture dell'estremo superiore della tibia. Arch. Putti, 2:64, 1952.
409. Guilleminet, M., Faysse, R., Blanchet, A., and Lapras, A.: À propos du traitement chirurgical des fractures des plateaux tibiaux. Lyon Chir., 53:431–437, 1957.
410. Guillen Giner, M.: Consideraciones sobre algunos aspectos en las fracturas de la tuberosidad externa de la tibia. Acta Ortop. Traum. Iber., 1:546–551, 1953.
411. Gumbel, T.: Isolierter bruch des condylus internus tibiae. Dtsch. Z. Chir., 107:617–619, 1910.
This case report involves a 22 year old with a medial condylar fracture and a lateral ligament avulsion from the femur.
412. Gumbel, T.: Die bruche des schienbeinkopfes. Dtsch. Z. Chir., 103:107–136, 1910.
This author provides a detailed analysis of 39 plateau fractures.
413. Gurau: Ein fall von compressionsfractur des condylus externus tibiae. Dtsch. Z. Chir., 41:181–188, 1895.
Two case reports of plateau fractures are cited. One patient with a plateau fracture was aspirated, placed in traction for 4 weeks, and then in a cast. The other patient died of abdominal injuries. The post mortem findings were described.
414. Gylling, U., and Lindholm, R.: (Fractures of the tibial condyle.) Ann. Chir. Gynecol. Fenn., 42:229–235, 1953.
Forty-seven plateau fractures were treated, 37 of which were closed and 10 were operated. The results were reported.
415. Hadengue: Fracture de l'extrémité supérieure du tibia. Bull. Mem. Soc. Radiol. Paris, 1920.
416. Hadjistamoff, B.: Ein operationsverfahren zur behandlung schwerer schienbeinkopfbruche. Z. Orthop., 95:45–53, 1962.
The author describes a T incision that is centered at the joint line and takes up the tibial tubercle to expose both condyles. Eight patients were treated with fairly good results.
417. Haggart, G., and Clemmons, H. M.: The surgical treatment of fractures of the lateral tibial condyle. Surg. Clin. North Am., 29:893–903, 1949.
The authors advocate surgery mainly for fractures displaced more than ½ inch but the authors do use it sometimes for ¼ inch displacement. Comminuted fractures did not lend themselves to open reduction and internal fixation.
418. Haldeman, K. O.: The healing of joint fractures. J. Bone Joint Surg., 20:912–922, 1938.
The author studied joint defects in rabbits and human cartilage injuries and noted that there was a lack of repair unless the injury penetrated into the subchondral bone.
419. Hamant, A., and Durand, E.: Les fractures articulaires des tuberosités tibiales. Rev. Med. de Nancy, 64:442–447, 1936.
420. Hambury, H. J., and Davis, D. M.: Symposium on fractures of the head of the tibia (Abstract). J. Bone Joint Surg., 45B:223, 1963.
In a symposium on plateau fracture treatment, the author presented 55 fractures that were treated in traction with early movement of the knee.
421. Hamel, M.: Contribution à l'Étude des fractures de l'Extrémité Superieure du Tibia. Paris, Thesis, 1884.
422. Han-Ting, C.: Fracture of the tibial plateau. J. Formos. Med. Assoc., 60:138–147, 1961.
423. Handelberg, F., DeRoeck, P., Vandkerckhove, P., et al: Arthroscopic assessment and treatment of tibial plateau fractures: Results of a multicentre study. J. Bone Joint Surg., 75B(Suppl. II):202, 1993.
The authors report arthroscopy in 67 plateau fractures in whom 54 arthroscopically controlled reductions were carried out. Of the fractures, 48 had screw fixation and 19 had bone grafts. Two

fractures had a plate, and three had an external fixator. A continuous passive motion machine was started immediately. Forty-nine percent of the results were excellent, and 24% were good with 1 year follow-up.

424. Harper, M. C., Henstorf, J. E., Vessely, M. B., et al: Closed reduction and percutaneous stabilization of tibial plateau fractures. Orthopedics, 18:623–626, 1995.
Twenty-eight plateau fractures were managed by closed reduction and percutaneous fixation with pins or screws. Six bicondylar fractures were treated by fixation wires and an external fixator. This method yields good results in fractures without central depression and with large fragments.
425. Hartenson, L., and Lagerquist, U.: Tomographic study of posterior fractures of the tibial plateau. Acta Orthop. Scand., 31:240, 1961.
426. Hartmann, G.: (Surgical therapy of recent and old fractures of the tibial head following faulty reposition.) Arch. Orthop. Unfallchir., 44:359–364, 1951.
427. Hasler, C.: (Proximal intra-articular tibial fractures in skiers.) Z. Unfallchir. Versicherungsmed., 86:169–177, 1993.
The author studied 56 intra-articular tibial fractures in skiers and noted that they all had valgus compression forces. The author used four x-ray views and computed tomography scans to make the diagnosis. A cast-brace was used after rigid internal fixation.
428. Heerfordt, J., and Mouritzen, V.: Follow-up on 50 cases with fractures of the lateral tibial condyle treated predominantly by operation (Abstract). Acta Orthop. Scand., 42:430–431, 1971.
The authors noted, after treating 122 plateau fractures by open reduction, that fractures depressed more than 10 mm did well generally. Fractures with a depression of 3 to 10 mm did better with closed treatment.
429. Hell, K., and Muller, C.: Spaetkontrollen nach operativ behandelten tibiakopffrakturen. Hefte Unfallheilk., 120:132–136, 1975.
430. Hell, K., Muller, C., and Ruedi, T.: Nachkontrolle von 50 operativ behandelten tibiakopffrakturen. Helv. Chir. Acta, 42:27–29, 1975.
The authors used an AO system to treat 50 plateau fractures with 70% good to excellent results. They found that plates were especially useful.
431. Henkemeyer, H., Albrecht, K., and Passler, H.: Die aussagekraft des rontgenbildes bei der operatikven versorgung von tibiakopffrakturen im hinblick auf das entstehen posttraumatischer gonarthrosen. Hefte Unfallheilk., 110:192–194, 1972.
X-rays were noted to be unreliable in portraying the true articular displacements after a plateau fracture. Tomography was superior to the x-ray and was recommended for routine use.
432. Henkert, K., Brewka, N., and Winter, H.: Tibiakopffrakturen und ihre behandlung. Beitr. Orthop., 17:273–290, 1970.
433. Herbert, J. J., Andre, P., and Fenies, M. T.: À propos des fractures de l'extrémité supérieure du tibia. Ann. Chir., 13:1387–1398, 1959.
434. Herbert, J. J., Paillot, J., and Fenies, M. T.: A propos des fractures de l'extrémité supérieure du tibia. Mem. Acad. Chir., 85:488–493, 1959.
435. Herold, Z.: Fractures of the tibial plateau (Abstract). J. Bone Joint Surg., 45B:805, 1963.
This abstract reports on 25 plateau fractures that were treated by bandaging and non–weight-bearing movement with 2- to 8-year follow-up. All patients were stable: two patients had pain, and 23 of 25 patients had normal motion and alignment.
436. Herzog, E. C.: Fractures of the tibial plateau. Am. J. Osteopath. Assoc. 57:314–317, 1958.
437. Hess, T., Rupp, S., Hopf, T., et al: Lateral tibial avulsion fractures and disruptions of the anterior cruciate ligament. Clin. Orthop., 303:193–197, 1994.
The authors noted that the Segond fracture is an avulsion of the meniscotibial ligament that occurs with flexion and internal tibial rotation after rupture of the anterior cruciate ligament. Of 151 anterior cruciate ligament ruptures, 9% had Segond fractures. Of 133 other knee ligament injuries, only one possible Segond fracture occurred.
438. Heucher, L.: Deux cas de fractures du plateau tibial traités par greffe de rotule. Acta Chir. Belgica, 60:804–816, 1961.
These case reports involve two severe plateau fractures in which the patella was substituted for the articular surface, thus salvaging satisfactory results.
439. Heydenreich, A.: Des Fractures de l'Extrémité Supérieure de Tibia. Paris, Thesis, 1877.
The author studied specimens of many different proximal tibial fractures and proposed a classification: upper epiphyseal fracture, tubercle fracture, medial or lateral condyle fracture, and comminuted fracture.
440. Hierholzer, G.: Arthrodese nach schienbeinkopfbruchen. Hefte Unfallheilk., 126:283–289, 1975.
The author discusses arthrodesis as a salvage method for failed treatment in plateau fractures.
441. Hierholzer, G., Voorhoeve, A., Kleining, R., and Kehr, H.: Reintervention nach scheinbeinkopfbruchen. Chirurg., 46:352–358, 1975.
The authors discuss indications for and techniques of salvaging malaligned and unstable knees after a plateau fracture. Osteotomies and ligament reconstructions are explored and illustrated.
442. Hinz: Zentralbl. Chir., 52:82, 1925.
443. Hinz: (Discussion.) Zentralbl. Chir., 65:614, 1938.
This discussion suggests that more internal fixation should be used in bicondylar fractures, but the author mainly uses closed reduction and traction.
444. Hirsch, G., and Sullivan, L.: Experimental knee joint fractures. Acta Orthop. Scand., 36:391–399, 1965.
The authors applied mechanical forces to 32 cadaver knees and noted no combined bone and ligament injuries. Compression fractures occurred with the knee in flexion and split fractures in extension. The depression occurred before the split.
445. Hoffmann, H. G.: Tibiakopffrakturen. Zentralbl. Chir., 68:1342–1354, 1941.
446. Hoffmann, R.: Z. Org. Ges. Chir., 47:669, 1929.
447. Hoffmann, R.: Le traitement conservateur des fractures du plateau tibial. Rev. d'Orthopédie, 16:313–332, 1929.
448. Hohl, M.: Tibial condylar fractures. J. Bone Joint Surg., 49A:1455–1467, 1967.
The author provides a general discussion of all aspects of diagnosis, associated ligament and bony injuries, treatment methods, complications, results, and sequelae.
449. Hohl, M.: A point system for grading results after knee fracture or surgery. Unpublished, 1970.
A 100-point rating system was developed for grading results after knee fractures or surgery. Forty-five points were allowed for function, 25 points for anatomic restoration, and 30 points for subjective factors.
450. Hohl, M.: Tibial condylar fractures: Long term follow-up. Tex. Med., 70:46–56, 1974.
The author followed 300 plateau fractures for 2 years or more. Seventy-one percent were acceptable. Less than 55% of patients achieved 120 degrees of movement, whereas 15% had moderate or severe deformity and 14% had moderate or severe instability. A point rating system (developed by Hohl) showed a mean of 75 points. Sequelae were discussed.
451. Hohl, M.: Treatment methods in tibial condylar fractures. South. Med. J., 68:985–991, 1975.
This general discussion is about the advantages and disadvantages of the various methods of treatment for tibial plateau fractures. The author studied 915 plateau fractures in relation to the methods of treatment used.
452. Hohl, M.: Management of tibial condylar fractures. *In* AAOS Symposium on Reconstructive Surgery of the Knee. St. Louis, C.V. Mosby, 1978.
This general discussion covers all aspects of the diagnosis, classification, and treatment of plateau fractures.
453. Hohl, M.: Fractures about the knee. *In* Rockwood, C., and Green, D., (Eds.): Fractures. Philadelphia, J.B. Lippincott, 1984.
This chapter deals with the general topics of plateau fractures, diagnosis, and treatment.
454. Hohl, M.: Complications of treatment of fractures and dislocations of the knee. *In* Epps, C., (Ed.): Complications in Orthopaedic Surgery. Philadelphia, J.B. Lippincott, 1994.
This chapter deals with the complications encountered in treating plateau fractures as well as the late sequelae. Suggestions are made to avoid complications and to anticipate and prevent sequelae.
455. Hohl, M.: Surgical exposures and fractures about the knee. *In* Lauren, C. A., Riley, L. H., and Roy-Camille, R. (Eds.): Atlas of Orthopaedic Surgery. Paris, Masson, 1992.
These chapters illustrate in detail surgical exposures and techniques for treating tibial plateau fractures surgically.

456. Hohl, M.: Arthroscopic assisted reduction of tibial plateau fractures (Abstract). Orthopedic proceedings. J. Bone Joint Surg., 76B:108, 1994.
Thirty-one patients with plateau fractures were treated with arthroscopic-assisted reduction. Local compression fractures were most easily reduced. Split compression fractures and total depression fractures also derived benefit from arthroscopic reduction, supplemented by bone grafts or screw fixation. There were six minor complications, including the loss of 1 to 2 mm of reduction in three patients. The mean point rating after 1 year of follow-up was 96.
457. Hohl, M., and Hopp, E.: Ligament injuries in tibial condylar fractures (Abstract). J. Bone Joint Surg., 58A:279, 1976.
From a series of 917 plateau fractures, 164 patients were identified with injuries to collateral or cruciate ligaments. The incidence of ligament injury is higher than usually appreciated. Diagnosis and repair are suggested.
458. Hohl, M., Johnson, E. E., and Wiss, D.: Fractures of the knee. *In* Rockwood, C. R., Green, D. P., and Bucholz, R. W. (Eds.): Fractures. Philadelphia, J.B. Lippincott, 1991.
This chapter covers the general topic of tibial plateau fractures, classification, diagnosis, treatment, and results.
459. Hohl, M., and Luck, J. V.: Fractures of the tibial condyles. A clinical and experimental study. J. Bone Joint Surg., 38A:1001–1018, 1956.
This is a review of 726 plateau fractures with classification and follow-up analysis of 227 patients. Experimental joint defects in the knees of primates were noted to heal with adhesions when the knee was immobilized and with fibrocartilage when the monkey was allowed to walk in its cage.
460. Hohl, M., and Moore, T.: Articular fractures of the proximal tibia. *In* Evarts, C. M. (Ed.): Surgery of the Musculoskeletal System. New York, Churchill Livingstone, 1990.
This chapter covers all aspects of plateau fractures and includes a classification of fracture-dislocation of the knee.
461. Holle, F.: (A new nail for bone fractures.) Chirurg., 24:134–137, 1953.
462. Holle, F., and Hart, W.: Konservative oder operative behandlung der tibiakopfbruche. Mschr. Unfallheilk., 61:65–86, 1958.
The authors studied 65 plateau fractures and concluded that comminuted fractures do best with closed treatment. Compression fractures were not thought to do well with open treatment, but split compression fractures can do well with either treatment.
463. Holz, U.: Formen und einteilung der tibikopffrakturen. Chirurg., 46:341–344, 1975.
The author discusses proximal tibial fractures and their various classifications by several authors.
464. Holz, U.: Ursachen, formen, und begleitverletzungen der tibiakopffraktur. Hefte Unfallheilk., 120:99–113, 1975.
465. Holz, U., Welte, G., Marklin, H. M., and Weller, S.: Ergebnisse nach operativer versorgung von tibiakopffrakturen. Unfallheilkunde, 88:519–527, 1985.
The authors followed 48 of 146 plateau fractures that were mostly treated by the AO type of open reduction for 4 to 7 years. Despite operative complications, the authors concluded that open reduction and internal fixation was the best treatment.
466. Holzach, P., and Matter, P.: Arthroscopie und osteosynthese von tibiaplateaufrakturen. Arthroskopie, 1:74–76, 1988.
Arthroscopy is advocated to treat B02.2/B3.1 AO type plateau fractures. The advantages and disadvantages are mentioned without discussing results or cases in detail. This article is based on eight patients who were operated on for plateau fractures.
467. Holzach, P., and Matter, P.: (Arthroscopically guided osteosynthesis of lateral tibial plateau fractures.) Z. Unfallchir. Versicherungsmed., 1(Suppl.):157–164, 1993.
This prospective study involves 16 lateral plateau fractures caused by skiing accidents. These fractures were treated by arthroscopic-assisted reduction and by autografts with lag screws as necessary. Fifteen patients were followed 1 to 6.5 years, and all except two patients were at a preinjury activity level.
468. Holzach, P., Matter, P., and Minter, J.: Arthroscopically assisted treatment of lateral tibial plateau fractures in skiers: Use of cannulated reduction system. J. Orthop. Trauma, 8:273–281, 1994.
This prospective study involves 16 lateral plateau fractures in skiers (out of 87). Indications for surgery were B2.2 or B3.1 fractures with 2 mm or more displacement. The authors used arthroscopy and placed a threaded pin from the distal window into the depressed fragment and pushed it upward with a cannulated impactor. Twelve factors were anatomically reduced at follow-up, the other three were 1 to 2 mm step-offs. The OAK scores were 86 to 100.
469. Honkonen, S. E.: Indications for surgical treatment of tibial condyle fractures. Clin. Orthop., 302:199–295, 1994.
The author studied 131 plateau fractures for prognostic factors. If the fracture healed with a medial tilt, the result deteriorated; however, a lateral tilt of 5 degrees was well tolerated. A step-off of 3 mm and widening up to 5 mm had no adverse effects. Unsatisfactory results were found in 70% of unstable knees. The author concluded that accurate reduction and restoration of stability was important for a good result.
470. Honkonen, S. E.: Degenerative arthritis after tibial plateau fractures. J. Orthop. Trauma, 9:273–277, 1995.
Traumatic arthritis was found using Albeck's criteria and was found in 44% of 131 patients followed 3 to 13 years (an average of 7.6 years). Patients who had a meniscectomy had 74% arthritis. Knee angulation, varus, or excessive valgus increased the incidence of arthritis.
471. Honkonen, S. E., and Jarvinen, M. J.: Classification of fractures of the tibial condyles. J. Bone Joint Surg., 74B:840–847, 1992.
The authors analysed 131 plateau fractures using a classification by Schatzker. The follow-up averaged 7.6 years. The authors looked carefully at bicondylar fractures and noted that those medially tilted went into varus and laterally tilted went into valgus. The poorest results were of medially tilted bicondylar fractures. The authors concluded that bicondylar fractures should be subclassified as neutral, medial, and laterally tilted.
472. Hulten, O.: Uber die indirekten bruche des tibiakopfes nebst betragen zur rontgenologie des kniegelenks. Acta Chir. Scand., 66(Suppl. 15):1–167, 1929.
This thesis discusses types of fractures, mechanisms, ligament injury, and experimental fracture production. The author could not produce a combined fracture and ligament injury in the same specimen.
473. Hulten, O.: Ueber die behandlung der schalenformigen eindruckungen der gelenkflachen des tibiakopfes. Zentralbl. Chir., 59:344–349, 1932.
Two cases of local compression fracture were treated operatively by elevation and bone graft with good results. One was a medial plateau.
474. Hulten, O.: Chirurg., 10:525, 1938.
475. Hulten, O.: Uber die operative behandlung der schalenformigen tibiakondylenbruche. Zentralbl. Chir., 66:401–410, 1939.
The article includes case reports and a discussion of issues. The author favors wires for fracture fixation and suggests traction followed by cast in comminuted fractures and late open reduction and fixation if necessary.
476. Humbert, R.: Contribution à l'Étude des Fractures du Plateau Tibial par l'Extension au Fil de Kirschner. Lausanne, Thesis, 1939.
The author advocates use of skeletal traction and early knee movement in order to obtain satisfactory results. The author reviews controversies regarding treatment.
477. Humbert, R.: Contribution à l'étude du traitement des fractures du plateau tibial par l'extension au fil de Kirschner. Rev. Med. Suisse Rom., 59:641–666, 1939.
The author reviewed state-of-the-art treatment of plateau fractures as of 1939 and reported five fractures treated by Kirschner wire traction and early motion with satisfactory results.
478. Hvid, I., Christensen, P., Sondergaard, J., et al: Compressive strength of tibial cancellous bone. Acta Orthop. Scand., 54:819–825, 1983.
The authors compressed 12 cadaver knees in an Instron machine and measured the strength of cancellous bone in various areas. The medial plateau was stronger than the lateral plateau. The strongest areas were the anteromedial and posterolateral plateaus.
479. Hvid, I., and Hansen, S.: Trabecular bone strength patterns at the proximal tibial epiphysis. J. Orthop. Res., 3:464–472, 1985.
The authors tested compression strength of plateau trabecular bone of human specimens. The surface was tested with an indentor with the finding that the medial condyle was stronger than the lateral condyle, which was weakest near the margin.
480. Ibsen, J., and Mossing, N.: Conservative treatment of tibial condylar fractures. Acta Orthop. Scand., 42:431–432, 1971.

The authors used conservative treatment primarily and noted good results.

481. Ieanbreau: Frakture du condyle interne du tibia. Arch. d'Électricité Med. Experim. Clinique, October 1900.
482. Ilfeld, F. W., and Hohl, M.: Closed reduction treatment of tibial plateau fractures (Abstract). J. Bone Joint Surg., 42A:534–535, 1959.
The authors treated 20 plateau fractures by traction-reduction manipulation followed by traction. The method is especially applicable when fragments are large, and the method works well in bicondylar and comminuted fractures. The results showed that functional recovery was quite good and that anatomic recovery was satisfactory.
483. Imamaliev, A.: (Periarticular and intra-articular fractures of the knee joint in middle-aged and aged patients.) Ortop. Travmatol. Protez., 121:37–43, 1984.
484. Inclan, A.: El tratamiento quirurgico de las fracturas graves de las tuberosidades de la tibia. Cir. Ortop. Tramatol., 5:32–40, 1937.
485. Inclan, A.: El tratamiento quirurgico de las fracturas graves de la tuberositades de la tibia. J. Chir., 50:734, 1937.
486. Indelicato, P. A.: Nonoperative management of complete tears of the medial collateral ligament. Orthop. Rev., 18:947–952, 1989.
The author reports experience with nonoperative treatment of complete medial collateral ligament injuries by bracing in 30 degrees of flexion for 2 weeks, then 30 to 90 degrees of flexion for 4 weeks, followed by rehabilitation.
487. Insall, J.: A midline approach to the knee. J. Bone Joint Surg., 53A:1584–1586, 1971.
The author used a lateral parapatellar skin incision with splitting of the quadriceps tendon toward the medial side. The fat pad is divided, and the patella is dislocated laterally for exposure.
488. Insall, J. N., Dorr, L. D., Scott, R. D., and Scott, W. N.: Rationale of the knee society clinical rating system. Clin. Orthop., 248:13–14, 1989.
This rating system allows 50 points for pain, 25 points for range of knee motion, and 25 points for stability. From this figure are deductions for walking problems, difficulty climbing stairs, and use of a cane, crutch or brace.
489. Irvine, G. B., Dias, J. J., and Finlay, D. B.: Segond fractures of the lateral tibial plateau: Brief report. J. Bone Joint Surg., 69B:613–614, 1987.
The authors noted nine typical Segond fractures during 1985. Computed tomography scans demonstrated the avulsion that occurred half-way between Gerdy's tubercle and the fibular head, where an oblique band of the lateral collateral ligament attaches.
490. Ishiguro, T., Imai, N., Tomatsu, T., et al: A new method of closed reduction using the spring action of Kirschner wires for fractures of the tibial plateau—A preliminary report. Nippon Seikeigeka Gakkai Zasshi, 60:227–236, 1986.
The authors treated seven split compression fractures by percutaneous insertion of about six Kirschner wires into the split fragment from the medial side. The K wires were bent into a short leg cast, and motion was started with good results.
491. Itokazu, M.: (Use of arthroscopy in the treatment of tibial plateau fractures.) Jpn. J. Seikeigeka, 39:1415–1422, 1988.
The author noted 50% meniscal injury and 10 to 30% ligament injuries in plateau fractures. The arthroscope adds greatly to the diagnosis of soft tissue injuries and also allows treatment by percutaneous methods. Several case reports are cited. The author used external fixation in some fractures.
492. Itokazu, M., and Matsunaga, T.: Arthroscopic restoration of depressed tibial plateau fractures using bone and hydroxyapatite grafts. Arthroscopy, 9:103–108, 1993.
The authors treated 13 depressed plateau fractures by arthroscopic-assisted reduction. Three patients had autografts, and 10 patients had hydroxyapatite. After a follow-up at 18 months, there seemed to be no difference between the two graft materials. After reduction, the hydroxyapatite graft was shaped into a block and placed under the surface. Only one patient had a reduction that left more than a 3-mm depression. On biopsy, the hydroxyapatite grafts were incorporated.
493. Jackson, D. W.: The use of autologous fibula for a prop graft in depressed lateral tibial plateau fractures. Clin. Orthop., 87:110–115, 1972.
The author reports on two plateau fractures that were treated operatively using a segment of distal fibula to hold up the elevated articular surface.
494. Jacobs, J. E.: Patellar graft for severely depressed comminuted fractures of the lateral tibial condyle (Follow-up note), J. Bone Joint Surg., 47A:842–847, 1965.
The authors have done five more patellar graft articular replacements. One knee was shown in large microscopic section showing that articular cartilage did survive the transplant. Some long-term follow-ups were shown.
495. Jacobs, J. E., and Wilson, W. J.: Patellar graft for severely depressed comminuted fractures of the lateral tibial condyle. J. Bone Joint Surg., 34A:436–442, 1952.
496. Jaeger, M., Gasteiger, W., and Weseloh, G.: Die tibiakopffraktur des alten menschen. Bruchform, therapie und nachuntersuchungsergebnisse. Mschr. Unfallheilk., 73:228–236, 1970.
The author notes that plateau fractures are the eighth most frequent fracture in patients older than 60 years of age. He studied 45 plateau fractures in patients older than 60 years of age and noted that knee deformity was a frequent sequel.
497. Jakobsen, A.: Operative treatment of lateral tibial condyle fractures—A follow-up study of 68 cases. Acta Orthop. Scand., 23:35–50, 1953.
The author reports 69 operative reductions of lateral plateau fractures using screws or wire loops. Fifty-one were reported to have satisfactory results. Open reduction was advised.
498. Jalland, W. H.: Transverse fracture of the upper end of the tibia by indirect violence. B.M.J., 1:71, 1876.
This case report involves a patient who had fallen 6 to 8 feet and sustained a proximal tibial articular fracture.
499. Jancke: (Abstract). Zentralbl. Chir., 56:2857, 1929.
This case report involves a plateau fracture, and the result is good.
500. Janek: Les fractures intra-articulaires du genou. Slovansky Shortnikk Orthop., 13:5, 1938.
501. Jarge, and Landivar: Enfoncement unituberositaire du tibia, operation et guerison. Bull. Trav. Soc. Shir. de Buenos Ayres, 21:511, 1937.
502. Jeanne: Fracture du condyle interne du tibia droit. Normandie Med., 20:15–16, 1905.
This case report involves a medial total depression fracture that was tilted posteriorly.
503. Jeanne: Fracture du condyle externe du tibia; intervention, visage. Normandie Med., 31:242, 1919.
504. Jennings, J. E.: Arthroscopic management of tibial plateau fractures. J. Arthroscopy, 1:160–168, 1985.
Twenty-one plateau fractures were treated using arthroscopic methods with percutaneous fixation and followed for 1 to 5 years. The author noted that postoperative recovery was rapid and morbidity was minimized. He used screws, pins, and at times an external fixator frame. The results were good for all patients.
505. Jensen, D. B., Rude, C., Duus, B., and Bjerg-Nielson, A.: Tibial plateau fractures: A comparison of conservative and surgical treatment. J Bone Joint Surg., 72B:49–52, 1990.
The authors studied 61 patients who were treated by traction and movement and 48 who were treated by open reduction and internal fixation. The functional results were similar, and it was believed that traction is a valid alternative to open reduction. The average follow-up time was 6 years. Arthritis was more frequent after open reduction. Arthritis was observed more in patients who underwent meniscectomy.
506. Jensen, D. B., Bjerg-Nielsen, A., and Laursen, N.: (Tibial condylar fractures: Results of non-surgical treatment.) Uyeskr. Laeger., 15:924–926, 1988.
507. Jensen, D. B., Bjerg-Nielsen, A., and Laursen, N.: Conventional radiographic examination in the evaluation of sequelae after tibial plateau fractures. Skeletal Radiol., 17:330–332, 1988.
The authors followed 72 conservatively treated plateau fractures for 5¾ years. The residual depression was the same in 47 of 55 cases. Arthritis was present in 10 of 72 cases. The results were acceptable in 84% of lateral fractures and 67% of medial fractures. The authors concluded that persistent articular depression has no clinical significance.
508. Jensen, D. B., Johansen, T. P., Bjerg-Nielsen, A., and Hendrikson, O.: Magnetic resonance imaging in the evaluation of sequelae after tibial plateau fractures. Skeletal Radiol., 19:127–129, 1990.
The author did magnetic resonance imaging (MRI) studies on patients a mean time of 8 years after these patients sustained depressed plateau fractures. The minimum depression was 10

mm, and the treatment was traction and early motion. The MRI findings showed that the defects filled with tissue and often cartilage or fibrous or synovial tissue appeared. These patients had a residual valgus deformity.

509. Jensenius, H., Jensen, I., and Nielsen, F. K.: Tibiakondylfrakturer. Nord. Med., 66:1573–1579, 1961.
These authors studied 184 plateau fractures and followed 165 patients for 2 to 9 years. Results were acceptable in 71% of cases. Fifty-three patients were operated on and 89 patients were treated nonoperatively.
510. Johanssen, S.: Ein operierter fall von spaltbruch den schienbeinkopfes. Acta Chir. Scand., 67:476–481, 1930.
This case report involves a split compression fracture that would not reduce with manipulation. The knee was opened, and the meniscus was found to be imbedded in the fracture cleft, thus preventing reduction. The meniscus was removed for reduction.
511. Johnson, L.: Lateral capsular ligament complex: Anatomical and surgical considerations. Am. J. Sports Med., 7:156–160, 1979.
The author reports seven Segond-type capsular avulsions. The author did anatomic dissections and concluded that the lateral capsular ligament is important for knee stability.
512. Jonasch, E.: Mschr. Unfallheilkunde, 59:1, 1958.
513. Jonasch, E.: Die randabbruche von schienbeinkopf. Z. Orthop., 97:321–326, 1963.
The author discusses marginal avulsion fractures about the knee and suggests that large avulsions indicate a collateral ligament injury whereas smaller ones can be ignored.
514. Jonasch, E.: Einfache methode zur behandlung der unikondylaren scienbainkopfbruche. Arch. Orthop. Unfallchir., 57:5–7, 1965.
The author describes the use of a window in the tibial flare through which an impactor is used to elevate depressed articular fragments.
515. Jones, R., and Smith, S. A.: On rupture of the crucial ligaments of the knee and on fractures of the spine of the tibia. Br. J. Surg., 1:70–89, 1913.
Two plateau fractures with associated tibial spine fractures are described. The authors suggested an operative attachment of cruciates because ligament laxity caused the disability.
516. Jopson, J.: Ann. Surg., 42:617, 1905.
This case report involves a split fracture that was treated for 6 weeks in plaster.
517. Joulie: Contribution à l'Étude des Fractures Unituberositaires Externes de l'Extrémité Supérieure du Tibia. Toulouse, Thesis, 1960.
518. Jozsa, L., Jarvinen, M., and Kannus, P.: Fine structural changes in the articular cartilage of the rat's knee following short-term immobilization in various positions: A scanning electron microscopical study. Int. Orthop., 11:129–133, 1987.
The authors immobilized the knees of 36 rats in either flexion or extension. Some were sacrificed at 1, 2, or 3 weeks, and the knees were studied. After 1 week there was cartilage disruption, and after 2 weeks there was disintegration at points of contact. At 3 weeks in extension there was localized disruption, and in flexion there was more generalized disruption.
519. Junghanns, H.: Die bruche des knienahen unterschenkelabschnittes (schienbeinkopfbruche). Langenbecks Arch. Klin. Chir., 276:242–253, 1953.
The author discusses the mechanism of injury, classification, and associated injuries and analyses the results. He suggests retention of the meniscus.
520. Junghanns, H.: Zentralbl. Chir., 78:730, 1953.
521. Juvara, E.: Procede d'osteosynthese par boulon amovible. Presse Med., 28:605, 1920.
522. Kaiser, J.: Unfallmedizinische studie uber die fraktur des tibiakopfes. Rev. Suisse des Accidents de Travail, 21:193, 1927.
523. Kalb, R. L., and Gosman, J.: Primary prosthetic replacement for depressed tibial plateau fractures. Orthop. Rev., 11:77–87, 1982.
The authors did primary Sbarbaro plateau replacements for six comminuted depressed fractures. Acceptable results were noted in four patients.
524. Kaplan, E.: Avulsion fracture of proximal tibial epiphysis. Bull. Hosp. Jt. Dis., 24:119, 1963.
This case report involves a 14-year-old boy who caught his foot in parallel bars. The tibial tubercle was avulsed with a good part of the plateaus as well. The injury was treated with open reduction, and the result was good.
525. Kappis, M.: Uber die behandlung der schienbeinkopfbruche. Zentralbl. Chir., 62:194–201, 1931.
The author noted better results than were expected after studying 52 plateau fractures. He suggested closed reduction, and, if the result was not satisfactory, open reduction. The author described known sequelae of injury.
526. Kappis, M.: Ergebnisse der operativen behandlung des schalenformigen einbruchs am scheinbeinkopf. Zentralbl. Chir., 61:1116, 1934.
The author in a brief note discusses the operative treatment of plateau fractures.
527. Karitsky, B.: Chirurg., 5:202, 1954.
528. Karpinski, M. R., and Botting, T. D.: Patellar graft for late disability following tibial plateau fractures. Injury, 15:197–202, 1983.
Three case reports are given with a 3-year follow-up after patellar grafts were used at a late stage to replace the damaged articular surface.
529. Karas, E. H., Weiner, L. S., and Yang, E. C.: The use of anterior incision of the meniscus for exposure of tibial plateau fractures. Orthop. Trans., 18:944, 1994.
The authors did a late arthroscopic examination on 10 of 27 plateau fractures that had been exposed previously by anterior meniscal approach or peripheral detachment and were repaired. All menisci were stable and healed.
530. Kasper, M.: Erfahrungen mit der bohlershen knochenbruchbehandlung am uber 1000 fallen. Bruns. Beitr., 157:225–238, 1933.
531. Katzenstein, M.: Berl. Klin. Wchr., 15:1914.
532. Katzenstein, M.: Demonstrationen aus der Gelenkchirurgie. Zentralbl. Chir., 59:495–496, 1932.
The author reported three operated plateau fractures.
533. Kearns, R., Mendelow, G., Soltes, G., et al: Radiographic view and quality in the assessment of the tibia/plateau fracture: Are we missing something? Orthop. Trans., 13:756, 1989.
These authors present an abstract of an experimental study on cadaver knees in which four different depressions were created in the plateaus, and various x-ray views and techniques were used. Three-millimeter depressions were often missed, and the depth was most frequently underestimated in poor-quality films.
534. Keating, J. F., Kuo, R. S., and Court-Brown, C. M.: Bifocal fractures of the tibia and fibula: Incidence, classification and treatment. J. Bone Joint Surg., 76B:395–400, 1994.
The authors studied combined fractures of the proximal and distal ends of the tibia. They classified these into three types with different characteristics and prognoses.
535. Keinbock: Ein fall von abbruch de tuberositas tibiae samt teil des condylus. Forsch. Roentgen., 1910.
536. Keller: Tibiakopffrakturen. Zurich, Medical Thesis, 1958.
537. Kemke, H.: Zentralbl. Chir., 64:2424, 1937.
538. Kennedy, J. C., and Bailey, W. H.: Experimental tibial-plateau fractures. J. Bone Joint Surg., 50A:1522–1534, 1968.
The authors used 44 cadaver knees and a force machine to study the mechanism of plateau fracture production. Abduction fractures were split, rim, or total depression types of fracture. Compression fractures were the local compression type. Mixed fractures were the split compression type. Explosive fractures were bicondylar and comminuted types.
539. Kennedy, W. R.: Fractures of the tibial condyles: A preliminary report on supplementary fixation with methyl methacrylate. Clin. Orthop., 134:153–157, 1978.
Filled defects that were created by elevation of the depressed articular surfaces with methyl methacrylate in seven patients. Six results were acceptable, and one result was unacceptable. The authors found no adverse effects from the methacrylate.
540. Keogh, P., Kelly, C., Cashman, W. F., et al: Percutaneous screw fixation of tibial plateau fractures. Injury, 23:387–389, 1992.
The authors treated 13 plateau fractures by closed reduction and percutaneous pin or screw fixation. Two patients had arthroscopic reduction. Eleven patients were treated with a Schatzker I and II. Eleven patients had excellent results. One patient had a fixation failure and lost reduction.
541. Keppler, P., Meinig, R., Suger, G., and Kinzl, L.: Long-term results of the operative reconstruction of the bicondylar tibial plateau fractures. Orthop. Trans., 19:141, 1995.
542. Keyser, J.: Die Tibiakondylenbruche. Z. Chir., 251:281–297, 1938.

543. Kindersley, C. E.: Fractures of the tibial tuberosities. Proc. R. Soc. Med., 30:1255–1257, 1937.
This case report of a 40-year-old man with a plateau fracture that was treated by closed reduction using 40 to 50 lb traction and manipulation. Pins were placed above and below and incorporated into a cast.

544. King, G. J., and Schatzker, J.: Nonunion of a complex tibial plateau fracture. J. Orthop. Trauma, 5:209–212, 1991.
The authors report on the sixth plateau nonunion in the literature. They discuss the Schatzker VI fracture with abandoned open reduction and internal fixation and treatment involving traction with a continuous passive motion machine. The subcondylar fracture failed to unite and reconstruction was carried out successfully after 8 months.

545. Klapp, R.: Über den spaltbruch des sheinbeinkopfes und eine behandlung. Zentralbl. Chir., 54:2883, 1927.

546. Klopper, P. J.: Conservative behandlung van tibiaplateaufracturen, Ned. Tidschr. Geneesk., 106:572–580, 1962.

547. Knaggs, R.: A case of fracture of the upper end of the tibia from indirect violence. Lancet, 2:88–89, 1906.
This case report involves a 45-year-old person who was struck by a heavy weight on the side of the leg and sustained an "entire" type of fracture of the medial condyle. Traction for 10 weeks restored good motion. The tip of the fibula was avulsed.

548. Knight, R. A.: Treatment of fractures of the tibial condyles. South. Med. J., 38:246–255, 1945.
The author reviewed 134 fractures that were treated by various methods. He mentions the repair of collateral ligament injuries. Of 134 fractures, 53 were operated on and 81 were treated with closed reduction.

549. Knoblauch, H.: Beitrag zur operativen behandlung der tibiakopfgelenbruche. Mschr. Unfallheilk., 56:340–347, 1953.

550. Koch, F.: (Intra-articular fractures of the knee joint.) Arch. Klin. Chir., 191:12–28, 1938.

551. Kock: V. Nordiske Arbejderforsikringsmode, 1922.

552. Kode, L., Lieberman, J. M., Motta, A. O., et al: Evaluation of tibial plateau fractures: Efficacy of MR imaging compared with CT. Am. J. Roentgenol., 163:141–147, 1994.
The authors evaluated 22 plateau fractures with both magnetic resonance imaging (MRI) and computed tomography (CT). Both techniques were equal in diagnostic ability in 14. MRI was superior in five cases, and CT was successful in three cases (complex and comminuted). MRI showed 12 complete ligament injuries, 15 incomplete ligament injuries, and 55% meniscal injuries. MRI was considered to be the preferable imaging technique.

553. Koechlin, P., Nael, J. F., Bonnet, J. C., et al: (Ligament injuries associated with fractures of the tibial plateau.) Acta Orthop. Belg., 49:751–760, 1983.
Thirty-one ligament injuries were found in 348 plateau fractures. The diagnosis was made by stress film, preoperatively or intraoperatively. Fifteen of 31 were repaired, and 12 of 15 were stable at follow-up. Only six of the 11 patients who were treated nonoperatively were stable.

554. Koeppel, W.: Z. Org. Chir. 87:238, 1936.

555. Kohnlein, H., and Weller, S.: Uber frakturen im bereich des kniegelenks. Zentralbl. Chir., 86:849–852, 1961.
This general article involves plateau fractures.

556. Kohut, M., and Leyvraz, P.: (Importance of meniscal and ligamentous lesions in the long-term prognosis of fractures of the tibial plateau.) Rev. Med. Suisse Romande, 112:685–689, 1992.
The authors studied 250 plateau fractures and followed 146. Twenty-one percent had ligament injuries, and 16% had meniscal lesions. Eighty-three percent had good or excellent results. The conclusion is that restoration of normal knee anatomy is the key for a good result and for minimization of arthritic changes.

557. Konig, E.: Behandlung der bruche im scheinbeinkopf. Zentralbl. Chir., 55:578, 1928.
This case report involves a split compression fracture that was treated by 3 weeks of traction and then a cast with preservation of a good final position.

558. Konig, W.: Erfahrungen uber tibiakopffrakturen der letzen 5 jahre an der leipziger chirurgischen klinik. Dtsch. Z. Chir., 223:420–428, 1930.
The author treated 42 plateau fractures by Steinmann pin traction and reports the usual range of motion to be 75 to 180 degrees.

559. Koralewski, F.: Beitrag zur behandlung der scheinbeinkopfbruche. Chirurg., 66:707–709, 1953.
The author proposes a method of percutaneous fixation of bicondylar fractures by using traction and Kirschner wires placed in the sagittal plane and twisted together to exert compression. A cast is then applied.

560. Koss, B., and Felder, K.: Spatergebnisse der behandlung von scheinbeinkopfbruchen. Mschr. Unfallheilk., 68:348–361, 1965.
The authors treated 64 plateau fractures and followed 45 patients. They noted that 53% had good results; 31% had fair results; and 16% had poor results. The best results involved split compression fractures.

561. Koval, K. J., and Helfet, D. L.: Tibial plateau fractures: Evaluation and treatment. J. Am. Acad. Orthop. Surg., 3:86–94, 1995.
This review article summarizes the goals of treatment of plateau fractures, emphasizing open and external fixation techniques.

562. Koval, K. J., Sanders, R., Borelli, J., et al: Indirect reduction and percutaneous screw fixation of displaced tibial plateau fractures. J. Orthop. Trauma, 6:340–346, 1992.
The authors did indirect reduction and percutaneous screw fixation in 20 displaced plateau fractures. Successful reduction occurred in 18 of 20; the other two failed because they were local compression fractures. Thirteen of 18 were anatomically reduced, and five of 18 were nonanatomic and were mainly local compression fractures. Six were excellent, and 10 had good results. None lost reduction. The authors did arthroscopy in three patients. Postreduction treatment involved a hinged cast.

563. Kozhukh, B. S.: (Injuries of the knee joint in fractures of the head of the fibula and metaphyseal fractures of the tibia.) Ortop. Travmatol. Protez, 23:61–63, 1962.

564. Krackow, K. A., and Vetter, W. L.: Knee motion in a long leg cast. Am. J. Sports Med., 9:233–239, 1981.
The author studied movements within long-leg casts and noted that there is significant valgus-varus and flexion-extension movement within a long-leg cast.

565. Kramer, G.: Zur frage der unterfutterung aufgerichteter imprimate des scheinbeinkopfes. Hefte Unfallheilk., 126:259–261, 1976.

566. Krieg, H., Chmielewski, W., and Sarvestani, H.: Die versorgung der impressionsfrakturen am tibiakopf durch plattenosteosynthese. Hefte Unfallheilk., 126:256–257, 1976.
The authors discuss operative treatment of compression fractures with the use of T plates and screws.

567. Krull, F.: (Surgical treatment of tibial head fractures.) Arch. Orthop. Unfallchir., 41:114–116, 1953.

568. Krull, F.: (Use of Andreesen's double threaded wire.) Mschr. Unfallheilk., 59:305–310, 1956.

569. Kuhlmann, K.: Tibiakopffrakturen (Abstract). Zentralbl. Chir., 78:731, 1953.
This abstract indicates that the author treated 125 plateau fractures—90% by traction or closed methods and 10% by open reduction.

570. Kuhlmann, W.: Tibiakopffrakturen. Langenbecks Arch. Klin. Chir., 276:257–260, 1953.

571. Kummer, A.: Eine neue behandlung des hohen bis ins kniegelenk durchschlaufenden tibiakopfbruches auf operativem wege. Zentralbl. Chir., 62:503–513, 1935.
The author reports on 15 plateau fractures, 12 of which were treated with closed reduction and three operatively. He used a large cortical graft that was placed under the elevated condyle for internal fixation.

572. Kuntscher, G.: Zentralbl. Chir., 75:1320–1324, 1950.
The author illustrates a device that can be inserted and then expanded by twisting a screw, thus elevating and supporting a depressed plateau.

573. Kuppermann, W.: Zur operativen behandlung der schienbeinkopfbruchen. Zschr. Orthop., 90(Suppl.):91–94, 1962.

574. Kurt, H.: Langenbecks Arch. Klin. Chir., 279:443, 1954.

575. Kus, W. M.: (Use of the arthroscope in the treatment of fractures of the proximal tibial epiphysis with lowering of the joint surface.) Chir. Narzadow Rucha Orthop. Pol., 52:296–301, 1987.

576. Kuss, B.: Bemerkenswerte eigenschaften des schienbeinkopfbruche und ihre bedeutung fur die wahl des behandlung. Zentralbl. Chir., 43:1569–1576, 1966.
The author used the AO system in eight open reductions and concluded that it was better than other available methods.

577. Kuss, B.: Zur indikation und technik des osteosynthese von schienbeinkopfbruchen. Arch. Orthop. Unfallchir., 61:297–314, 1967.

The author discusses an early study of the use of cancellous screws and anterior oblique plates in the fixation of plateau fractures.

578. Kuss, B., and Felder, K.: Spatergebnisse der behandlung von scheinbeinkopfbruchen. Mschr. Unfallheilk., 68:348–361, 1965.
The authors classified 45 plateau fractures and noted that 60% had satisfactory results.
579. Kuss, B., Felder, K., and Philip, R.: Zur problematik des behandlung von tibiakopffrakturen. Arch. Orthop. Unfallchir., 60:293–305, 1966.
The authors reviewed plateau fractures that were treated closed and noted a higher incidence of arthritis in patients older than 40 years of age. They concluded that open reduction and internal fixation would be better in patients older than 40 years of age.
580. Kuss, G.: (Fractures of the external plateau.) Mem. Acad. Chir., 73:680–681, 1947.
581. Labey: Fracture unicondylienne interne du tibia. Bull. Mem. Soc. de Paris, 49:195, 1923.
582. Lachiewicz, P. F., and Funcik, T.: Factors influencing the results of open reduction and internal fixation of tibial plateau fractures. Clin. Orthop., 259:210–215, 1990.
The authors analysed 43 plateau fractures that were treated by open reduction and internal fixation and evaluated the results on a 100-point scale after 2.7 years. Despite 10 complications, 35 results were excellent; five were good; three were fair; and there were no poor results. Implants were removed in 14 cases. Bicondylar fractures averaged 18 degrees less motion than did other types.
583. Laduron, E.: Le traitement des fractures du plateau tibial. J. Chir. Soc. Belge Chir., 31:156–165, 1932.
584. Laduron, E.: Le traitement des fractures du plateau tibial. Le Scalpel, 1109–1121, 1932.
585. Landelius, E.: (Traitement operatoire des fractures condyliennes.) Zentralbl. Chir., 63:2009, 1936.
The author gives a brief discussion of plateau fracture fixation.
586. Landelius, E.: Die operative behandlung der spaltbruche des proximalen tibiaendes. Acta Chir. Scand., 82:90–98, 1939.
The author used a method of fixing split fragments by using a strong wire tied over the os purum. Twelve fractures that were treated in this manner obtained good results.
587. Landelius, K.: Nord. Med. Tidsskr., 557, 1938.
588. Landelius, K.: Die operative behandlung der spalbruche des proximalen tibiaendes. Acta Chir. Scand., 53:111–138, 1967.
The author reports on 12 plateau fractures that were treated operatively by closed reduction and fixed by drilling wires through the bone and twisting the ends over pieces of os purum. The knee was exercised early.
589. Landivar, A. F., and Leoni-Iparraguirre, C. A.: Aplatissement unitubérositaire du tibia: Operation et guerison. Bol. Trab. Soc. Chir. de Buenos Aires, 21:501–510, 1937.
590. Landois: Zentralbl. Chir., 52:81–82, 1925.
This case report involves an open reduction that required the removal of the meniscus for fracture elevation.
591. Lange, S.: Obscure fractures discovered by roentgen examination. Lancet-Clinic, 58–60, 1908.
592. Langer, G., and Lang, H.: Indications and contraindications in the use of the MacIntosh prosthesis. Zentralbl. Chir., 106:408–412, 1981.
The authors used a MacIntosh prosthesis to substitute the damaged surface in some old and some new plateau fractures.
593. Lanos, J.: Fractures de l'extrémité supérieure du tibia. Documents Med. Perm. Med. Pract., 52(Suppl. Concours Med.):110–115, 1960.
594. Lansinger, O., Bergman, B., Korner, L., and Andersson, G. B.: Tibial condylar fractures: A twenty year followup. J. Bone Joint Surg., 68A:13–19, 1986.
The authors again followed as many of Rasmussen's original 260 plateau fractures as possible. With a 20-year mean follow-up, they noted no further deterioration of results, further validating the concept of using clinical instability as a criterion for surgical reduction.
595. Lataste, J.: Les fractures bicondyliennes du tibia. Presse Med., 66:116–119, 1958.
The author treated eight bicondylar fractures, seven by open reduction and internal fixation (ORIF) and one closed. Five of the seven cases of ORIF did well using bolts, pins, and screws. One poor result required fusion. The author subclassified the bicondylar fractures.
596. Lataste, J.: Les fractures bicondyliennes du tibia: Document. Med. Perm. Med. Prat. 52(Suppl. Concours Med.): 110–115, 1960.
597. Le Page: (Fractures of the upper end of the tibia: Late results of surgical therapy—three cases.) Bull. Mem. Soc. Chir., 25:635–646, 1933.
598. Leadbetter, G. W., and Hand, F. W.: Fractures of the tibial plateau. J. Bone Joint Surg., 22:559–568, 1940.
The authors consider intra-articular damage to be a sufficient indication to justify operative exposure. They reported 23 plateau fractures, 16 of which were operated on. The patients who were operated on had much better results than did the patients who were not operated on.
599. Lecher, W.: Rekonstruktion veralteter scheinbeinkopfbruchen. Hefte Unfallheilk., 126:272–275, 1976.
The author reports four reconstructions of old plateau fractures using plates and rigid fixation with restoration of a good position.
600. Lee, H. G.: Fractures of the tuberosities of the tibia. N. Engl. J. Med., 204:584–594, 1931.
The authors tabulated the 263 plateau fractures reported in the literature up to 1931 and reported on 21 new cases.
601. Lee, H. G.: Osteoplastic reconstruction in severe fractures of the tibial condyles. Am. J. Surg., 94:940–944, 1957.
The author reports two plateau fractures with severe articular damage in which a large full-thickness wedge of anterior ilium was used as an articular substitute. The defect under the graft is also filled with iliac chips. The 1- and 2-year results on these patients were good.
602. Lefkoe, T. P., Walsh, W. R., Anastasatos, J., et al: Remodeling of articular step-offs. Is osteoarthritis dependent on defect size? Clin. Orthop., 314:253–265, 1995.
The authors created 2- to 5-mm offsets on rabbits and sacrificed them at various intervals. It was noted that significant articular incongruity was required for development of osteoarthritis.
603. Lehmann: (Fracture par depression centrale du condyle tibial.) Zentralbl. Chir., 63:2672–2674, 1936.
This author describes five open reductions for depressed plateau fractures.
604. Lehmann: Chirurg., 656, 1936.
605. Lehmann: Fractures fissuraires du tibia. Bruns Beitr. Klin. Chir., 165:4, 1937.
606. Lehmann, A., and Noesberger, B.: Reconstruction of the tibial plateau. Helv. Chir. Acta, 43:439–441, 1976.
These authors used plates to reconstruct a comminuted plateau and upper tibial fractures.
607. Lembcke, W.: Tibiakoppffrakturen (Abstract). Zentralbl. Chir., 78:731, 1953.
In this brief note the author suggests the use of traction and sideways compression in the treatment of plateau fractures.
608. Lembcke, W.: Tibiakopffrakturen. Langenbecks Arch. Chir., 276:256–257, 1953.
The author treated 39 plateau fractures by operation and noted infection in 11 cases.
609. Lemercier: Fractures Unicondyliennes du Tibia. Paris, Thesis, 1913.
610. Lemon, R. A., and Bartlett, D. H.: Arthroscopic assisted internal fixation of certain fractures about the knee. J. Trauma, 25:355–358, 1985.
This case report involves an entire plateau fracture that was arthroscoped. Pins were placed in the large fragment to aid in reduction, and fixation was secured by percutaneous screws with an excellent result.
611. Lenormant, C.: Sur le traitement opératoire des fractures sous-articulaires par écrasement du plateau tibial. Rev. Path. Physiol. Travail, 4:173–185, 1934.
612. Lenormant, C.: Fracture du condyle externe du tibia: Reduction sanglant et greffe osseuse. Mem. Soc. Nat. Chir., 1190, 1935.
613. Lentz, W.: Hefte Unfallheilk, 43:213, 1952.
614. Lentz, W.: Ergebnisse der behandlung von schweren tibiakopfbruchen mit der spongiosafeder. Chirurg., 27:252–257, 1956.
Fifty plateau fractures were operated on and followed for 6 to 60 months. The results were generally satisfactory; 39 showed no complications, and 38 showed good postoperative reduction.
615. Leriche, R.: Résultat eloigné d'une reduction sanglante sui-

vie de greffes osteoperiostiques dans une fracture de la partie externe du plateau tibial avec destruction étendue de tissu spongieux. Mem. Acad. Chir., 60:2–4, 1934.

616. Leriche, R.: À propos de 8 observations de traitement sanglant de fractures du plateau tibial; Arthrotomie ou nou? Greffe ou vissage? Mem. Acad. Chir., 63:639–644, 1936.
617. Leriche, R., and Jung, A.: Indications et résultats de l'osteosynthese dans les fractures du plateau tibial. Rev. Chir., 10:321–349, 1930.
618. Levitin, J.: March fracture of tibial articular surface: Relation to osteoarthropathy. Radiology, 46:273–275, 1946.
619. Levy, O., Solai, M., Ganel, A., et al: The operative results of tibial plateau fractures in older patients: A long-term followup and review. Bull. Hosp. Joint Dis., 53:15–16, 1993.
The authors treated 19 patients who were 65 years and older by operative means and followed these patients for an average of 11 years. Twelve patients had buttress plates, three plates, and six screws or bolts. Early motion was used. There were five complications. Seventy-nine percent were excellent or good. Over 90 degrees of motion were present in 15 cases and over 120 degrees were present in nine cases. Limited motion was present in four cases.
620. Lexer, E.: Algemeines zur behandlung von knochenbruchen. Munch. Med. Wochenschr., 70:1024–1026, 1923.
621. Lexer, E.: Gelenksplastik bei schweren gelenkbruchen. Zentralbl. Chir., 57:2261, 1930.
This case report involves a plateau fracture that was treated operatively.
622. Lexer, E.: Die gesampte wiederherstellungschirurgie. 2:816, 1931.
623. Lexer, E.: Die richtigstellung der scheinbeingelenkflache durch hebung mit knockenkeilen. Zentralbl. Chir., 59:642–643, 1932.
The author discusses the technique of treating fractures in spongy bone.
624. Lexer, E.: Bermerkung zu der mitteilung von Dr. S. Zimmer: Die richtigstellung der scheinbeingelenkflache durch hebung mit knockenkeilen. Zentralbl. Chir., 59:1227–1228, 1932.
The author gives a brief description of a treatment technique.
625. Lichtblau, S.: Fractures into the knee. Med. Trial Techn. Q., 10:65–74, 1963.
626. Lichtenauer, F.: (Surgical therapy of central cup-shaped fractures of the tibial head.) Zentralbl. Chir., 251:1–11, 1938.
627. Lichtenauer, F.: Zur blutigen behandlung der sheinbeinkopfbruche mit centraler (sogenannter schalenformiger) depression ennes gelenkanteiles. Dtsch. Z. Chir., 241:1–11, 1939.
The author reports on 11 plateau fractures that were treated by using a wire loop that was tightened and tied over buttons. Postoperative support is provided by suspension.
628. Linder, E., Perey, O., and Palmer, I.: (Intra-articular fractures of the tibia at the knee joint.) Nord. Med., 45:320–321, 1951.
629. Lindholm, R. V.: Treatment of fractures of the tibial condyles by active movement therapy. Acta Orthop. Scand., 23:320–323, 1954.
This case report emphasizes the use of a simple suspension apparatus to foster early active knee motion after a fracture.
630. Lindgren, U.: Nord. Med. Tidsskr., 557, 1938.
631. Liniger: Zwei falle einer seltenen knieverletzung. Mschr. Unfallheilk., 2:289–292, 1895.
One case report involves a plateau fracture that presented initially with varus and that healed in varus after 6 weeks of cast treatment. Another was a lateral compression plateau fracture treated closed with valgus deformity late.
632. Liphardt, H.: Ein weiterer fall von abrissfraktur des fibulakopfchens. Zentralbl. Chir., 78:1638–1640, 1953.
This case report involves an entire plateau type of fracture accompanied by fibular head avulsion. The result was a varus deformed knee because of medial plateau depression.
633. Lippmann, R. K.: Surgical treatment of depressed fractures of the plateau. J. Mt. Sinai Hosp., 17:761–768, 1951.
This author describes a technique to hold up elevated articular fragments by using a prop graft of cortical bone.
634. Llinas, A. M., Lovasz, G., and Park, S. H.: Effect of joint incongruity on the opposing articular surface. Presented at the AAOS Meeting, New Orleans, February 1994.
These authors created 0.5-mm and 1-mm coronal offsets on the femoral condyles of rabbits and studied the tibial articular surface after immobilization, intermittent active motion, or continuous passive motion (CPM) at 12 weeks. The rabbits' articular thickness was 0.5 mm. Offsets of 0.5 mm were well accommodated with only minor changes, but the 1-mm offset created degenerative changes especially after CPM.
635. Llinas, A. M., McKellop, H. A., Marshall, J., et al: Healing and remodeling of articular incongruities in a rabbit fracture model. J Bone Joint Surg., 75A:1508–1523, 1993.
One-half millimeter and 1-mm articular offsets were created in rabbits' knees in 54 animals. Some animals were immobilized; others were allowed movement; and still others were given continuous passive motion (CPM). The results were studied after 12 weeks. Cartilage on the high part tapered and thinned, while the opposite side thickened slightly. CPM did not seem to help. If step-off is near cartilage thickness there should be concern.
636. Lobenhoffer, P., and Tscherne, H.: Tibial plateau fractures: Improved techniques and results of open reduction/internal fixation. Orthop. Trans., 15:806, 1991.
This follow-up study involves 190 of 244 plateau fractures. The authors noted improved results but did have 8% wound infection.
637. Locht, R. C., Gross, A. E., and Langer, F.: Late osteochondral allograft resurfacing for tibial plateau fractures. J. Bone Joint Surg., 66A:328–335, 1984.
The authors performed osteochondral allografts on 17 patients with arthritic knees after tibial plateau fractures. Three patients collapsed, and one lost cartilage space. Others did well. The procedure is useful in younger patients.
638. Longhi, G., et al: (Use of delitala pressor in fracture of the tibial plateau.) Minerva Med., 56:2667–2670, 1965.
639. Loock, P.: Les Fractures Articulaires de l'Extrémité Supérieure du Tibia: À propos de 217 Cas. Lille, Medical Thesis, 1977.
640. Lopez Duran Lozano, L.: Le fratture del piatti tibiali. Rev. Ortop. Traum., 6:73, 1962.
641. Lortat-Jacob, A., Mazel, C., Frank, A., et al: La fixation epiphysaire par fixateur externe: Étude bio-mechanique et clinique. Rev. Chir. Orthop., 70:207–217, 1984.
The authors used an external fixator in 51 fractures of the distal femur, upper tibia and distal tibia. One half of the patients with plateau fractures who were treated with the device did well because of early knee movement. Infection was not a problem.
642. Lory, G., and Thouvenin, R.: Fracture fissuraire de l'extrémité supérieure du tibia. Bull. Mem. Soc. Anat. Paris, 1920.
643. Low: Dtsch. Z. Chir., 44:442, 1897.
This case report is about a 68-year-old woman who fell downstairs after which valgus knee deformity was noted. Treatment was given by bandage and massage. After healing, the medial joint was open slightly. Another plateau fracture was treated by traction, after which the fracture healed.
644. Low-Beer: Virchows Arch., 273:191, 1929.
645. Lucht, U., and Pilgaard, S.: Fractures of the tibial condyles. Acta Orthop. Scand., 42:366–376, 1971.
The author treated 109 plateau fractures of which 28% were minimally displaced. Forty-seven percent were operatively reduced and immobilized in plaster. Functional results were 87% satisfactory.
646. Luck, J. V.: Traumatic arthrofibrosis. Bull. Hosp. Jt. Dis., 12:394–403, 1951.
The author called attention to a fibrous reaction that occurred frequently following joint trauma. This reaction included pannus formation and capsular contracture due to scarring.
647. Lukasik, S.: (Surgical treatment of articular fractures of the upper end of the tibia.) Chir. Narzad. Ruchu. Ortop. Pol., 28:461–465, 1963.
648. Maatz, R.: Z. Orthop., 80:643, 1951.
649. Maatz, R.: Die behandlung des tibiakopfbruches mit der spongiosafeder. Chirurg., 27:247–249, 1956.
The author used a corkscrew-like fixation device to support elevated fragments and exert pressure on split fragments.
650. MacAusland, W. R. Jr.: Fractures of the tibial plateau. *In* Reynolds, F. C. (Ed.): Instructional Course Lectures. Am. Acad. Orth. Surg., 17:87–91, 1961.
This general discussion concerns the diagnosis and treatment of plateau fractures in which open reduction is emphasized. Early motion and preservation of the meniscus are advocated.
651. MacDonald, G.: Tibial condylar fractures (Abstract). J. Bone Joint Surg., 43B:612–613, 1961.

The author reports 77 plateau fractures, divided into stable or unstable categories. The stable fractures did well with closed treatment. The 37 unstable fractures were treated by open reduction and a Barr bolt, and 82% of the results were acceptable.

652. MacIntosh, D. L.: Hemiarthroplasty of the knee using space occupying prostheses for painful varus and valgus deformities (Abstract). J. Bone Joint Surg., 40A:1431, 1958.
The author reports 13 MacIntosh prosthetic replacements for malaligned knees after a plateau fracture or arthritis.
653. Magerl, F.: The surgical treatment of fractures of tibial condyles. Excerpta Med. Amsterdam, 377:79–84, 1976.
654. Magistroni, C., and Ferrero, A.: Le fratture articolari dell'epifisi prossimale della tibia: Considerazioni clinico-statistiche. Minerva Ortop., 14:663–679, 1963.
The author discusses history, classification, mechanism of injury, and information about the treatment of 185 plateau fractures.
655. Magnus, G.: Indikationen und kontraindikationen in der frakturbehandlung. Arch Klin. Chir., 177:265–289, 1933.
The author treated 92 plateau fractures with pin fixation and plaster.
656. Magnuson, P. B., and Coulter, J. S.: Fractures of both bones of the leg extending into the knee joint. Int. Clin., 4:191, 1920.
657. Maheson, M., and Colton, C. L.: Fractures of the tibial plateau in Nottingham. Injury, 19:324–328, 1988.
The authors treated 45 patients, using open reduction in 25 patients and closed treatment in 20 patients. Thirty of 45 were evaluated using objective clinical, objective radiographic, and subjective results, usually with a 1:4 rating in each.
658. Mahomed, M. N., Beaver, R. J., and Gross, A. E.: The long term success of fresh, small fragment allografts used for intraarticular post-traumatic defect in the knee joint. Orthopedics, 15:1191–1199, 1992.
The authors performed 92 fresh allografts in 91 patients with post-traumatic knee defects. Some were residuals of plateau fractures. Of the unipolar grafts, 67% survived for 14 years. Joint malalignment must be corrected for best results.
659. Maisel, B., and Cornell, N. W.: Conservative treatment of fractures of the tibial condyles. Surgery, 23:591–598, 1948.
The authors explored a previously fractured knee and noted that the fractured condyle was covered by thick fibrocartilage tissue. They reported on three fractures that were treated with a splint and then mobilized with good results.
660. Malabarba, G., and Poggi, U.: Posterior marginal fracture of the tibial plateau due to ligament tear. Minerva Ortop., 18:388–390, 1967.
661. Malatray, and Bastien: Le traitement des fractures du plateau tibial: Résultats eloignés à propos de 24 observations personnelles. Rev. Chir. Paris, 77:45–74, 1939.
662. Malerba, F., and Zagra, A.: Sulla terapia delle fratture del piatto tibiale. Minerva Ortop., 21:569–573, 1970.
663. Mallik, A. R., Covall, D. J., and Whitelaw, G. P.: Internal versus external fixation of bicondylar tibial plateau fractures. Orthop. Rev., 21:1433–1436, 1992.
The authors treated 11 bicondylar fractures, seven by open reduction and fixation (ORIF) and three by the Monticelli-Spinelli circular fixation. The other fracture was by closed reduction and cast-brace. Varus deformity was present in one third of the patients. The authors believe that external fixation is an acceptable alternative to ORIF because there are fewer complications. No joint infection was noted.
664. Mammi, I.: Le nostre esperienze nel trattamento delle frattura del piatto tibiale. Minerva Ortop., 18:354–355, 1967.
In this brief note the author discusses methods of closed and open treatment of plateau fractures.
665. Manfredi, L.: Terapia ed esiti di fratture dei condili tibiali. Riv. Infort. Mal Prof., 47:407–412, 1960.
666. Manfredi, L.: Sulle fratture del condili tibiali. Atti S.O.T.I.M.I., 5:246, 1960.
667. Manhold, E.: Ein fall von keiltormigem langsbruch am oberen tibiaende. Mschr. Unfallheilk., 16:107–110, 1909.
This case report involves a split compression fracture that was treated by the closed method.
668. Manninger, J., Salacz, T., and Fekete, K.: Impresszios tibia condylus tores mozgasstabil szintezise modositatt lemezzel. Magy Traumatol. Orthop. Helyreallito, Sebesz., 24:108–120, 1981.
669. Manzotti, G., and Pina, C.: Sul trattamento delle fratture scomposte del piatto tibiale. Minerva Ortop., 18:398–401, 1967.
The authors discuss treatment of comminuted bicondylar fractures.
670. Marie, E.: Des Fractures de l'Extrémité Supérieure du Tibia et de Leur Prognostic. Paris, Thesis, 1867.
671. Marino, V., and Moscato, P.: Considerazioni sul trattamento di alcuni casi di fratture intrarticolari del ginocchio. Ort. Traum. App. Mot., 22:551, 1954.
672. Marion, J., and Grezard, L.: (Posterior glenomarginal fracture of the external tibial plateau; transperoneal reposition with graft; use of tomography and oblique radiography.) Lyon Chir., 46:763–764, 1951.
673. Marique, P., and Collard, R.: Les fractures des tuberosites tibiales. Bull. Soc. Belge d'Orthop., 9:241, 1937.
674. Marottoli, O. R.: (Therapy of fractures of the external tibial condyle; Barr technique.) Bol. Soc. Cir. Rosario, 17:218–226, 1950.
675. Marottoli, O. R.: (Therapy of fractures of the external tibial condyle; Barr technique.) An. Chir., 15:128–136, 1950.
676. Marsh, J. L., Do, T. T., and Smith, S. T.: Outcome of severe tibial plateau fractures. Orthop. Trans., 19:141, 1995.
677. Marsh, J. L., Smith, S. T., and Do, T. T.: External fixation and limited internal fixation for complex fractures of the tibial plateau. J. Bone Joint Surg., 77A:661–673, 1995.
The authors treated 21 complex tibial plateau fractures by closed reduction, percutaneous screw fixation, and a half pin external fixator. All fractures healed. There were 7 pin tract infections and 2 knees with septic arthritis. All obtained at least a 115 degree arc of motion. The Iowa score averaged 87.
678. Marsili, E., and Bardo, G.: Considerazioni sul trattamento delle fratture del piatto tibiale. Arch. Inst. Osp. Corona, 29:439, 1964.
679. Martin, A. F.: The pathomechanics of the knee joint. I: The medial collateral ligament and lateral tibial plateau fractures. J. Bone Joint Surg., 42A:13–22, 1960.
This author used the knees of cadavers to study the effect of a plateau fracture on the medial collateral ligament (MCL) and the clear space medially. The clear space only opens when there has been injury to the MCL. Stress testing, which shows more than 1 mm of medial opening, suggests a MCL injury.
680. Martin, P. L., and Planes, A.: Considerations radiologiques sur l'évolution des fractures articularaires de l'extrémité supérieure du tibia. J. Radiol. Electro., 45:561–562, 1964.
681. Martini, M., et al: (A propos of articular fractures of the upper tibia.) Tunis. Med., 41:55–67, 1963.
682. Marwah, V., Gadegone, W. M., and Magarkar, D. S.: The treatment of fractures of the tibial plateau by skeletal traction and early mobilisation. Int. Orthop., 9:217–221, 1985.
This author studied 50 plateau fractures that were treated by traction and early mobilization with 94% good results in a 2-year follow-up period.
683. Marwege, H.: (A contribution to the care of extensive longitudinal fracture of the head of the tibia.) Mschr. Unfallheilk., 63:65–67, 1960.
684. Masse, Y., and Mazas, F.: Devenir à long terme des fractures des plateaux tibiaux. Rev. Chir. Orthop., 63:203–207, 1977.
Of 232 patients with plateau fractures, the authors were able to follow 56 patients for 10 to 24 years. The results were excellent in 33 cases, good in 13 cases, and fair or poor in 10 cases.
685. Matti, H.: Die knochenbruche und ihre behandlung. 1922.
686. Matzen, F.: Wiederherstellung nach frakturen im knieberich. Z. Orthop., 96(Suppl.), 1962.
687. Mauclaire: Bull. Mem. Soc. Chir. Paris, 44:272, 1918.
688. Mauer, I., and Friedman, A.: Hinged casts in the treatment of tibial plateau fractures. Bull. Hosp. Joint Dis., 20:61–68, 1959.
The authors reduced eight fractures manipulatively and applied a cast for 1 week. A new hinged cast was then applied to allow knee movement.
689. Maurer, G.: (Fractures of the knee joint). Zentralbl. Chir., 65:1463–1467, 1938.
690. Mazas, F.: Contribution à l'Étude des Fractures des Plateaux Tibiaux. Paris, Thesis, 1959.
691. McAndrew, M. P., Gorman, P. W., and Lange, T. A.: Tricalcium phosphate as a bone graft substitute in trauma: Preliminary report. J. Orthop. Trauma, 2:333–339, 1988.
The authors used ceramic tricalcium phosphate (TCP) to fill traumatic bone defects in 43 patients. Absorption of TCP was 10% per month. TCP was used in at least one plateau fracture that did well.

692. McConkey, J. P., and Meeuwisse, W.: Tibial plateau fractures in alpine skiing. Am. J. Sports Med., 16:159–164, 1988.
Eighteen skiers sustained plateau fractures that were thought to have been caused by hyperextension and valgus forces. Forty-four percent were of the local compression type.

693. McDonnell, M. F., and Butler, J. F.: Osteochondral fracture of the tibial plateau in a ballerina. Am. J. Sports Med., 16:417–418, 1988.
This case report involves a 23-year-old ballerina who did a hyperextension move, felt a pop, and sustained a minor osteochondral fracture.

694. McEnery, K. W., Wilson, A. J., Pilgrim, T. K., et al: Fractures of the tibial plateau: Value of spiral CT coronal plane reconstruction for detecting displacement in vitro. Am. J. Roentgenol., 163:1177–1181, 1994.
The authors produced artificial fractures in cadaveric tibial plateaus. Several different displacements were created and spiral computed tomography scans done. The technique can detect clinically important plateau fractures.

695. McLeod, W., Moschi, A., Andrews, J., and Hughston, J.: Tibial plateau topography. Am. J. Sports Med., 5:13–18, 1977.
The authors studied topographic anatomy and cartilage thickness of the tibial plateaus. The cartilage was thicker anteriorly on the medial plateau and posteriorly on the lateral plateau.

696. Meerwein, H.: Die fraktur des condylus externus tibiae. Dtsch. Z. Chir., 102:522–531, 1909.
The author reported on four soldiers with split compression fractures. He also cited a plateau fracture that was given to him by H. Wilms, who opened a plateau fracture and fixed it internally with two nails without reducing the depressed fragment.

697. Meggitt, B. F., Broom, N. D., and Ross, P. M.: Hinged walking plaster for fractures around the knee (Abstract). J. Bone Joint Surg., 57B:393, 1975.
The authors treated 10 plateau fractures in traction until the fracture was stable and then applied a hinged cast for a few weeks. Load sparing of 25 to 50% was measured using load transducers. No fracture collapse occurred.

698. Melere, G.: Les Fractures Récentes des Plateaux Tibiaux. Lyon, Medical Thesis, 1976.
This thesis analyses 127 plateau fractures and provides a general review of the subject. The importance of early knee mobilization is emphasized.

699. Mendes, A.: Fractures of the tibial plateau (Abstract). J Bone Joint Surg., 51B:573, 1969.
The author advocates open reduction, grafting, and a tibial bolt for depressed fractures. He used a bolt and suspension with early motion for comminuted fractures.

700. Mennitti, D., and Rossi, A.: Le fratture inveterate del piatto tibiale e loro trattamento. Boll. Mem. Soc. Tosco-Umbra Chir., 24:891, 1963.

701. Mesa del Castillo, M.: Traitement des fractures articulaires de l'extrémité supérieure du tibia. Cir. y Gin. Urol., 4:338–349, 1964.

702. Mestdagh, H.: (Reconstruction of the lateral tibial plateau using a vascular pedicle patellar transplant.) Unfallchirurgie, 93:205–207, 1990.
The author reconstructed a lateral plateau with marked depression resulting from necrosis after a local compression fracture. The lateral portion of the patella was used as an osteochondral pedicle graft.

703. Meyers, M. H., Moore, T. M., and Harvey, J. P.: Traumatic dislocation of the knee joint. J. Bone Joint Surg., 57A:430–433, 1975.

704. Middeldorpf: Beitrage zu der lehre von den knochenbruchen. Breslau, 1853.
This case report concerns a 42-year-old man who fell 8 feet. The examination showed crepitus in the knee. After the autopsy, an impression fracture of the lateral plateau with a fibular fracture was identified.

705. Mikhailova, N. M.: (Treatment of intra-articular fractures of the proximal end of the tibia.) Vestn. Khir., 81:93–99, 1958.

706. Mikkelsen, O.: Intraartikulare frakturen des obersten tibiaendes. Acta Chir. Scand., 73:1–42, 1933.
The author studied 248 plateau fractures that were treated predominantly with the closed method. A follow-up of 128 cases after 1 to 19 years showed that only 12 patients were unable to work. He emphasized the value of early knee motion.

707. Milch, H.: Cortical avulsion fracture of the lateral tibial condyle. J. Bone Joint Surg., 18:159–164, 1936.
Three patients with avulsion fractures of the lateral plateau are described. The avulsion was caused by pull of the iliotibial band.

708. Milev, T., and Mourgues, G. de: Du traitement des fractures des condyles du femur et du tibia par embrochages. Lyon Chir., 61:89–92, 1965.
The authors used pins to fix some plateau fractures with moderate success.

709. Milgram, J. W.: Injury to articular cartilage joint surfaces—Displaced traumatic fractures of the underlying bone. Proc. Orthop. Res. Soc., 211, 1985.
The author studied 32 injured joint specimens and documented the response of the joint to articular surface repair. No repair took place unless the marrow was violated.

710. Millard, I.: Fracture of the lateral tibial plateau. J. Ark. Med. Soc., 78:132–133, 1981.
This short review article is about the principles of open reduction.

711. Mink, J.: Occult cartilage and bone injuries of the knee: Detection, classification, and assessment with MR imaging. Radiology, 170:823–829, 1989.
The author discusses magnetic resonance imaging findings after occult fracture. Fracture lines and bone bruises can be seen.

712. Miroux, J.: Traitement Chirurgical des Fractures Récentes des Plateaux Tibiaux (À Propos de 56 Cas Inédits). Paris, Thesis, 1958.

713. Mitchell, N., and Shepard, N.: Healing of articular cartilage in intra-articular fractures in rabbits. J. Bone Joint Surg., 62A:628–634, 1980.
The authors created intra-articular defects in rabbits. Those reduced accurately healed with a hyaline-like cartilage. The rabbits that were left displaced healed with a fibrocartilage-like material. The authors recommend accurate reduction and rigid fixation.

714. Moller, D.: Uber bruche des tibiakopfes. Kiel, Thesis, 1875.

715. Mollowitz, G., and Thiemann, K. J.: Kniegelenksarthrographie nach scheinbeinkopfbruchen. Hefte Unfallheilk., 126:230–231, 1976.
The authors discuss the role of arthrography in fresh and old plateau fractures but noted that it is of more use in old fractures.

716. Molsberger, C., et al: Chip fracture of the lateral tibial condyle—A roentgen sign of anterior cruciate ligament injury. Sportverletz. Sportschaden, 3:120–123, 1989.

717. Monceau: Fracture de l'extrémité supérieure du tibia. Bull. Soc. Anat. Paris, 31:75, 1856.
This case report involves a patient with a total condylar type of fracture. The fracture was initially an open fracture that became infected with a septic joint and the patient died.

718. Monticelli, G.: L'osteosintesi delle fratture articolari e para-articolari. Ort. Traum. App. Mot., 20:125, 1952.

719. Monticelli, G., and Pizzetti, M.: Sulle lesioni meniscali e legamentose nelle fratture del piatto tibiale. Atti Sotimi, 3:326–330, 1958.

720. Mooney, V.: Cast bracing. Clin. Orthop., 102:159–166, 1974.
The author studied cast-bracing and noted that about 50% of weight sparing could be obtained with a cast-brace. Fifty patients with comminuted plateau fractures were treated, primarily those with little displacement. The brace held reduction satisfactorily in these patients.

721. Mooney, V., Nickel, V., and Snelson, R.: Ambulatory care of lower extremity fractures (Abstract). J. Bone Joint Surg., 52A:832–833, 1980.
The authors noted that 50% of weight sparing could be obtained in a cast-brace that was stressed into a valgus or varus position. The authors treated a few plateau fractures in traction for 2 to 3 weeks and then applied a cast-brace for 8 weeks.

722. Moons: Overgedruekt nit de handelingen van het 18e vlaamsch Natur en Genneeskundig Congres. Antwerpen, 1919.

723. Moore, T. M.: Fracture-dislocation of the knee. Clin. Orthop., 156:128–140, 1981.
The author found 128 articular fractures that were characterized by joint instability. These fractures had increased neurovascular injury and required open reduction in 83%. A classification of fracture-dislocation was presented.

724. Moore, T. M.: Management of tibial plateau fractures. *In* Symposium on Trauma to the Leg and Its Sequelae. St. Louis, C.V. Mosby, 1981.
This general discussion involves the classification and management of plateau fractures based on 1000 fractures studied pro-

spectively. Meniscal injury and traumatic arthritis are discussed in detail.

725. Moore, T. M., and Harvey, J. P.: Roentgenographic measurement of tibial plateau depression due to fracture. J. Bone Joint Surg., 56A:155–160, 1974.
The authors noted measurement inconsistencies using plain x-rays and suggested the tibial plateau view, 10 degrees caudal projection, for measuring depression.
726. Moore, T. M., and Meyers, M. H.: Apparatus to position knees for varus-valgus stress roentgenograms. J. Bone Joint Surg., 59A:984, 1977.
The authors describe an apparatus to apply valgus or varus knee stress to take x-rays. This apparatus provides consistent and reliable stress.
727. Moore, T. M., Meyers, M. H., and Harvey, J. P.: Collateral ligament laxity of the knee: Long term comparison between plateau fractures and normal. J. Bone Joint Surg., 58A:594–598, 1976.
The authors made bilateral valgus-varus stress x-rays after plateau fracture healing in 208 patients. They found no increased ligament laxity on the fractured side, but they did find 16 ligament calcifications.
728. Moore, T. M., Patzakis, M. J., and Harvey, J. P.: Tibial plateau fractures: Definition, demographics, treatment rationale, and long-term results of closed traction management or operative reduction. J. Orthop. Trauma, 1:97–119, 1987.
Data on 753 plateau fractures gathered prospectively were studied. Open reduction and internal fixation was carried out in 44%, and the remainder were treated in traction. A follow-up of 1 to 10 years (average of 3.7 years) was possible in 320 patients. The complication rate was 8% in patients with closed traction management and 19% in operated patients. Anatomic reduction and early motion led to good results.
729. Morandi, M., Watson, J. T., Blake, R., et al: Treatment of complex tibial plateau fractures with circular external fixators. Orthop. Trans., 17:1056, 1994.
The authors treated 31 Schatzker type VI complex fractures with circular small pin external fixators. They concluded that the method was good for complicated bicondylar fractures.
730. Moreau, J.: Fractures de l'extrémité supérieure du tibia. Ann. Soc. Belg. Chir., 12:63–80, 1912.
731. Moreau, J.: Fractures de l'extrémité supérieure du tibia. Clin. Brux., 27:241, 1913.
732. Moreau, L.: Deux cas de fractures rares de l'extrémité supérieure du tibia. Bull. Mem. Soc. Chir. Paris, 42:2628–2639, 1916.
733. Moreau, L.: Des fractures tuberositaires de l'extrémité supérieure du tibia. Rev. Orthop. Chir. l'Appareil Moteur, 15:193–224, 1928.
The author reviewed 22 plateau fractures that were treated by splint or plaster cast. There were nine lateral, two medial, and five bicondylar fractures.
734. Moreau, L.: Fracture du plateau tibial. Bull. Mem. Soc. Radiol. Med. France, 25:372–374, 1937.
735. Moreau, L.: Un cas curieux de fracture de la tuberosité interne du tibia. Bull. Mem. Soc. Electro-radiol. Med. France, 27:99–100, 1939.
736. Morini, G.: Intraarticular fractures of the knee: Arthroscopic diagnosis and treatment. Chir. Organi Mov., 80:39–44, 1995.
737. Morisi, M., Galli, P., and Riquier, G.: Sull'impiego di un dispositivo a pressione nel trattamento delle fratture del piatto tibiale. Arch. Ortop. Milano, 71:206–219, 1958.
738. Morisi, M., Gibelli, G., and Tiberio, G.: Il Trattamento chirurgico delle fratture recenti monocondiloidee depressee della epifisi prossimale della tibia. Arch. Ortop. Milano, 72:1349–1358, 1959.
739. Morisi, M., Tiberio, G., Gibelli, F., and Forti, P.: Considerazioni a proposito del trattamento delle fratture del piatto tibiale. Arch. Ortop., 72:491–517, 1959.
740. Mortensen, T.: Treatment of fractures of the condyles of the tibia. Ugeskr. Laeger, 131:1976–1980, 1969.
741. Mouchet, A.: Fracture isolée de la tuberosité extrème du tibia. Paris Med., 9:160, 1910.
742. Mourgues, G. de, and Chaix, D.: Traitement des fractures des plateaux tibiaux. Rev. Chir. Orthop., 50:103–122, 1964.
The authors studied 125 plateau fractures that were treated mainly by the traction-mobilization method.
743. Mourgues, G. de, and Chaix, D.: Traitement des fractures des plateaux tibiaux. Note de catamnese après 5 ans. Rev. Chir. Orthop., 55:575–576, 1969.
The authors reported on 259 plateau fractures using the traction-mobilization treatment. The follow-up of 137 patients showed 70% satisfactory results after 5 years.
744. Mourgues, G. de, Fischer, L. P., Moyen, B., et al: Les fractures des plateaux tibiaux: Leur traitement par la méthode de traction-mobilization. Chirurg., 105:142–146, 1979.
Skeletal calcaneal traction and early knee mobilization were used for more than 22 years. An 8-year follow-up study showed that 50% of patients had good to excellent functional results.
745. Mourgues, G. de, Venouil, J., Rey, A., et al: Les fractures des plateaux tibiaux. Presse Med., 77:2037–2039, 1969.
746. Molloy, L.: A rare, if not unique, fracture of the tibia. Lancet, 2:1198, 1898.
This case report involves a 65 year old who slipped, fell, and sustained a split compression fracture. Healing occurred with widening of the upper tibia but with acceptable function.
747. Moutier, G.: Fracture de la tuberosité externe du tibia reduction manuelle: Excellent résultat functionnel. Rev. Orthop., 14:145, 1927.
748. Moutoussy, P.: Les Fractures par Tassement du Pilier Antérieur du Tibia. Toulouse, Thesis, 1970.
749. Mueller, K.: Ersebnisse und posttraumatische arthrose nach operativ versorsten tibiakopffrakturen. Acta Traumatol., 6:55–60, 1976.
750. Muezzinoglu, U. S., Guner, G., and Gurfidan, E.: Arthroscopically assisted tibial plateau fracture management: A modified method. Arthroscopy, 11:506–509, 1995.
The authors describe a technique of harvesting and using a core graft to maintain reduction of depressed fractures.
751. Muggler, E.: Die tibiakopffraktur, problematik, operative therapie und resultate. Unfallchirurgie, 4:157–178, 1978.
752. Muggler, E., Huber, D., and Burri, C.: Ergebnisse nach operativer versorgung von 225 tibiakopffrakturen. Chirurg., 46:348–352, 1975.
The authors treated 225 plateau fractures by open reduction, emphasizing fixation and early knee movement. One pseudoarthrosis occurred. Arthritis was noted in 120 patients at follow-up.
753. Muhr, G.: (Conservative treatment of fractures of the tibial head.) Chirurg., 61:767–771, 1990.
754. Muller, and Thomas, T.: Impacted fracture of the upper end of the fibula and tibia. Ann. Surg., 74:107–108, 1921.
This case report pertains to closed treatment of a plateau fracture.
755. Muller, H., and Morach, M.: Uber die verwendung lyophilisierter, homologer spongiosa bei der tibiakopffrakturen. Helv. Chir. Acta, 45:43–47, 1978.
The authors operated on 30 plateau fractures using 19 allografts and 11 autogenic grafts. Identical results were noted. Two wound infections occurred.
756. Muller, M. E., Allgower, M., Schneider, R., and Willenegger, H.: Manual of Internal Fixation. New York, Springer-Verlag, 1979.
In this textbook on treatment of fractures, the authors discuss the principles and techniques of management of plateau fractures by open reduction. A classification of plateau fractures is illustrated.
757. Muller, M. E., Nazarian, S., Koch, P., and Schatzker, J.: Classification of Fractures. New York, Springer-Verlag, 1990.
This volume gives the complete AO classification scheme. It is organized by bone, location in bone, severity, and by type (e.g., 1, 2, and 3) to denote different types of fracture. It is based on the files of the Association for Study of Internal Fixation.
758. Muller, W.: Behandlungsergebnisse bei scheinbeinkopfbruchen. Dtsch. Militirarzt., 6:134, 1941.
759. Muller, W.: Behandlungsergebnisse bei scheinbeinkopfbruchen (Abstract). Zentralbl. Chir., 68:1462, 1941.
This abstract indicates the treatment of 33 plateau fractures by Bohler's method of manipulation and cast or traction.
760. Murphy, C. P., D'Ambrosia, R., and Dabezies, E. J.: The small pin circular fixator for proximal tibial fractures with soft tissue compromise. Orthopedics, 14:273–280, 1991.
761. Musculo, D., and Pacias, E.: (Treatment of fractures of the tibial tuberosities.) Rev. Ortop. Traumatol., 22:8–11, 1952.
762. Myint, K., Igbal, Q., and Kanagasunthereram, R.: Common peroneal nerve palsy due to posterolateral displacement of

fractured lateral tibial plateau. Med. J. Malaysia, 35:61–63, 1980.
This case report involves a split compression fracture with immediate peroneal nerve palsy. At surgery, the nerve was noted to be stretched around the displaced split fragment. Nerve recovery was noted after 1 year.

763. Nael, J. F.: Étude des Indications, Therapeutics et die Pronostic des Fractures des Plateaux Tibiaux a Propos d'une Serie de 132 Cas. Paris, Thesis, 1980.
764. Nael, J. F., Apoil, A., Koechlin, P., et al: Anatomie pathologique et indications therapeutiques des fractures des plateaux tibiaux: À propos d'une series de 132 cas. Ann. Chir., 36:5–12, 1982.
765. Naficy: Contribution à l'Étude Bibliographique des Fractures du Plateau Tibial et Reduction Therapeutique. Paris, Thesis, 1957.
766. Nagy, E.: Advantage of tomography in the estimation of the site and extent of tibial head fractures. Magy Traumatol. Orthop. Helyreallite Sebesz., 28:234–243, 1985.
767. Namba, R. S., Kabo, J. M., Dorey, F. J., and Meals, R. A.: Continuous passive motion versus immobilization: The effect on posttraumatic joint stiffness. Clin. Orthop., 267:218–223, 1991.
Rabbits' ankles were penetrated by Steinmann pins to create intra-articular injuries. One ankle was immobilized, the other was placed in a continuous passive motion (CPM) machine for 3 weeks. At 3 weeks there was no increased stiffness in the knees treated with CPM, but the immobilized knees were 2.6 times as stiff compared with preinjury stiffness.
768. Neviaser, J. S., and Eisenberg, S. A.: Diagnostic and therapeutic obstacles encountered in tibial plateau fractures. Bull. Hosp. Jt. Dis., 17:48–57, 1956.
The authors provide a general review of diagnostic and therapeutic problems encountered in the treatment of plateau fractures.
769. Newberg, A. H.: Computed tomography of joint injuries. Radiol. Clin. North Am., 28:445–460, 1990.
The author relies on high-quality computed tomography scanning for evaluation of tibial plateau fractures and others.
770. Newberg, A. H., and Greenstein, R.: Radiographic evaluation of tibial plateau fractures. Radiology, 126:319–323, 1978.
The authors propose tomography as the best method of demonstrating the extent and severity of a plateau fracture.
771. Ney, H. R.: (New clamp and unusual screw for reposition and fixation of fractures of the tibial head.) Chirurg., 26:334–335, 1955.
772. Nicolet, A.: Die meniscus verletzung bei tibiakopffrakturen. Langenbecks Arch. Klin. Chir., 313:544–549, 1965.
The author performed pneumoarthrograms after plateau fractures were healed. Meniscal problems were noted in approximately 40%. He concluded that arthrotomy might be indicated because of the incidence of meniscal problems.
773. Nicosi, A. V., and Parenti, G.: La fratture di piatto tibiale: Terapia chiruregia e recupero funzionale. Osp. Ital. Chir., 4:157, 1961.
774. Niederle, B.: Zentralbl. Chir., 78:554, 1953.
775. Niederle, B., and Vlcek, J.: (Fractures of the tibial condyle.) Rozhl Chir., 31:185–200, 1952.
776. Niethard, F. U., and Plaue, R.: (Experimental investigations regarding the limitations of radiological demonstration of fractures of the head of the tibia.) Fortschr. Geb. Roentgenstr. Nuklearmed. Erganzungsbd., 125:136–140, 1976.
777. Niethard, F. U., and Plaue, R.: Rontgenologische und morphologischen untersuchungen am experimentall erzeugten scheinbeinkopfbruchen. Arch. Orthop. Unfallchir., 85:71–80, 1976.
The authors produced plateau fractures in the knees of 12 cadavers using only axial loading. Local compression and split compression fractures were produced and illustrated.
778. Niethard, F. U., and Plaue, R.: Experimentelle untersuchunsen zur belastbarkeit typischer formen des scheinbeinkopfbruches. Orthop. Praxis, 10:764–768, 1977.
779. Noesberger, B., Lehmann, A., and Ganz, R.: Die rekonstruktion des tibiaplateaus. Hefte Unfallheilk., 126:281–283, 1975.
The authors discuss osteotomy and various methods to substitute for the articular surface.
780. Noesberger, B., Lehmann, A., and Ganz, R.: Die rekonstruktion des tibiaplateaus. Z. Unfallmed. Berufskr., 69:92–95, 1976.
The authors briefly discuss osteotomy and various articular substitutes to treat severe plateau fractures.
781. Nonnemann, H.: Die federosteosynthese nach maatz bei tibiakopffrakturen. Zentralbl. Chir., 95:729–739, 1970.
782. Novachenko, N. P.: (Fractures of the tibial tuberosities.) Ortop. Travmatol., 9:51–63, 1935.
783. Novello, A., and Gasparetto, G.: (Considerations on fractures of the tibial plateau.) Chir. Ital., 3(Suppl.):100, 1967.
784. Novikov, N.: (Treatment tactics in fractures of the tibial condyle combined with injuries to the menisci.) Ortop. Travmatol. Protez., 33:17–21, 1972.
The author recommends meniscectomy prior to osteosynthesis because of the frequency of meniscal injury. The results were generally good.
785. Nuboer, J. F.: Fractura condyli tibiae. Ned. Tijdschr. Geneeskd., 78:5768, 1934.
786. Nyga, W.: Tibiakopffrakturen behandlung. Ergebnisse. Chir. Praxis, 14:291, 1970.
787. O'Donoghue, D.: Chondral and osteochondral fractures. J. Trauma, 6:469–480, 1966.
788. O'Dwyer, K. J., and Bobic, V. R.: Arthroscopic management of tibial plateau fractures. Injury, 23:261–264, 1992.
The author treated eight plateau fractures by arthroscopic-guided internal fixation. Two fractures were only inspected and washed out. Most of the results were good, and seven cases were reviewed after a mean of 38 months. The only complication was one case of deep venous thrombosis that was confirmed by venography. The authors concluded that local compression fractures were not suitable because bone grafting was needed.
789. Oenicke, K. F.: Ein fall von compressionsfraktur des oberen tibiaendes. Griefswald, Inaugural Dissertation, 1888.
790. Ohashi, T.: (Fractures of the tibial condyles.) Saigai Igaku, 9:706–718, 1966.
791. Olaussen, T.: Intraarticular fractures in the upper end of the tibia and lower end of the femur. Acta Chir. Scand., 84:407–428, 1946.
The author treated 51 proximal tibial fractures, and the results were good in most cases. Bad results were due to knee instability.
792. Olerud, S.: Osteotomy on the tibial tuberosity in fractures of the tibial condyle. Acta Orthop. Scand., 42:432–435, 1971.
The author used a tibial tubercle osteotomy, reflecting the patellar mechanism proximally, to expose the articular surfaces for reduction in two cases. Reattachment was done by using a screw and wire.
793. Oleson, V.: (Therapy of tibial condyle fractures by operative reduction and screw osteosynthesis.) Ugeskr. Laeger, 117:644–647, 1955.
794. Ollerenshaw: Articular fractures of the knee. B.M.J., 20:9, 1930.
795. Oprandi, C., and Sette, F.: Fratture del piatto tibiale. Clin. Ortop., 13:563, 1961.
796. Orfanou, N.: Il Nostro metodo per il trattamento delle fratture della extremita prossimale della tibia. Ortop. Travmatol. Protez, 9:68, 1964.
797. Ostapowicz, G.: (Fracture of the lower leg.) Dtsch. Gesundh., 16:170–183, 1961.
798. Osterland: Spontanfrakturen bei soldaten nach reichsheilbeobachtungen. Arch. Klin. Chir., 179:567–588, 1934.
799. Otnes, W.: Traitement des fractures bi-condyliennes en Y. Norsk Mag. Laegevidenskapen, 97:169–172, 1936.
800. Ott, W., and Tschui, E.: Zur behandlung von frakturen im bereich des kniegelenkes. Helv. Chir. Acta, 26:583–587, 1959.
801. Ottolenghi, C.: Vascular complications in injuries about the knee joint. Clin. Orthop., 165:148–156, 1982.
The author reviewed 1377 severe knee injuries and noted 28 vascular complications: Fifteen were in the 387 plateau fractures (3.8%).
802. Paal, E.: Ein fall von traumatische (subcutaner) epiphysenlosung oberen tibiaende. Arch. Orthop. Chir., 31:399–402, 1932.
803. Paas, H. R.: Erreurs de diagnostic radiologique dans les fractures intra-articulaires de lat tête tibiale. Zentralbl. Chir., 65:2097–2098, 1938.
This brief discussion is about the diagnosis and closed reduction of plateau fractures.
804. Pachner, E.: Esiti di fratture articolari dell'epifisi superiore della tibia. Arch. Ortop., 50:1115–1134, 1934.
805. Padanilam, T. G., Ebraheim, N. A., and Frogameni, A.:

Meniscal detachment to approach lateral tibial plateau fractures. Clin. Orthop., 314:192–198, 1995.
The authors evaluated 18 patients over an average of 13 months after open treatment of lateral plateau fractures in which the meniscus was detached and repaired anteriorly. No patient had meniscal symptoms, and the five patients who had a late arthroscopic examination showed healing. The results were excellent in 13 patients and good in five patients. The exposure was safe and excellent.

806. Padeano: L'Osteosynthèse par Cadrage des Fractures des Plateaux Tibiaux. Paris, Thesis, 1964.
807. Paezer, E.: Chirurg., 309, 1935.
808. Palagi, P.: Sopra un caso di frattura indiretta dei condyli tibiali tratata con l'osteosintes precoce. Atti d. Accad. Med. Fis. Firenze, 30, 1912.
809. Palmer, I.: Nord. Med. Tidsskr., 556, 1938.
810. Palmer, I.: Compression fractures of the lateral tibial condyle and their treatment. J. Bone Joint Surg., 21:674–680, 1939.
The author concluded that the only way to reduce compression fractures was surgery. Os purum was used to fill defects under the elevated plateau. Early knee motion was instituted with late weight-bearing.
811. Palmer, I.: Fractures of the upper end of the tibia. J. Bone Joint Surg., 33B:160–166, 1951.
The author discusses the classification, treatment indications, surgical technique, and results in three patients. He advocates meniscal repair.
812. Palmer, I.: Z. Org. Ges. Chir., 123:252, 1952.
813. Pankovich, A.: Arthroscopic management of tibial plateau fractures (Letter). Arthroscopy, 2:132–134, 1986.
This letter is critical of Jenning's article on the arthroscopic treatment of plateau fractures.
814. Parisien, J. S.: The role of arthroscopy in the treatment of postoperative fibroarthrosis of the knee joint. Clin. Orthop., 229:185–192, 1988.
The author treated 21 knees with postoperative arthrofibrosis after previous surgery. He used arthroscopic lysis of adhesions and manipulation and noted that 12 of 21 had more than 120 degrees of motion. Six of eight had no further extensor lag. He concluded that arthroscopy was useful in adhesion lysis.
815. Patania, A., and Rapisarda, P.: Risultati nelle fratture del piatto tibiale trattate con avvitamento. Minerva Ortop., 18:409–415, 1967.
The author used a Lippman screw in 21 open reductions.
816. Paterson, D.: The international documentation and evaluation system (IDES). Orthop., 16:11–14, 1993.
The author gives the background and philosophy of a universal system of documentation and evaluation of results in orthopedics.
817. Pawlik, Z.: (Results of the treatment of fractures of the proximal end of the tibia.) Chir. Narzadow Ruchu Ortop. Pol., 53:307–312, 1988.
818. Peraire: Paris Chirurg., 14:107, 1922.
819. Perey, O.: Depression fractures of the lateral tibial condyle. Acta Chir. Scand., 103:154–157, 1952.
The author treated 103 plateau fractures and followed 30 patients who had been operated on using cortical grafts to prop up the plateau.
820. Perkins, G.: Zentralbl. Chir., 678, 1947.
821. Perry, C. R., Evans, L. G., Rice, S., et al: A new surgical approach to fractures of the lateral tibial plateau. J. Bone Joint Surg., 66A:1236–1240, 1984.
The author describes the inframeniscal approach and adds transection of the anterior portion of the lateral meniscus for improved visualization.
822. Persch, W. F., and Birkner, H.: Erkennung, einteilung, diagnostik und begutachtung von tibiakopfbruchen. Monatsschr. Unfallheilk., 78:315–320, 1975.
823. Persich, G., and Retta, G.: Considerazioni statistico dinamiche sul carico negli esiti di frattura del piatto tibiale. Minerva Ortop., 18:359–363, 1967.
The authors discuss biomechanics as it pertains to the treatment of plateau fractures.
824. Pfaehler, E.: Zur behandlung von tibiakopfbruchen auf grund von 179 fallen aus dem krankengut der schweizerischen unfallversicherungsanstalt der jahre 1950–1954. Z. Unfallmedd. Berufskr., 55:325–360, 1962.
825. Picard, J. J.: Forme particulière de calvicieux de l'extrémité supérieure du tibia. Montpellier Chir., 14:164–166, 1957.
826. Picard, J. J., and Rapp, P. E.: Fracture de l'epiphyse tibiale supérieure avec troubles vasculaires. Rev. Orthop., 44:102–106, 1958.
827. Picque, L.: Fracture cuneiforme de l'extrémité supérieure du tibia. Bull. Soc. Anat. Paris, 58:524–526, 1883.
This case report is about a very unstable plateau fracture. The patient died, and the fracture was later identified as a comminuted fracture.
828. Piercey, M.: Tibial plateau fracture. Nurse Pract., 3:40, 1978.
This case report illustrates the diagnosis of a fracture.
829. Pierra, C.: (Comminuted fractures of the upper end of the tibia with posterior-internal luxation of the knee; reduction by resection and nailing.) Case report. Mem. Acad. Chir., 79:104–107, 1953.
830. Pietu, G.: (Triplane fractures of the head of the tibia. (A propos of 2 cases). Rev. Chir. Orthop., 77:121–124, 1991.
831. Pilih, R.: An armature made of Kirschner's wires in the reconstruction of compressions of the plateau of the tibial condyle. Acta Chir. Iugosl., 31:33–38, 1984.
832. Pillet, J.: Fractures du plateau tibial externe chéz les sujets de plus de cinquante ans. J. Chir. (Paris), 75:72–86, 1958.
833. Pineiro Sorondo, J., and Ferre, R. L.: (Fractures of the external tuberosity of the tibia.) Rev. Asoc. Med. Argent., 59:1057–1061, 1945.
834. Pineiro Sorondo, J., and Ferre, R. L.: (Surgical therapy of fractures of the external tuberosity at the knee.) Bol. Soc. Arg. Cir., 6:540–551, 1945.
835. Pino, A. E.: The role of arthroscopy in the diagnosis and treatment of fractures about the knee (Abstract). Orthop. Trans., 10:633, 1986.
The author treated eight plateau fractures percutaneously using arthroscopic fracture visualization. The results were generally good, and the method was recommended.
836. Piotet, G.: Traitement des fractures de l'epiphyse supérieure du tibia avec dislocation des condyles tibiaux. Rev. Med. Suisse Romande, 54:455–462, 1934.
837. Pique, J. A.: (Bone grafts in fractures of the tibial tuberosities.) Rev. Asoc. Med. Argent., 64:302–305, 1950.
838. Pique, J. A.: Z. Org. Ges. Chir., 118:429, 1951.
839. Pironneau, A.: Les Fractures du Plateau Tibial Externe. Paris, Thesis, 1951.
The author reviews the literature and presents 19 plateau fractures treated by open reduction and bolt fixation.
840. Pironneau, A., and Gosset, J.: Le traitement chirurgical des fractures du plateau tibial externe avec separation et enfoncement. Semin. Hôp. Paris, 27:55–56, 1951.
841. Pisani, A. J.: New type of fastener for joint separations and oblique fractures. Am. J. Surg., 73:624–628, 1947.
842. Planes, A.: La Mobilisation Précoce et l'Extension Continue dans le Traitement des Fractures Articulaires de l'Extrémité supérieure du tibia. Bordeaux, Thesis, 1963.
843. Plaue, R.: Behandlung schwerer schienbeinkopfbruche durch patella implantation. Arch. Orthop. Unfallchir., 61:240–246, 1967.
Four severe compression plateau fractures were treated by articular replacement using the patella. The results were satisfactory after a short follow-up.
844. Plaue, R., and Niethard, F.: Experimentelle untersuchungen uber die grenzen der rontgenologischen darstellung von impressionsbruchen des tibia plateau. Hefte Unfallheilk, 126:224–225, 1975.
The authors recommend tomography for the diagnosis of the type of fracture and displacement based on experimental work.
845. Politis, A. M.: Les Fractures Fermées et Récentes du Plateau Tibial. Paris, Thesis, 1935.
846. Politis, A. M.: Sur le traitement des fractures du plateau tibial. Bull. Soc. Chir. de Marseille, 9:377, 1935.
847. Pollosson, E., and Violet: A propos des fractures du plateau tibial. Lyon Chir., 33:71–75, 1936.
848. Porter, B. B.: Treatment of fractures of the lateral tibial table (Abstract). J. Bone Joint Surg., 51B:569, 1962.
This abstract cites a study of 138 crush lateral plateau fractures to determine factors influencing results and indications for surgery.
849. Porter, B. B.: Crush fractures of the lateral tibial table. J. Bone Joint Surg., 52B:676–687, 1970.
The author studied 138 crush fractures of the lateral plateau and followed 66 patients for a minimum of 3 years (average of 6 years). Those patients with less than a 10-mm depression were

treated mainly by early movement, and 28 of 29 had satisfactory results. Of those with 10 mm or more, half were treated with the closed method and half with the open method. The patients who were operated on had much better results.

850. Porzelt: Uber compressionsfrakturen am kniegelenk. Bonn, Inaugural Dissertation, 1897.
851. Poshvin, V.: Lateral compression osteosynthesis in fractures of the condyles of the knee joint. Vestn. Khir., 106:93–94, 1971.
852. Postel, M., Mazas, E., and de la Caffiniere, J. Y.: Fractures separation posterieure des plateaux tibiaux. Rev. Chir. Orthop., 60(Suppl. II):317–323, 1974.
The authors draw attention to the coronal plane split type of fractures and some complex bicondylar configurations.
853. Potapov, V.: Functional treatment of intra-articular fractures of the knee. Sov. Med., 1:81–83, 1988.
854. Potherat, E.: Fracture isolée de la tuberosité externe du tibia de cause indirecte. Bull. Mem. Soc. Chir. Paris, 32:140, 1906.
This case report discusses a 56 year old with a lateral plateau fracture.
855. Potherat, E.: Fracture de la tête du pérone avec fracture communicative de la tuberosité externe du tibia. Bull. Mem. Soc. Chir. Paris, 1919.
856. Poulsen, J. O., and Tophoj, K.: Konservativ behandling af tibiakondylfrakturer. Nord. Med., 82:1243–1246, 1969.
This follow-up study involves 47 plateau fractures that are mainly treated with the closed method. Only eight fractures were operated on. The authors found no evidence that joint incongruity invariably led to traumatic arthritis.
857. Pouyanne, L.: Grave fracture des plateaux tibiaux traitée par extension continue associée à la compression latérale. Bordeaux Chir., 4:181, 1963.
858. Pouyanne, L., and Honton, L.: Consequences artérielles des fractures de l'extrémité supérieure du tibia. Bordeaux Chir., 2:74–76, 1963.
859. Power, D.: Simple comminuted fracture of the head of the tibia. Tr. Path. Soc. London, 39:237, 1887.
860. Prestat, J.: Les Fractures des Plateaux Tibiaux. Nancy, Thesis, 1955.
861. Primo, G.: Traitement opératoire des fractures du plateau tibial. Acta Chir. Belg., 52:720–735, 1953.
862. Putz, P., Gebhaert, M., and Bremen, J.: (The treatment of fractures of the tibial condyles.) Acta Orthop. Belg., 54:465–473, 1988.
The authors treated 95 plateau fractures by either closed or open treatment. The results indicated that anatomic reconstruction with fixation and early mobilization produced the best results.
863. Quenee, and Quenee: Fracture parcellaire et médiane du plateau tibial: Blocage permanent en demi-flexion. Echo Med. du Nord, 38:20, 1935.
864. Rafii, M., Firooznia, H., Golimbu, C., and Bonamo, J.: Computed tomography of tibial plateau fractures. Am. J. Roent., 142:1181–1186, 1984.
The authors studied 20 plateau fractures by x-ray and also by computed tomography (CT) scans. The CT scan gave much more information about the fracture and altered treatment planning.
865. Rafii, M., Lamont, J., and Firooznia, H.: Tibial plateau fractures: CT evaluation and classification. Crit. Rev. Diagn. Imaging, 27:91–112, 1987.
The authors noted that the fat level may be seen on a horizontal lateral x-ray when there is bloody effusion. They also noted that tomography needs to be in both the arteroposterior and lateral planes, but computed tomography is easier on the patient and gives more accurate spatial information.
866. Rangitsch, M. R., Duwelius, P. J., and Colville, M. R.: Limited internal fixation of tibial plateau fractures: A prospective protocol. Orthop. Trans., 18:9, 1993.
Sixty-three plateau fractures were treated using instability as the reason for surgery. There were 23 C3 fractures, 18 B3 fractures, and 22 lesser fractures. Acceptable results were obtained in all unoperated patients and in 87% of those operated on. Nineteen patients had arthroscopic inspection. The complication rate was 7%, and there were no infections. Poor outcomes occurred in the C3 fractures.
867. Rappold, G.: (Traumatic lesions of the proximal tibial epiphysis.) Unfallchirurg., 18:154–161, 1992.
The authors studied 36 proximal tibial epiphyseal fractures in children of an average age of 13 years. The fractures were associated with medial ligament and anterior cruciate ligament injuries. Premature epiphyseal closure occurred in three patients.
868. Rasheed, M.: Tibial Plateau Fractures. Ain Shams, Egypt, Thesis, 1984.
This comprehensive thesis contains a review of anatomy, biomechanics, diagnosis, treatment, and results of treatment of plateau fractures.
869. Rasmussen, P. S.: Lateral condylar fracture of the tibia (Abstract). Acta Orthop. Scand., 42:429, 1971.
The author suggests that his study of plateau fractures has led him to use clinical findings of stability as an indication for surgery rather than displacement as noted by x-ray.
870. Rasmussen, P. S.: A Functional Approach to Evaluation and Treatment of Tibial Condylar Fractures. Gothenburg, Sweden, Thesis, 1971.
871. Rasmussen, P. S.: Tibial condylar fractures as a cause of degenerative arthritis. Acta Orthop. Scand., 43:566–575, 1972.
The author studied 260 plateau fractures and followed 204 patients for 4 to 11 years (7.3 years). He took x-rays of both knees in 162 patients. Ahlback's criteria for arthritis were used with special emphasis on standing joint narrowing to indicate arthritis. Cases of arthritis were divided into none, doubtful, moderate, and severe. Twenty-one percent of cases had arthritic change in the injured knee, and only 2% had arthritic change in the uninjured knee. Varus deformity and instability in extension were major factors in arthritis.
872. Rasmussen, P. S.: Gonarthrose nach tibiakopffrakturen. Z. Orthop., 111:509–512, 1973.
The author followed 192 plateau fractures and found moderate to severe arthritis with varus deformity, instability in full extension, and in bicondylar fractures. There was very little correlation with age or with local compression fractures. The author believes that biomechanical problems are responsible for the arthritic condition.
873. Rasmussen, P. S.: Tibial condylar fractures. J. Bone Joint Surg., 55A:1331–1350, 1973.
The author studied 260 plateau fractures using instability of 10 degrees or more as tested in full extension as the indication for surgery. Eighty-seven percent had acceptable function, and arthritis was noted in 17%.
874. Rasmussen, P. S., and Sorensen, S.: Tibial condylar fractures: Non-operative treatment of lateral compression fractures without impairment of knee-joint stability. Injury, 4:265–271, 1973.
The authors studied 40 local compression fractures that were usually stable in extension despite a depression of 5 to 20 mm. All were treated by early motion and weight-bearing after a few weeks. Further depression was rare. The results were excellent in 21 cases, good in nine cases, and fair in two cases.
875. Rehbein, F., and Busse, K. A.: Gesichtspunkte fur die behandlung der scheinbeinkopfbruche. Chirurg., 20:118–132, 1949.
The authors treated 36 plateau fractures—15 with open reduction and internal fixation and 21 closed. They did a follow-up of half of the patients for 19 years. Drawings are used to document the results.
876. Rehbein, F., and Busse, K. A.: (Screwing of fractures of the head of the tibia.) Beitr., 180:409–418, 1950.
877. Rehn, J.: Die operative behandlung der scheinbeinkopfbruche. Zentralbl. Chir., 102:905–911, 1977.
The author suggested that open treatment should bring stability to the fracture. He recommended grafts of spongy bone for compression fractures.
878. Rehn, J., and Willenegger, H.: Indikationen zur konservativen und operativen knochenbruchbehandlung. Langenbecks Arch. Chir., 337:389–397, 1974.
Of 220 plateau fractures treated, 159 were followed. One hundred and two plateau fractures were treated by the closed method and 57 by the AO method of open reduction and internal fixation (ORIF). Of closed cases, 63% were satisfactory, and 84% of ORIF were satisfactory. The authors advocated closed treatment for very complex fractures. They use ORIF only when results are better than with closed treatment.
879. Reibel, D. B., and Wade, P. A.: Fractures of the tibial plateau. J. Trauma, 2:337–352, 1962.
The authors studied 120 plateau fractures of which 92 were treated by the closed method, often with a hinged cast. Some had early motion. Open reduction was performed in 28 patients, and one half were started on early motion. Hinged casts were used for suspension or traction. Early motion was the key to good results.
880. Reiner, M. J.: The arthroscope in tibial plateau fractures: Its use in evaluation of soft tissue and bony injury. J. Am. Osteopath. Assoc. 81:704–705, 1982.

The author describes three plateau fractures that were visualized through the arthroscope. The joint was only inspected and irrigated.

881. Reiner, S., Rinott, M., and Kaufman, B.: Trans-arthroscopic monitoring of reduction and percutaneous internal fixation of minimally displaced intraarticular fractures about the knee (Abstract). Orthop. Trans., 10:98, 1986.
The authors reported on four plateau fractures that were visualized arthroscopically and internally fixed using Steinman pins or percutaneous screws with immediate knee movement. No complications were noted.
882. Renard, J.: Devenir à Plus de Huit Ans de Recul des Fractures des Plateaux Tibiaux Traitées par Traction-mobilisation Immédiate. Lyon, Thesis, 1978.
883. Reschauer, R.: Zur problematik der operativen versorgung der tibiakopffrakturen. Congressber. Oester. Ges. f. Chir., 1979.
884. Rhinelander, F. W.: Minimal internal fixation of tibial fractures. Clin. Orthop., 107:188–220, 1975.
The author describes a percutaneous technique of plateau fracture treatment using wires and pins.
885. Ricchioni, L.: Considerazioni sui risultati del trattamento delle fratture del piatto tibiale. Clin. Ortop., 15:268, 1963.
886. Riccio, L.: Lesioni meniscali associate a fratture del plateau tibiale. Orizz. Ortop. Odierna e Riabilit., 3:235–244, 1958.
887. Rich, C., and Dabezies, E. J.: Tibial plateau fractures. Orthopedics, 10:1455–1458, 1987.
This case report involves a split compression fracture that was treated by reduction, graft, and screw fixation. The authors briefly review the treatment for all types of plateau fractures.
888. Richard: Lyon Chirurg., Sep. 1929.
889. Richet: Fracture incomplète de l'extrémité supérieure du tibia. France Med., 27:169–170, 1880.
An autopsy report is given of a young man who sustained serious bone and soft tissue injuries and had an amputation. Dissection of the specimen showed a medial total condylar depression fracture with rupture of the lateral capsule and ligament.
890. Richter, H., and Hofer, D.: Unsere erfahrungen in der unterfutterung der tibiakopfimpressionen mit heteroplastischer spongiosa. Mschr. Unfallheilk., 72:311–316, 1969.
The authors operated on 75 compression types of plateau fractures, pushing the fragments up from the opposite side and using bank bone grafts. They followed 59 patients of whom 54% had good results, 29% had fair results, and 17% had poor results. The results were better with split and impression fractures.
891. Ricklin: Helv. Chir. Acta, 9:96, 1958.
892. Riedl, H.: Eine seltene kompressionsfraktur der tibia. Mschr. Unfallheilk., 14:229–233, 1907.
The author reported a split compression fracture that was irreducible by closed means and was operated only to find a wedge of depressed bone that, when disimpacted and elevated, allowed reduction. The second reported open reduction.
893. Riedl, H.: Verrentrungsbruch des oberen scheinbein mit erhaltung des wadenbeins eine typische verletzung. Zentralbl. Chir., 42:33–41, 1915.
This case report involves a bicondylar displaced fracture that was treated surgically due to the failure of closed reduction. A good result was obtained and illustrated.
894. Ries, M. D., and Meinhard, B. P.: Medial external fixation with lateral plate internal fixation in metaphyseal tibia fractures: A report of 8 cases associated with severe soft tissue injury. Clin. Orthop., 256:215–223, 1990.
The authors treated six plateau fractures by half pin external fixation. Five of the six were open fractures. There was one infection and two compartment syndromes. All healed with a range of at least 110 degrees.
895. Rieunau, G.: Les Fractures de l'Extrémité Supérieure du Tibia avec Subluxation et Accrochage Condylien. Toulouse, Medical Thesis, 1971.
896. Rieunau, G., Ficat, P., Utheza, G., and Chandeclerc, D.: Le traitement des fractures articulaires de l'extrémité supérieure du tibia. Rev. Chir. Orthop., 57:209–218, 1971.
897. Rinaldi, C., and Vacirca, M.: Le fratture del piatto tibiale. Arch. Putti, 17:470–490, 1962.
898. Rinonapoli, E.: Modalita di trattamento nei vari tipi di fratture del piatto tibiale. Boll. Mem. Soc. Tosco-Umbra Chir., 20:801–817, 1959.
899. Rinonapoli, E.: Le lesioni del menisco nelle fratture del piatto tibiale. Arch. Putti Chir. Organi Mov., 16:319–334, 1962.
Meniscus lesions were identified in 86% of 101 operated plateau fractures. The author believes that scar tissue may hold torn menisci to prevent locking in nonoperated plateau fractures. He advises open reduction to care for meniscal lesions.
900. Rinonapoli, E.: (Studies on the treatment of fractures of the tibial plateau.) Minerva Ortop., 18:381–383, 1967.
901. Rinonapoli, E., and Aglietti, P.: (Comparison of treatment by open and closed reduction of comparable cases of articular fractures of the proximal tibia.) Ital. J. Orthop. Traumatol., 3(Suppl.):99–116, 1977.
The authors used Insall's evaluation in 128 plateau fractures treated. Fractures minimally displaced (42) were satisfactory in 93%. Displaced fractures (35) treated with closed reduction had 63% satisfactory results, whereas those treated with the open method had 73% satisfactory results. Instability was found in 45%, and deformity was present in 41%.
902. Rivington: Fracture of the external tuberosity of the tibia. B.M.J., 2:654, 1872.
This case report involves a 60 year old who fell. Crepitus and swelling were noted, and the treatment was by ice applications.
903. Roberts, J. M.: Fractures of the condyles of the tibia. J. Bone Joint Surg., 50A:1505–1521, 1968.
The authors classified 230 plateau fractures into nondisplaced, local compression, or displaced fractures with knee instability. Fifty-six were bicondylar; 141 were lateral; and 33 were medial. Ligament tears were noted in 17 cases; two medial collateral ligaments were repaired, but nine were not. The authors followed 100 patients and concluded that open reduction should be done in displaced unstable fractures followed by early knee motion.
904. Robin: Lyon Med., 128:391, 1919.
905. Rocher, H. L., and Souchet: Fracture des deux extrémitiés supérieures tibiales. J. Med. Bordeaux, 41:809, 1911.
906. Roffi, R. P., and Merritt, P. O.: Total knee replacement after fractures about the knee. Orthop. Rev., 19:614–620, 1990.
The authors performed knee replacement for traumatic arthritis after knee fractures. Problems to be anticipated are the posterior tibial tilt. The results are similar to revisions rather than primary replacements.
907. Rohan, C.: Fracture des plateaux tibiaux sans tendance à la consolidation traitée par greffe tibiale. Lyon Med., 41:457–458, 1946.
908. Rohrbeck, R., and Troeger, H.: (Tibial plateau fractures—Indications for and results of surgical and functional-conservative therapy.) Beitr. Orthop. Traumatol., 37:148–157, 1990.
The authors treated 56 patients with tibial plateau fractures. They treated one-third operatively and two-thirds nonoperatively. They followed patients clinically and radiographically.
909. Rolfi, D.: Algunas consideraciones sobra la frattura de les platillos tibiale. Arch. Ortop. Traumat., 4:217, 1951.
910. Rombold, S.: Depressed fractures of the tibial plateau. J. Bone Joint Surg., 42A:783–797, 1960.
The author operated on one half of plateau fractures seen, primarily only those with significant deformity. Indications were more than 5 mm of depression, 1 cm of horizontal displacement, or more than 5 degrees of deformity. The author used contoured plates on each side for bicondylar fractures to achieve stability. The author believed that converting an unstable or deformed fracture to a stable one and starting movement was the best approach.
911. Roques, P.: Fracture du plateau tibial externe (tassement central en ecuelle) traitée par reposition sanglante et greffe osseuse fixee par une synthèse metallique. Soc. Nat. Chir., 61:1146–1155, 1935.
A 35-year-old man fell onto his flexed knee. Stress testing showed knee instability. Open reduction and internal fixation was performed with elevation, grafting, screw fixation, and meniscectomy with a good result.
912. Roques, P.: Fracture marginale du plateau tibial interne; reduction sanglante et greffes. Bull. Soc. Chir. Marseille, 10:206, 1936.
913. Ruedi, T.: Die operative behandlung der tibiakopfbruche. Hefte Unfallheilk., 126:248–253, 1976.
The author discusses indications and techniques for open reduction and fixation of plateau fractures, emphasizing the use of plates and cancellous screws. The author also suggested to begin knee motion the day after surgery for the best results.

914. Ruf, P.: Beitrag zur behandlung der schienbeinkopfbruche. Mschr. Unfallheilk., 69:74–80, 1966.
The author reviewed 107 plateau fractures that were treated mainly by closed means. There were sufficient meniscal problems to suggest early open reduction and internal fixation and management of any meniscal problems noted.

915. Ruggieri, P., Biagini, R., Ruggieri, N., et al: Complex fractures of the tibial plateau. Chir. Organi Mov., 76:209–215, 1991.
From 142 plateau fractures, 48% were considered complex and treated surgically. The results were good or excellent in 69%. The most unfavorable prognostic factors were comminution of the fracture and residual widening of the tibia. Seven complications were noted.

916. Ruju, A.: Considerazioni sulle fratture del bordo posterior del piatto tibiale. Atti S.O.T.I.M.I., 8:12, 1963.

917. Ruther, A., and Burri, C.: Tibiakopffrakturen. Discussion. Hefte Unfallh., 120:145, 1975.

918. Ryd, L., and Tokevig-Larsen, S.: Stability of the elevated fragment in tibial plateau fractures: A radiographic stereophotogrammetric study of postoperative healing. Int. Orthop., 18:131–134, 1994.
The authors treated five split compression fractures by elevation, grafting, and screw fixation. They placed tantalum markers in the depressed fragment and in the metaphysis for x-ray analysis. They found that three of the five elevated fragments redepressed 2.8 mm in the first month despite non-weightbearing and a long leg cast.

919. Sabella, P.: Le fratture dell'extremo superiore della tibia. Policlinico, 18:745–749, 1911.

920. Sakakida, K.: Tibial condylar fractures: A followup study of 80 cases. J. Kyoto Pref. Univ. Med., 85:653–659, 1976.

921. Salacz, T., Manninger, J., and Fekete, K.: (Functional stability in the fixation of impression fractures of the tibial condyle using a modified bone plate. II. [8-year healing results in 105 cases].) Magy. Traumatol. Orthop., 25:243–255, 1982.
The authors followed 105 of 155 plateau fractures treated for 2 to 9 years after injury. Bicondylar fractures developed a lot of arthrosis. The authors noted that the better the fixation, the earlier movement could start and the better the result.

922. Salacz, T., Nemes, G., and Wagner, J.: (Postoperative treatment of knee ligament injuries using a hinged plaster cast.) Magy. Traumatol. Orthop., 27:199–203, 1984.

923. Salas Heredia, J.: (Callahan operation for fractures of the tibial plateau.) An. Med., 3:53–56, 1942.

924. Salem, G., and Wurnig, P.: Die gelenfrakturen am oberen tibiaende und ihre behandlung. Arch Orthop. Unfallchir., 45:600–616, 1953.

925. Salmon, M.: Affaisement traumatique du pilier antérieur tibial-genou recurvatum-subluxation postérieure du tibia-reduction greffe. Rev. Chir. Orthop., 47:109–110, 1961.

926. Salomon, D.: Uber fracturen am oberen ende der tibia. Arch. Klin. Chir., 99, 1912.

927. Salter, R. B., Hamilton, H. W., Wedge, J. H., et al: Clinical application of basic research on continuous passive motion for disorders and injuries of synovial joints. J. Orthop. Res., 1:325–342, 1984.
The authors reported on nine joint fractures treated by continuous passive motion, and they concluded that the method was well tolerated without untoward results.

928. Salter, R. B., Simmonds, D. F., Malcolm, B. W., et al: The biological effect of continuous passive motion on the healing of full thickness defects in articular cartilage. J. Bone Joint Surg., 62A:1232–1252, 1980.
The authors describe a new concept of continuous passive movement (CPM) of synovial joints in knee joints of rabbits compared with immobilization and intermittent active motion. Healing of articular defects was more rapid and complete with CPM compared with control immobilization or active movement.

929. Salvagni, A.: Particolare technica di riduzione di aleune fratture de piatto tibiale. Minerva Ortop., 10:1–5, 1959.

930. Salvi, V., Tos, L., and Tessore, A.: (Direct pressure on the skeleton according to the dentitala method in the treatment of fractures of the tibial plateau.) Minerva Ortop., 17:633–666, 1966.

931. Salvini, E., and Zucali, R.: (Roentgen cinematographic study of articulation mechanics of the knee in the sequelae of fractures of the tibial plateau.) Minerva Radiol., 12:70–71, 1967.

932. Sandberg, R., Balkfors, B., Nilsson, B., and Westlin, N.: Operative versus non-operative treatment of recent injuries to the ligaments of the knee. J. Bone Joint Surg., 69A:1120–1126, 1987.
A prospective randomized consecutive series of 200 patients with medial collateral ligament (MCL) or anterior cruciate ligament (ACL) injuries treated for 6 weeks in a cast. The MCLs did as well as those treated by operative suture. The ACLs were not good when treated in a cast.

933. Sandberg, R., Nilsson, B., and Westlin, N.: Hinged cast after knee ligament surgery. Am. J. Sports Med., 15:270–274, 1987.
The authors randomly studied 113 patients with knee ligament injuries in whom either a cast or a hinged cast was used. There was no difference in final stability, but patients who moved early had a shorter recovery time.

934. Sanders, R. W., Gregory, P., Jersinovich, I., and Koval, K.: The treatment of combined tibial plateau and shaft fractures: Is there still a role for plates and screws? Orthop. Trans., 18, 1995.
The authors used plates to treat 26 Schatzker VI bicondylar fractures. They recommend delaying surgery until the swelling goes down and avoiding a triradiate incision. Stable internal fixation and immediate postoperative motion produce good results. Twenty patients were followed for an average of 31 months. There was 90 degrees or more motion in 85%.

935. Sanguinetti, C., and DePalma, L.: (Indications in the treatment of tibial plateau fractures.) Arch. Putti Chir. Organi Mov., 32:275–282, 1982.

936. Sankhala, S. S., Gupta, S. P., Sharma, J. C., and Agarwal, S.: Tibial condylar fractures treated with traction and early mobilization (report on study of 75 cases). J. Indian Med. Assoc., 88:309–311, 1990.
The authors treated 75 plateau fractures, irrespective of type, by below-knee skin traction for 3 weeks in hospital and 5 to 9 weeks of traction-mobilization at home. Sixty-seven of 75 were satisfied subjectively, and 72 were acceptable results. They concluded that traction-mobilization is an acceptable treatment.

937. Santacroce, A.: Frattura bilaterale della superficie retrospinale della tibia. Clin. Ortop., 5:1, 1953.

938. Santo Tomas Cobos, E.: (Inveterate subluxation of the knee with fractures of the tibial shelf; arthroplasty.) Rev. Espana Cir. Traumatol. Ortop., 7:30–36, 1947.

939. Sardi, A.: Proporta di un metodo di pressore su filo per le reduzione e contenzione delle fratture del piatti tibiali. Minerva Ortop., 18:355–358, 1967.
The author describes a technique of passing wires through a cannula to maintain plateau fracture reduction.

940. Sarmiento, A., Kinman, P., and Latta, L.: Fractures of the proximal tibia and tibial condyles: A clinical and laboratory comparative study. Clin. Orthop., 145:136–145, 1979.
The authors studied 38 plateau fractures treated in the functional brace clinic. They used a cast for 3 weeks, then a brace. More condylar subsidence was noted in medial condyle fractures and bicondylar fractures when the fibula was intact. The authors did experimental studies on 40 cadavers' knees, and the results supported the clinical observations.

941. Savoie, F. H., and Vander Griend, R. A.: Tibial plateau fractures: Treatment using AO technique. Surg. Rounds Orthop., 1:25–32, 1987.
The authors discuss preoperative planning, exposures, fixation techniques, and postoperative care. Fifty-two plateau fractures that were treated by this method achieved 90% satisfactory results.

942. Savoie, F. H., Vander Griend, R. A., Ward, E. F., and Hughes, J. L.: Tibial plateau fractures: Treatment using AO technique. Orthopedics, 10:745–750, 1987.
The authors analysed 52 AO open reductions of 80 fractures. Continuous passive motion was used, and the results were satisfactory in 92% of the surgically treated group and in 66% of the traction–cast-brace group.

943. Scarfi, G., Bassi, P. B., and D'Arienzo, M.: (Fractures of the tibial plateau. Case studies.) Arch. Putti Chir. Organi Mov., 31:413–420, 1981.

944. Schafer, H.: Uber die operative behandlung von knockenbruchen. Z. Chir., 181:238–255, 1923.

945. Schall, O.: Behandlungmethoden und deren ergebnisse bei tibiakopfbruchen. Hamburg, 1938.

946. Scharf, S., and Christophidis, N.: Fractures of the tibial

plateau in the elderly as a cause of immobility. Aust. N. Z. J. Med., 24:725–726, 1994.

947. Schatzker, J.: Fractures of the tibial plateau. *In* Schatzker, J., and Tile, M. (Eds.): The Rationale of Operative Fracture Care. Berlin, Springer-Verlag, 1987.

948. Schatzker, J.: Anterior approach to the knee with osteotomy of the tibial tubercle for bicondylar tibial fractures (Letter). J. Bone Joint Surg., 70A:1575–1576, 1988.
This letter comments on the Fernandez tibial tubercle osteotomy for a comprehensive approach for plateau fractures. The author believed that it was risky to take up the tubercle in bicondylar or comminuted fractures because of the inability to refix solidily and also the likelihood of avascular changes. He instead recommends Z tenotomy of the patellar tendon. Fernandez replied that if all conditions for use are met, the procedure is successful.

949. Schatzker, J.: Fractures of the tibial plateau. *In* Chapman, M. (Ed.): Operative Orthopedics. Philadelphia, J.B. Lippincott, 1988.
Closed treatment is indicated if the joint is stable, alignment is good, and the joint is congruous; otherwise open reduction with accurate articular reduction and rigid internal fixation is indicated. Early motion is the key to a good result. He presents ideas about methyl methacrylate under plateaus.

950. Schatzker, J., McBrown, R., and Bruce, D.: The tibial plateau fracture. The Toronto experience. Clin. Orthop., 138:94–104, 1979.
The authors describe a new classification based on the AO, and they analyse each type of fracture in detail. AO treatment was used primarily. It was noted that experienced surgeons did best to obtain rigid fixation. Osteoporosis was a factor in obtaining fixation.

951. Schatzker, J., and Schulak, D. J.: Pseudoarthrosis of a tibial plateau fracture. Clin. Orthop., 145:146–149, 1979.
This case report involves an elderly patient with a medial plateau entire plateau depression type of fracture that was treated with 3 months of bedrest. The result was a 25-degree varus nonunion that was operatively corrected using anterior oblique fixation with healing and a good result.

952. Schautz, R.: Die wiederherstellung des tibiakopfes nach kompressions frakturen mit knochenspanen. Hefte Unfallheilk., 81:102–103, 1965.
The author discusses the timing of open reduction and techniques of closed reduction.

953. Schauwecker, F., and Weller, S.: Die operative behandlung der tibiakopf-und subkondylaren tibiafrakturen. Mschr. Unfallheilk., 73:114–126, 1970.
The authors describe the inframeniscal approach and the technique of open reduction. They recommend a postoperative exercise device.

954. Scheibe, G.: Vergleichende resultate konzervative und operative behandlung der scheinbeinkopfbruche. Zentralbl. Chir., 81:374–382, 1956.
Ninety-three plateau fractures were subclassified by when treated. Fractures treated before 1950 were mostly managed with closed treatment and a few with open treatment. Those seen after 1950 were treated with the closed method, since it produced better results.

955. Scherpe, O.: Uber frakturen der tibia am oberen ende. Leipzig, Inaugural Dissertation, 1903.
In this thesis, 16 plateau fractures are reported. Treatment was by plaster and bandaging with a variety of results.

956. Schindera, G.: Was wird aus unseren kniegelenksbruchen. Zentralbl. Chir., 64:112–114, 1937.
The author describes four operated plateau fractures.

957. Schioler, G.: Tibial condylar fractures with a particular view to the value of tomography. Acta Orthop. Scand., 42:462, 1971.
The author compares conventional radiography with tomography in plateau fractures and concludes that the diagnosis is incomplete without tomography.

958. Schmidt, G.: Operative treatment of tibial plateau fractures. Zentralbl. Chir., 65:613–614, 1938.
Operative approaches and techniques are described briefly. The Y incision and others were used. The author suggests immobilization for 4 to 9 weeks postoperatively.

959. Schmit-Neuerburg, K. P.: Zur behandlung des schienbeinkopfbruches. Actuel Traumatol., 2:101–108, 1972.
The author discusses surgical approaches and rigid techniques of fracture fixation using anterior oblique equipment.

960. Schneider, J.: Unsere technik bei der einrichtung schwer zu stellender tibiakopffrakturen. Zentralbl. Chir., 66:1613–1616, 1939.
The author used a device to impact fracture fragments during open reduction and internal fixation. Internal fixation was used. Two cases are described.

961. Schnepp, J.: Utilisation des platres pendants dans les fractures des plateaux tibiaux. Lyon Chir., 62:254–256, 1966.
The author used a below-knee cast with medial and lateral extensions to support the knee after a few days of traction.

962. Schnute, W.: Fractures of the tibial plateau (Abstract). J. Bone Joint Surg., 45A:432, 1963.
In this abstract, the author favors open reduction with early knee motion.

963. Schrecker: Z. Orthop., 86:547, 1907.
This case report involves a 38 year old with hemarthrosis that was treated by traction. The patient was seen at 12 months with 40% weakening of the knee.

964. Schuber, J.: Zur diagnostik begleitender seitenbandlasionen bei scheinbeinkopfbruchen. Münster, Medical Dissertation, 1981.

965. Schulak, D. J., and Gunn, D. R.: Fractures of the tibial plateaus: A review of the literature. Clin. Orthop., 109:166–177, 1975.
The authors reviewed literature concerning all of the problems of managing plateau fractures and concluded that early knee movement was the key to improved results and that in unstable fractures knee alignment must be secured and maintained.

966. Schulitz, K. P., and Dustmann, H. O.: Late complications following tibial head fractures. Hefte Unfallheilk., 126:318–321, 1975.

967. Schulitz, K. P., Dustmann, H. O., and Puhl, W.: Die entwicklung der posttraumatischen arthrose am beispiel des schienbeinkopfbruches. Arch. Orthop. Unfallchir., 77:136–148, 1973.
The authors followed 161 plateau fractures and noted that 50% had arthritis at 5 years. When motion was started within the first month or with younger patients, there was less arthritis. The type of fracture was not significant.

968. Schulze: Z. Orthop. Chir., 66:311, 1937.

969. Schurch: Unfallmed. Berufskr., 37:228, 1944.

970. Schutte: Ueber compressionsfrakturen am obern ende der tibia. Greifswald, Inaugural Dissertation, 1898.

971. Schwartzman, V., Martin, S. N., Ronquist, R. A., and Schwartzman, R.: Tibial fractures. The Ilizarov alternative. Clin. Orthop., 278:207–216, 1992.
The authors report on two plateau fractures treated by Ilizarov. The first was an open fracture that extended to the midshaft. Three weeks after the fracture, the Ilizarov alternative method was used for 2 months, then a cast-brace. There was some valgus deformity at the shaft fracture and 90 degrees of motion at follow-up.

972. Scotland, T. R., and Wardlaw, D.: The use of cast-bracing as treatment for fractures of the tibial plateau. J. Bone Joint Surg., 63B:575–582, 1981.
The authors treated 23 plateau fractures with a cast-brace. There were seven wedge, two bicondylar, and 20 compression fractures. Patients were allowed as much weight-bearing as possible. No change in valgus or varus occurred with use of the brace.

973. Scupola, G.: Contributo alla studio delle fratture rare del piatto tibiale. Clin. Ortop., 10:538, 1958.

974. Sebellin, O., and Lazzari, A.: L'osteosintesi nelle fratture recenta del piatto tibiale. Clin. Ortop., 16:206, 1964.

975. Sechehaye, L.: Les tassements unituberositaires du tibia. J. Chir., 45:561–590, 1935.

976. Segal, D., Franchi, A. V., and Campanile, J.: Iliac autograft for reconstruction of severely depressed fracture of a lateral tibial plateau: Brief note. J. Bone Joint Surg., 67A:1270–1272, 1985.
Two case reports are presented of severely depressed fractures of the lateral plateau that were replaced by the iliac crest held in place by a buttress plate. Postoperatively, the patient was placed in a cast-brace. The results were good.

977. Segal, D., Mallik, A. R., Wetzler, M. J., et al: Early weight bearing of lateral tibial plateau fractures. Clin. Orthop., 294:232–237, 1993.
This prospective study involves 134 consecutive plateau fractures. Operative treatment was used for more than 5 mm of depression or displacement. All had early motion and weight-

bearing in cast-brace. Local compression fractures did better with surgery. Early weight-bearing caused further depression of no more than 2 mm.

978. Segond, P.: Recherches cliniques et expérimentales sur les épanchements sanguins du genou par entorse. Progrès Med., 7:297–299, 1879.
In this experimental study, cadavers knees were subjected to lateral stress and hyperextension, which produced a few plateau fractures or ligament injuries.

979. Sever, J. W.: Fracture of tuberosities of the tibia: A report of three cases. Am. J. Orthop. Surg., 14:299–302, 1916.
Three plateau fractures were treated in a cast. The author in retrospect thought that open reduction might have produced better than fair results in one of the patients.

980. Sever, J. W.: Fractures of the tibial spine combined with fractures of the tuberosities of the tibia. Surg. Gynecol. Obstet., 35:558–564, 1922.
Eight plateau fractures in which the fracture lines extended into the region of the intercondylar notch are described, and a short follow-up is given noting knee instability.

981. Seyffarth, G., and Richter, J.: Die funktionnelle behandlung der tibiakopffrakturen. Zentralbl. Chir., 88:1973–1982, 1965.
The authors treated 17 plateau fractures by heel pin traction and mobilization on a fracture frame. Most patients were reported to be doing well.

982. Shelton, M. L., Neer, C. S., and Grantham, S. A.: Occult knee ligament ruptures associated with fractures. Trauma, 11:853–856, 1971.
Twenty-six patients with a variety of pelvic and lower extremity fractures were noted to have 34 knee ligament injuries. Eleven patients had plateau fractures.

983. Shimizu, T., Videman, T., Shimazaki, K., and Mooney, V.: Experimental study on the repair of full thickness articular cartilage defects: Effects of varying periods of continuous passive motion, cage activity, and immobilization. J. Orthop. Res., 5:187–197, 1987.
This short-term study of cartilage healing involves immobilized rabbits' knees and knees with passive motion or cage ambulation.

984. Shires, P. R.: Tibial condylar fractures: The late results of conservative treatment. Postgrad. Med. J., 40:543–548, 1964.
The author treated 115 plateau fractures and followed 40 for an average of 9 years. All were treated with the closed method, many by traction and early knee movement.

985. Shortley, H. F., and Tracey, J.: A study of the treatment of plateau fractures of the tibia. Milit. Med., 129:551–553, 1964.
The management and outcome of 27 plateau fractures are discussed. Seventeen of the 19 fractures treated with the closed method were satisfactory and five of eight open reductions did well except for one that became infected and was arthrodesed.

986. Shybut, G. T., and Spiegel, P. G.: Tibial plateau fractures (Editorial). *In* Symposium on Rigid Internal Fixation of Fractures. Clin. Orthop., 138:12–17, 1979.
This editorial is about the need for standardizing reporting and results of fracture series. A plea is made for a standard classification, such as Schatzker's classification.

987. Sierra Cano, L. de la, and Arguelles Blanco, M.: Tratamiento de las fracturas del condilo tibial externo. Cirugia del Appar. Locom., 9:48–56, 1952.

988. Sisk, T. D.: Autogenous patella transplantation for severe tibial plateau fractures. Jefferson Ortho., 9:23–28, 1980.
The author treated 13 plateau fractures with severe articular damage by using the lateral patellar facet as an articular surface replacement. The results were satisfactory in 12 of 13 patients after 9 years of follow-up.

989. Slee, G. C.: Fractures of the tibial condyles. J. Bone Joint Surg., 37B:427–437, 1955.
The author reviewed 60 plateau fractures of which 10 were operated on. The author proposed indications for operative treatment and cited the need to immobilize ligament injuries.

990. Smillie, I.: Injuries of the Knee Joint, 4th ed. Baltimore, Williams & Wilkins, 1970.

991. Smith, L.: A concealed injury of the knee. J. Bone Joint Surg., 44A:1659–1660, 1962.

992. Smith, S., Marsh, J. L., and Found, E. M.: External fixation for severe tibial plateau fractures. Orthop. Trans., 16:631, 1993.

993. Soderberg, L.: End results in conservatively treated compression fractures of the lateral tibial condyle. Acta Orthop. Scand., 29:49–58, 1959.

994. Solonen, K. A.: Fractures of the tibial condyles. Acta Orthop. Scand., 63(Suppl.):7–32, 1963.
The author followed 53 plateau fractures and analysed the results by type of fracture and treatment.

995. Sonntag, O.: Uber die fracturen am oberen ende der tibia. Bruns. Beitr. Klin. Chir., 1:430, 1906.
The author collected 34 compression fractures of the plateau.

996. Soupault, R.: L'Osteosynthèse dans les Fractures du Genou. Paris, Thesis, 1921.

997. Sovio, O. M., Boyle, M. R., and Meek, R. N.: Bicondylar tibial plateau fractures (Abstract). J. Bone Joint Surg., 68B:850, 1985.
This abstract involves treatment of bicondylar fractures with AO plate fixation. The authors noted that 22 of 28 with displacement and comminution did poorly despite early knee mobilization.

998. Sparano, V.: Contribution au traitement des fractures intra-articulaires du plateau tibial. Minerva Med., 49:3106–3108, 1958.

999. Specchia, L., Masetti, G., Montanari, G., and Sasbalat, S.: (Unreduced fractures of the tibial plateau: Surgical treatment.) Chir. Organi Mov., 73:323–327, 1988.

1000. Spier, W., and Burri, C.: Behandlungsprinzipien bei tibiakopffrakturen. Chirurg., 46:345–347, 1975.
The author discusses classification, approaches, and postoperative care.

1001. Spier, W., and Muggler, E.: (Injuries to the tibial plateau.) Langenbecks Arch. Chir., 345:409–414, 1977.
The authors studied two different series of plateau fractures, one with 163 and the other with 179 fractures. Each had a different percentage of open reduction and internal fixation (ORIF). The series with more ORIF (17%) did better than did the group with 6% ORIF. Buttress plates and early motion were recommended. The results were good in 91% of cases.

1002. Spigelman, L.: Positive pressure in the reduction of fractures of the tibial condyle: A preliminary report. J. Bone Joint Surg., 35A:696–700, 1953.
A Moore pin is inserted across the reduced large fragment of tibial plateau and bent to exert positive pressure as the bolt is tightened. Case reports are cited.

1003. Spina, G. M.: La fratture monocondeloide e de tibia e il loro trattamento cruente. Minerva Med., 16:333–340, 1961.

1004. Sprague, N. F., O'Connor, R. L., and Fox, J. M.: Arthroscopic treatment of postoperative knee fibroarthrosis. Clin. Orthop., 166:165–172, 1982.

1005. Sprengell, H.: Ergeb. Chir. Orthop., 34:397, 1943.

1006. Spring, R.: Spaetersebnisse der operativen therapie von tibiakopffrakturen. Helv. Chir. Acta, 43:437–438, 1976.
The author treated 238 plateau fractures, 163 with the open method and 75 with the closed method. The results are not discussed in any detail.

1007. Squazzini-Viscontini, C.: Clinical results of treatment of recent fractures of the tibial plateau. Minerva Ortop., 18:390–394, 1967.

1008. Stahel, R.: Zur beurteilung traumatischer intraartikularer veranderungen mit der roentgenschichtaufnahme. Helv. Chir. Acta, 39:339–345, 1972.
The author briefly describes advantages of tomography in the diagnosis of plateau fractures.

1009. Stainier, H.: Trajtment des fractures des plateaux tibiaux. Rev. Med. Liege, 18:730–737, 1963.

1010. Stallenberg, B., Gevenois, P. A., Sintzoff, S. A., et al: Fracture of the posterior aspect of the lateral tibial plateau: Radiographic sign of anterior cruciate ligament tear. Radiology, 187:821–825, 1993.
From 750 magnetic resonance knee studies, 25 with fresh anterior cruciate ligament injuries were studied. Eleven had fracture of the posterior lateral plateau, two had an impacted fracture of the lateral femoral condyle, three had a Segond fracture, and two had an avulsion of the tibial attachment of the anterior cruciate ligament. The frequency of posterolateral fracture makes this an indirect sign of an anterior cruciate ligament injury.

1011. Stamer, D. T., Schenk, R., Staggers, B., et al: Bicondylar tibial plateau fractures treated with a hybrid ring external fixator: A preliminary study. J. Orthop. Trauma, 8:455–461, 1994.
Twenty-three knees with Schatzker VI plateau fractures were treated with the hybrid ring external fixator with tension wires proximally and half pins distally. Six were open injuries. Eight also had limited open reduction. Thirteen had excellent results; three had good results; one had fair results; and six had poor results.

1012. Stamm, T. T.: Treatment of injuries. Proc. R. Soc. Med., 28:1047, 1935.

1013. Stanek, W. F.: Internal derangements and fractures involving the knee. J. Bone Joint Surg., 27:86–94, 1945.
The author reports on four soldiers who obtained inferior results after treatment that required their discharge from the service. There were two medial and two lateral plateau fractures.

1014. Stern, W. G., and Papurt, L. E.: Healing of the newer bumper fractures of the tibia. J.A.M.A., 105:2147–2150, 1935.
The author noted a change in fracture pattern from plateau to shaft as the bumper height decreased.

1015. Steuer, H. S.: Fractures of the tibia involving the knee. Ann. Surg., 89:580–590, 1929.
The author studied skeletons from the medical school and found 16 with plateau fractures. Photographs and diagrams of the fractures are presented.

1016. Stills, M., Christensen, K., and Bucholz, R.: Cast bracing of bicondylar tibial plateau fractures after combined internal and external fixation. J. Pros. Orthop., 3:106–113, 1991.

1017. Stocker: Zentralbl. Chir., 67:132, 1940.

1018. Stokel, E. A., and Sadasivan, K. K.: Tibial plateau fractures. Standardized evaluation of operative results. Orthopedics, 14:263–270, 1991.
One surgeon treated 20 patients operatively using AO techniques and classified the results using a 100-point rating system.

1019. Streli, R.: Zur therapie der tibiakopffrakturen neue kondylenplatte. Mschr. Unfallheilk., 73:127–146, 1970.
The author describes the technique employed in the use of a new condylar plate that is inserted under the articular surface and has perforations in it.

1020. Streli, R.: Gabelplatte bei scheinbeinkopfbruchen. Hefte Unfallheilk., 126:253–255, 1976.
The author describes a special broad-bladed plate for use in plateau fractures.

1021. Stropeni, L.: Contributo alla conoscenza delle fratture monocondyloidee della tibia con special regardo al loro meccanismo di produzione. Clin. Chir. Milano, 22:2315–2338, 1915.

1022. Struben, P. J.: The tibial plateau. J. Bone Joint Surg., 64B:336–339, 1982.
The author experimented with cadavers' knees and clay modeling of the articular surfaces. He concluded that the knee joint was a closed kinematic chain and that one component is dependent on the shape of the others.

1023. Stubenrauch: A propos du decollement épiphysaire traumatique de l'extrémité supérieure du tibia. Arch. Klin. Chir., 164:621–640, 1931.

1024. Stubinger, K.: Kniegelenksbruche. Zentralbl. Chir., 64:2490–2493, 1937.
This case report involves a 27-year-old victim of an automobile accident with operated plateau fractures that became infected leaving only 70 degrees of knee movement.

1025. Stumpfegger, L.: Meniscusvernarbung nach schienbeinkopfbruchen. Arch. Klin. Chir., 189:226–234, 1937.
The author noted intra-articular adhesions that covered the meniscus and were adherent to the cruciates and the fat pad. There was an observed decrease in tibiofemoral rotation because of the adhesions.

1026. Suckert, R.: Knockenplastische operation mit gebrauchsfertigen ampullenspan bei scheinbeinkopfbruchen. Beitrag. Z. Orthop., 96:107–108, 1962.

1027. Sudkamp, N. P., Lobenhoffer, H. P., and Tscherne, H.: (Fracture of the tibial head: Classification, diagnosis, therapy [Review].) Acta Chir. Orthop. Traumatol. Cech., 58:129–141, 1991.

1028. Surace, A., and Mineo, G.: (Problems in fractures of the tibial plateau.) Chir. Ital. 31(Suppl.):249–263, 1979.
The authors discuss classification and treatment of tibial plateau fractures.

1029. Swete-Evans, W.: Unusual case of fracture of the tibia involving the knee joint. J. R. Army Med. Corps, 44:46, 1925.
This case report involves a soccer player whose plateau fracture was treated by screw fixation with a good result at 1 year.

1030. Swett, P. P., McPherson, S. H., and Pike, M. M.: Fracture of the tibia into the knee joint. N. Engl. J. Med., 204:749–756, 1931.
The authors treated 50 plateau fractures by closed reduction and a cast with generally good results.

1031. Syller, B.: Munch. Med. Wochenschr., 77:1586, 1930.

1032. Tammes, A.: Intra-articulaire tibiafracturen. Amsterdam, Thesis, 1953.

1033. Tanton, J.: Fractures: Nouveau Traité de Chirurgie. Paris, J. B. Bailliere, 1916.
The author collected 63 reported plateau fractures and discussed these fractures in this book.

1034. Taparelli, A.: Due casi non frequenti di frattura completa della tuberosita externa della tibia. Radiol. Med., 3:64, 1916.

1035. Tegaldo, G.: Contributo clinico sul trattamento delle fratture articolari del ginocchio. Minerva Ortop., 205–208, 1963.
The author discussed the operative treatment of femoral condylar and tibial plateau fractures.

1036. Terrillon: Fracture de l'extrémité supérieure du tibia; Chondrité subaigue ulcerante. Bull. Soc. Anat. de Paris, 47:49, 1872.

1037. Tessari, L., and Spina, G.: Le lesioni meniscali e legamtose quali complicanze di fratture del piatto tibiale. Clin. Ortop., 13:573, 1961.

1038. Thamhayn, C.: Interesanter bruch des condylus tibiae. Z. Dtsch. Chir., 6:327–329, 1852.
This is the first report of a plateau fracture in the literature. The patient was injured when a horse fell on him. Reduction was by direct pressure; the knee was bandaged and healed.

1039. Theodoresco, M., and Negresco, G.: (Treatment of plateau fractures.) Rev. Chir. Bucharest, 40:99–102, 1937.

1040. Thiboumery, M.: Fracture en écaille du plateau tibial. Rev. Chir. Orthop., 40:229–231, 1954.

1041. Thiele, K.: Schienbeinkopfbruche. Bruchformen, behandlung, spatergebnisse bei 486 fallen. Hefte Unfallheilk., 95:1–126, 1968.
This thesis covers all aspects of plateau fractures and uses 378 plateau fractures as the basis of the research.

1042. Thomas, M., Schofield, C. B., and Unwin, A. J.: Tibial plateau fractures followed by stress fractures. J. Bone Joint Surg., 73B:1005, 1991.
The authors report on three elderly patients who had tibial plateau fractures and developed a stress fracture of the tibia below the plateau area. The authors consider this to be a potential complication.

1043. Thomson, W.: Comminuted fracture of the head of the tibia. Trans. Acad. M. Ireland, 2:446–451, 1883.

1044. Thornton, L., and Sandison, C.: Fracture of the knee. Am. J. Surg., 44:178–186, 1939.

1045. Titze, A.: (Variations in the slope of the proximal articular surface of the tibia.) Z. Orthop., 80:436–444, 1951.

1046. Titze, A.: Ersatz der zertrummerten gelenkflache des scheinbeinkopfes durch die kniescheibe. Chirurg., 33:360–362, 1962.
The author used surgery for impression fractures and found that the patella was a satisfactory articular substitute.

1047. Tixier, and Pollosson: À propos des résultats eloignes des fractures articulaires de l'extrémité supérieure du tibia. Lyon Chir., 720, 1929.

1048. Trabucco, A.: Contributo allo studio delle fratture dell'estremita superiore della tibia. Chir. Organi Mov., 16:306–323, 1931.
This author reports on eight plateau fractures that were treated by traction and early motion.

1049. Trabucco, A.: Die bruche am oberen tibiaende. Z. Orthop. Chir., 56:463, 1932.

1050. Traina, G. C., Martella, P., Fioravanti, S., and Marchiodi, L.: Interpretazione critica sulla evoluzione delle fratture scomposte del piatto tibiale. Chir. Organi Mov., 68:41–49, 1982.
The authors followed 50 operated plateau fractures for 5 years and noted 33 satisfactory results and traumatic arthritis in 14. The authors concluded that it was best to restore articular anatomy as well as possible.

1051. Tralles, D., Wojczik, H., and Hildebrandt, T.: (Fractures of the head of the tibia: Evaluation of an East German multicenter study 1981–1985.) Zentralbl. Chir., 115:635–643, 1990.
The authors gathered 1954 plateau fractures from centers in East Germany and concluded that closed and open treatment produced similar results.

1052. Trauma Rounds, Montreal General Hospital: Fractured tibial plateau. Can. Med. Assoc. J., 106:583–584, 1972.
The author describes the treatment of bicondylar fracture (Y) type using a tibial bolt. The medial plateau subsided leaving a varus deformity of the knee.

1053. Trauma Symposium Rizzoli Institute: Trattamento chirurgico delle fratture del piatto tibiale. Chir. Organi Mov., 61:637–643, 1974.
The author summarizes a symposium on plateau fractures held at the Rizzoli Institute in 1973. Indications, methods of treatment, and types of internal fixation are described.

1054. Travaini, E., and Vignati, E.: La fisiochinesiergoterapia negli esiti di fratture del piatto tibiale. Minerva Ortop., 18:366–373, 1967.
The authors discuss the uses of physical therapy following tibial plateau fractures.

1055. Trickey, E. L.: Injuries of the knee. *In* Wilson, J. N. (Ed.): Watson Jones Fractures and Joint Injuries, Vol. 2, 6th ed. Edinburgh, Churchill Livingstone, 1982.

1056. Trigo-Cabral, A., Lortat-Jacob, A., Ramadier, J., and Benoit, J.: Les fractures fraîches des plateaux tibiaux. Ann. Chir., 32:273–283, 1978.
The authors treated 113 plateau fractures, 47 closed and 66 open. Eighty-two were followed for 2.7 years average with 90% satisfactory results. The authors concluded that open treatment was most suitable.

1057. Trillat, A., and Charney, P.: Subluxation du genou, complication des fractures de l'extrémité supérieure du tibia. Lyon Chir., 2:623–625, 1953.

1058. Tscherne, H., and Lobenhoffer, P.: Tibial plateau fractures: management and expected results. Clin. Orthop., 292:87–100, 1993.
The authors classify plateau fractures as plateau fractures, fracture-dislocations, and comminuted fractures depending on the severity. Soft-tissue injuries associated with these fractures are graded from 0 to 3. The authors advocate comprehensive approaches and continuous passive motion after surgery. The authors treated 657 tibial plateau fractures (1970 to 1987) with 60% by open reduction. They noted 33% ligament injuries and 25% meniscal injuries. They thought that the rate of complication and the results were good.

1059. Tscherne, H., Lobenhoffer, P., and Russe, O.: Proximale intraartikulare tibiafrakturen. Unfallheilkunde, 87:277–289, 1984.
The author practices exact reconstruction of tibial articular surfaces and restoration of knee stability in order to get good results. The author did open reduction in 163 plateau fractures and followed 72 on a long-term basis.

1060. Tsoutis, N. G.: Traitement des fractures épiphysaires du genou. Rev. Chir., 75:706–720, 1937.

1061. Turner, V. C.: Fractures of the tibial plateaus. J.A.M.A., 169:923–926, 1959.
The author used closed treatment primarily but believed that anticipated deformity should be avoided by using open reduction.

1062. Tylman, D., Patyk, C., and Siwek, W.: (Intra-articular fractures in the knee area with considerable displacement of bone fragments: Methods of therapeutic management.) Wiad. Lek., 40:518–525, 1987.

1063. Uhl, R. L., Goldstock, L., Carter, A. T., and Lozman, J.: Hybrid external fixation for bicondylar tibial plateau fractures. Presented at the AAOS Meeting Feb. 1994.
Of 23 bicondylar fractures, 12 were treated operatively and 11 by limited open reduction and half-ring small wire external fixation. Forty-two percent of patients with open reduction and internal fixation developed significant infection but none of the externally fixed group had more than pin tract problems. The authors concluded that hybrid fixation gives fewer complications.

1064. Ulin, R.: Unusual etiology of "fender fracture." N. Engl. J. Med., 210:480–481, 1934.
Three case reports are given of slip and fall injuries that resulted in compression fractures. Axial weight-bearing and valgus were deemed to be the cause of the fractures.

1065. Valls, J., and Ottolenghi, C.: Hemiarthroplastia de rodilla por antigua fractura de platillos tibiales. Rev. Orthop. e Traum., 1:111–115, 1931.

1066. Valls, J., and Lagomarsino, E.: (Surgical therapy of plateau fractures.) Rev. Ortop. Traum., 7:315–324, 1938.

1067. Van Assen, M.: À propos des fractures des plateaux tibiaux. Rev. Chir. Orthop., 33:108–109, 1947.
Seven plateau fractures are reported, one fresh and six older.

1068. Vandenberghe, D., Cuypers, L., Rombouts, L., et al: Internal fixation of tibial plateau fractures using AO instrumentation. Acta Orthop. Belg., 56:431–442, 1990.
The authors retrospectively studied 76 plateau fractures, all of which were treated by AO method open reduction and internal fixation. They followed 50 on a long-term basis. The fractures were painless in 44%; 8% had severe pain. Two thirds lost an average of 17 degrees of flexion, and 25% lost 7.5 degrees of extension. Valgus averaged 10 degrees in 17 patients; a varus of 7.5 degrees was found in four patients. Seventy-four percent were stable; nine were bicondylar.

1069. Van Der Ghinst, M.: Les fractures du plateau tibial. J. Chir., 55:97–130, 1940.
The author reviewed the literature and analyzed 36 plateau fractures. He noted 80% good results at follow-up with little or no arthritis. A diagram is given of each fracture in this article.

1070. Van Der Slikke, W.: (Prognosis and treatment of fracture of the tibial condyle.) Arch. Chir. Neerl., 7:29–36, 1955.

1071. Vanek, J.: Posteromedial fracture of the tibial plateau is not an avulsion injury: A case report and experimental study. J. Bone Joint Surg., 76B:290–292, 1994.
This case report involves a 41 year old who fell from a ladder and twisted the knee. There was a posteromedial tibial plateau fracture and rupture of the anterior cruciate ligament (ACL). The same injury was produced in 16 cadavers' knees by varus and external rotation of the tibia. The ACL ruptured, the tibia came forward, and the continuing force fractured the plateau margin.

1072. Vangsness, C. T., Ghaderi, B., Hohl, M., and Moore, T. M.: Arthroscopic evaluation of meniscal injuries with tibial plateau fractures. J. Bone Joint Surg., 76B:488–490, 1994.
The authors arthroscoped 36 consecutive plateau fractures. Seventeen of the 36 had either a meniscal tear or a peripheral tear in all fracture types. Five had peripheral repair, and 10 had a partial meniscectomy. Open reduction and internal fixation were used in most cases, and arthroscopic-assisted reduction was done in 10 cases.

1073. Van Haelst, A.: Réflexions à propos du traitement des fractures du plateau tibial. Acta Orthop. Belg., 13:13–16, 1947.
The author discusses the dilemma of open versus closed treatment. He reports one plateau fracture that was treated in traction with late limitation of knee motion.

1074. Vanni, E.: Sulle fratture del piatto tibiale. Minerva Ortop., 14:224–234, 1962.
The author studied 99 plateau fractures and operated on 22 of these using screws for fixation. Closed reduction for displaced fractures was done, and a considerable number of good results were obtained.

1075. Vannoni, S., and Mezzadra, G.: La meccanica articolare del ginocchio nelle fratture del piatto tibiale. Minerva Ortop., 18:363–366, 1967.
Three case reports of plateau fractures are discussed. Of these reports, two were treated by bolt fixation. An x-ray study was done of the joint after reduction.

1076. Vasilevskii, N. N.: (Remote results of the treatment of fractures of the tibial condyle.) Ortop. Traum. Protez, 22:22–27, 1961.

1077. Vason, A., Wilbur, J., Lieberman, J., et al: A comparison of MRI versus CT scanning in evaluation of tibial plateau fractures. Orthop. Trans., 18:943–944, 1994.
The authors studied 22 plateau fractures by computed tomography (CT) and by magnetic resonance imaging (MRI) scans and noted that 64% of patients had soft tissue injuries. MRI gave better soft tissue information and was recommended for evaluation.

1078. Venezian, E.: Di un particolare tipo di frattura articolare del capitello tibiale: Le fratture della spina tibiale. Arch. Ortop., 43:211, 1927.

1079. Venouil, Fischer, Vuillard, and Baulieux: Fractures des plateaux tibiaux. Cah. Med. Lyonnais, 47:3517–3526, 1971.

1080. Vergara, G.: (Therapy of fractures of the tibial tuberosities.) Arch. Soc. Cirujano Hosp., 15:764–770, 1945.

1081. Vergoz, B.: (Four cases of fracture of the external tibial plateau.) Afrique Française Chir., 3–4:76–79, 1952.

1082. Vick, J.: Ergebnisse nach konzervativer behandlung von tibiakopffrakturen. Zentralbl. Chir., 90:1003–1011, 1965.
The author reported 251 plateau fractures and followed 171. There were 52% satisfactory results after mostly closed treatment. Only 13 cases of open reduction and internal fixation were done.

1083. Vierhout, P. A., Smulders, B. H. N., Hohmann, F. R., et al:

(Reconstruction of the tibial plateau fracture with arthroscopic monitoring without arthrotomy.) Ned. Tijdschr. Geneeskd., 135:893–896, 1991.
The authors performed 25 arthroscopically assisted plateau fractures with percutaneous fixation and grafts. There were 23 good results and two poor results, which were reported to be in bicondylar fractures. No infections or skin problems were noted. Rehabilitation was much faster.

1084. Vitali, H., Schellmann, W., and Klemm, K.: Behandlungsfehl-schlage bei tibiakopffrakturen. Mschr. Unfallheilk., 77:368–378, 1974.
After performing 104 open reductions for plateau fractures, it was believed that unsatisfactory results were due to poor diagnosis, prolonged immobilization, and unrecognized injuries.

1085. Vives, P., Massy, E., and Fichelle, G.: Réplacement du plateau tibial par la rotule pediculisée. Rev. Chir. Orthop., 61:543–546, 1975.
This case report involves a 23 year old who fell 10 feet and sustained a 3-cm fracture of the lateral plateau. The patella was used as articular replacement. There was a good result at the follow-up visit at 19 months with 100 degrees of motion.

1086. Vollmar, J., and Benz, K.: (Knee impacts and resulting injuries in automobile and motorcycle riders.) Arch. Orthop. Unfall-Chir., 52:438–459, 1960.

1087. Volpin, G., Dowd, G., Stein, H., and Bentley, G.: Degenerative arthritis after intra-articular fractures of the knee. J. Bone Joint Surg., 72B:634–638, 1990.
The authors reviewed 31 of 33 consecutive patients with intra-articular knee fractures 6 to 22 years later. Eleven were plateau fractures. On follow-up there was no difference in results between closed or open treatment. Age was the most important factor favoring arthritis.

1088. VonBahr, V.: Depressed and comminuted fractures of the lateral tibial tuberosity. Acta Chir. Scand., 92:139–149, 1945.
The author studied 27 depressed and comminuted fractures of the lateral tibial condyle that were treated by surgical elevation and grafting.

1089. Vorobev, N. A.: (Multiple comminuted intraarticular and periarticular fractures of the proximal segment of the leg.) Ortop. Traumatol., 11:50–57, 1935.

1090. Waddell, J. P., Johnston, D. W., and Neidre, A.: Fractures of the tibial plateau: A review of 95 patients and comparison of treatment methods. J. Trauma, 21:376–381, 1981.
The authors reviewed 95 plateau fractures that were treated by open or closed treatment. They concluded that fractures with depression or displacement of less than 10 mm were well tolerated and satisfactory results could ensue. If open reduction is done grafting and internal fixation are the best method of treatment.

1091. Wagner, H. E., and Jakob, R.: Zur problematik der plattenosteosynthese bei den bikondylen tibiakopffrakturen. Unfallchirurg., 89:304–311, 1986.
The authors analysed 40 operated bicondylar fractures and noted that 38% had wound complications and 15% had deep infections. They recommended that Y incisions should not be used and that double plates should be avoided.

1092. Wagner, W.: Uber compressionsfracturen des oberen tibiaendes. Ver. Dtsch. Ges. Chir., 15:116–126, 1886.
The author described nine plateau fractures that were treated by knee aspiration, massage, and distraction.

1093. Wagner, W.: Uber compressionsfracturen des oberen tibiaendes. Arch. Klin. Chir., 34:239–339, 1887.
This author described 9 plateau fractures or unicondylar fractures treated by traction and massage. Secondary arthritis developed after closed treatment in many cases.

1094. Wagner, W.: Arch. Klin. Chir., 44, 1897.

1095. Waldrop, J. I., Macey, T. I., Trettin, J. C., et al: Fractures of the posterolateral tibial plateau. Am. J. Sports Med., 16:492–498, 1988.
Of 196 plateau fractures, 28 were located on the posterior part of the lateral condyle. The authors suggested operative elevation and grafting to avoid late instability.

1096. Walker, P. S., and Erkman, M. J.: The role of menisci in force transmission across the knee. Clin. Orthop., 109:184–192, 1975.
The authors observed that the lateral meniscus bore 50% of weight and covered much of the articular surface, whereas the medial meniscus bore less than 50% of weight and covered less articular surface.

1097. Wallenbock, E., and Ledinski, C.: Indikation und grenzen der arthroscopischen versorgung von intraartikularen kniegelenksfrakturen. Akt. Traumatol., 23:97–101, 1993.
The authors treated 22 plateau fractures arthroscopically with three complications. They present a few illustrations and conclude that arthroscopic reduction can be used and is well tolerated by injured patients.

1098. Walther: 1852.
This is the first published autopsy of a tibial plateau fracture.

1099. Wassner, U. J.: Wann ist die behandlung der tibiakopffraktur mit der komprimierenden schraube indiziert? Chirurg., 26:536–537, 1955.
The author treated 27 plateau fractures, of which 12 were by bolt and cast, and provided a drawing of each. Only fair recovery of motion was noted.

1100. Watson, J. T.: High energy fractures of the tibial plateau. Orthop. Clin. North Am., 25:723–752, 1994.
The author studied 31 Schatzker type VI plateau fractures operatively with preoperative computed tomography scanning and a circular ring external fixator supplemented by internal fixation. He advocates the use of a femoral distractor medial and lateral and cannulated screws.

1101. Watson, J. T., Karges, D. E., and Moed, D. R.: The value of CT scanning for preoperative evaluation of tibial plateau fractures (Abstract). *In* Programs and Abstracts of the Annual Meeting of the Orthopedic Trauma Association, New Orleans, 1994.
The authors retrospectively reviewed 77 patients in a blinded fashion using plain x-rays and later computed tomography (CT) scans. Forty-seven percent of fractures had their classification changed and 66% had a change in preoperative planning as the result of CT scans.

1102. Watson, J. T., Morandi, M., Buckle, R., et al: Treatment of complex tibial plateau fractures with circular external fixators. Orthop. Trans., 18:8–9, 1994.

1103. Watson-Jones, R.: *In* Wilson, J. N. (Ed.): Fractures and Joint Injuries. London, Churchill Livingstone, 1982.

1104. Webb, R. C.: Fractures of the upper end of the tibia involving the knee joint. Minerva Med., 18:186–187, 1935.
The author reviews the treatment used generally, including plaster and traction. A bolt and washers were used in more severely displaced fractures.

1105. Weber, W. L.: Fractures of the tibial condyles. Calif. West. Med., 60:96–98, 1944.
Closed reduction using a C clamp is performed, and a hinged cast as described by Forrester is applied for early knee motion to retain muscle tone and strength.

1106. Weber, W. W., Neumann, C. H., Barakos, J. A., et al: Lateral tibial rim (Segond) fractures: Magnetic resonance imaging characteristics. Radiology, 180:731–734, 1991.
The authors studied 12 patients with Segond fractures for 1 to 21 days after trauma by magnetic resonance imaging. A fragment was seen only in four of 12. Eleven patients had an anterior cruciate ligament (ACL) injury, and seven had a medial cruciate injury. The lateral meniscus torn in four cases, and the medial meniscus was torn in one case. A high correlation exists between ACL tears and Segond fractures.

1107. Weiner, L. S., Kelly, M., Yang, E., et al: The use of combination internal fixation and hybrid external fixation in severe proximal tibia fractures. J. Orthop. Trauma, 9:244–250, 1995.
Forty-eight patients with 50 severe proximal tibial fractures were treated by limited internal fixation and external fixation. The follow-up was at 2 to 4 years with an average of 90 H.S.S. knee score and 82% excellent to good results and only 6% poor results.

1108. Weiner, L., Strauss, E., Yang, E., and Kelly, M.: Management of intraarticular and periarticular fractures of the proximal tibia. Orthop. Trans., 14:715, 1990.

1109. Weis, E. B. Jr., Pritz, H. B., and Hassler, C. R.: Experimental automobile-pedestrian injuries. J. Trauma, 17:823–828, 1977.
Simulated auto-pedestrian impacts were conducted on 15 cadavers' knees. Various fractures were produced, including six plateau fractures. The mechanism of injury to the lateral plateau was discussed. Axial compression and valgus were the major contributors.

1110. Weiss, J.: B. H. Z. Orthop., 96:95, 1962.

1111. Weissman, S. L., and Herold, Z. H.: Fractures of the tibial plateau. Clin. Orthop., 33:194–200, 1964.
The authors followed 25 consecutive plateau fractures for an average of 3 years looking at motion, alignment, and arthritis.

1112. Welte, G.: Fruh und spatergebnisse operativ versorgter tibiakopffrakturen. Tubingen, Thesis, 1984.

1113. Wendsche, P.: (Tibial condylar fractures—Conservative or surgical management? A retrospective study.) Beitr. Orthop. Traumatol., 36:512–517, 1989.
The authors treated 141 tibial plateau fractures. Fractures of both plateaus did better with conservative treatment. The infection rate was 13%. They recommended minimal internal fixation.

1114. Weyand, E.: Stellung und funktion bei unserer tibiakopffrakturen. Zentralbl. Chir., 79:1886–1895, 1954.
The author treated 80 patients and analysed the results by method of treatment. The best results were from use of traction for a while, followed by a cast.

1115. Wharton, H.: Fractures of the head of the tibia. Ann. Surg., 42:613–618, 1905.
Three plateau fractures treated in plaster are reported. One needed a peroneal nerve neurolysis for nerve pain. The author thought that limited motion was to be expected after these fractures.

1116. Wheeldon, T.: Sleeve wire fixation of fractures in which fragments are separated; 44 cases of fractures of the proximal end of the tibia. Virginia M. Monthly, 66:223–226, 1939.

1117. White, J. C.: T- and Y- fractures of the tibial condyles. Injury, 3:56–63, 1971.

1118. Wilhelm, K., Rueff, F. L., and Bedacht, R.: Die operative versorgung von tibiakopffrakturen. Mschr. Unfallheilk., 74:153–168, 1971.
The authors treated 171 plateau fractures, 124 closed and 47 by open reduction and internal fixation. They described treatment with elevation, fixation, screws, plate, and graft. No results are given.

1119. Willenegger, H.: Langenbecks Arch. Klin. Chir., 276:173, 1953.

1120. Williams, A.: An unusual fracture of the tibial plateau. Med. Biol. Illus., 15:266–268, 1965.

1121. Wilppula, E., and Bakalim, G.: Kiel bone in the surgical treatment of tibial condylar fractures. Acta Orthop. Scand., 43:62–67, 1972.
Kiel bone was used in 37 plateau fractures and compared with iliac bone that was used in 18 other plateau fractures.

1122. Wilppula, E., and Bakalim, G.: Ligamentous tear concomitant with tibial condylar fracture. Acta Orthop. Scand., 43:62–67, 1972.
The authors repaired ligament tears in 24 patients of 196 patients who were operated on. There were 18 medial collateral ligament, two lateral carpal ligament, 13 anterior cruciate ligament, and two posterior cruciate ligament tears. The authors believe that ligament repair was worthwhile to restore knee stability in the presence of plateau fractures.

1123. Wilson, W., and Jacobs, J.: Patellar graft for severely depressed comminuted fractures of the lateral tibial condyle. J. Bone Joint Surg., 34A:436–442, 1952.
The authors report five severely depressed lateral plateau fractures in which the patella and its articular cartilage was used as articular replacement with success. They found no evidence of avascularity in the graft. The method was not intended to be needed very frequently.

1124. Winkler, H., and Young, C. Jr.: Fractures of the tibial plateau. South. Med. J., 43:35–39, 1950.

1125. Wirth, C. R.: Meniscus repair. Clin. Orthop., 157:153, 1981.
The author describes the repair of menisci, emphasizing arthroscopic-assisted methods. The repairs were reported to be holding up well.

1126. Wise, R. A.: Combined traction-compression method for the treatment of bicondylar fractures of the tibia. Surg. Gynecol. Obstet., 72:778–780, 1941.
Under traction, a compression sleeve is inserted over a Kirschner wire and tightened to secure reduction. One plateau fracture, thus treated, is described.

1127. Withers, R. J.: Recent fractures of the upper end of the tibia. Ulster Med., 8:101–106, 1939.

1128. Witt, A.: Verh. Dtsch. Orthop. Ges., 41:180, 1954.

1129. Witt, U. N.: Der wert der tomographie zur beurteilung der spaetersebnisse der tibiakopfbruche. Hefte Unfallheilk., 126:228–230, 1976.
The author discusses the advantages of tomography in the diagnosis of articular displacement in older plateau fractures.

1130. Wittebol, P.: Treatment of fractures of the tibial plateau. Arch. Chir. Neerland., 23:253–267, 1968.
The author described the surgical approach used on 15 fractures and reviewed the literature about the indications, techniques, and treatment of different types of fractures.

1131. Witter, H.: Tibiakopfbruche als folge des verkehrsunfalles. Hefte Unfallheilk., 66:216–220, 1961.
The author used strong cortical lyophylized bone grafts as internal fixation after elevation of plateau fractures. The results were good.

1132. Wittmoser, R.: Zur behandlung der bruche des lateralen scheinbeincondyls. Zentralbl. Chir., 69:1814–1820, 1942.
The author described a posterior slope of the tibial condyles. He used pins in 12 fractures that were treated operatively.

1133. Wolf, L. R., Rothman, R. H., Hozack, W. J., et al: Primary total knee arthroplasty for displaced intraarticular knee fractures. Clin. Orthop., 276:229–236, 1992.
The authors report on one patient with an old depressed plateau fracture and a new femoral condyle fracture for which knee replacement was performed with a good result. A fresh tibial plateau fracture was replaced in a 58-year-old patient with rheumatoid arthritis and diabetes, and at 30 months the patient was doing well.

1134. Wolf, M. D., and White, E. H.: Depressed fractures of the tibial plateau. Surg. Gynecol. Obstet., 116:457–462, 1963.
Forty-nine fractures were treated by open reduction and were fixed by multiple Kirschner wires.

1135. Wolff, F.: Apport thérapeutique aux fractures articulaires de l'extrémité supérieure du tibia: À propos de 175 cas observés au centre de traumatologie de Strasbourg. Strasbourg Thesis, 76:1967.
The author reviewed the literature and 175 plateau fractures as the controversies in treatment were discussed in this thesis.

1136. Wondrak, E., and Sekaninova, J.: (On the treatment of fracture of the tibial condyle.) Acta Chir. Orthop. Traum. Czech., 28:491–498, 1961.

1137. Woo, S. L., Gomez, M. A., Inoue, M., and Akeson, W. H.: New experimental procedures to evaluate the biomechanical properties of healing canine medial collateral ligaments. J. Orthop. Res., 5:425–432, 1987.
Using canines, the authors observed that cut medial collateral ligaments that were repaired and immobilized for 3 weeks, then mobilized were more stable than were those similarly repaired and immobilized for 6 weeks.

1138. Woo, S. L., Gomez, M. A., Woo, Y. K., and Akeson, W. H.: Mechanical properties of tendons and ligaments. II: The relationships of immobilization and exercise on tissue remodeling. Biorheology, 19:397–408, 1982.

1139. Wood, J. P.: Major injuries in the region of the knee. Am. Osteo. Acad. Orthop., 64:958–962, 1965.

1140. Woods, G. W., Stanley, R. F., and Tullos, H. S.: Lateral capsular sign: X-ray clue to a significant knee instability. Am. J. Sports Med., 7:27–33, 1979.
The authors describe four patients who had avulsions of the meniscotibial ligament with a flake of bone from the lateral aspect of the plateau. Surgical exposure of the lesion showed that it was reparable.

1141. Wright, L. T.: Operative reduction and fixation by means of a specially devised blade plate for the treatment of supracondylar and T fractures of the lower end of the femur and T fractures of the upper end of the tibia. Harlem Hosp. Bull., 1:17–24, 1948.

1142. Wutherich, A.: Ueber die behandlung des tibiakopffrakturen. Arch. Orthop. Unfall. Chir., 40:71–78, 1939.

1143. Yang, E. C., Weiner, L., Strauss, E., et al: Metaphyseal dissociation fractures of the proximal tibia: An analysis of treatment and complications. Am. J. Orthop., 24:695–794, 1995.
The authors studied 44 dissociation fractures of which half were treated by conventional open treatment and plating and the other half were treated prospectively by external fixation and limited open reduction. The results were definitely better with external fixation and there were fewer complications.

1144. Yao, L., and Lee, J. K.: Avulsion of the posteromedial tibial plateau by the semimembranosus tendon: Diagnosis with MR imaging. Radiology, 172:513–514, 1989.
Two patients who were injured in sports accidents demonstrated avulsion of the posteromedial tibial plateau by the semimembranosus tendon as shown on magnetic resonance imaging.

1145. Yergason, R. M.: Simple clamp for reducing fractures of the calcaneum and tibial tuberosities. J. Bone Joint Surg., 17:225–227, 1935.

1146. Young, M. J., and Barrack, R. L.: Complications of surgical intervention in tibial plateau fractures. Orthop. Rev., 23:149–154, 1994.
A review was made of 48 consecutive displaced plateau fractures in 46 patients who were operated on at two university hospitals. The operative time and amount of hardware placed was directly proportional to the infection rate. No infection was noted when one buttress plate was used. A buttress plate plus multiple screws was used in 44% (8 of 18) and in 83% (five of six) two buttress plates were used.

1147. Younger, E. M., and Chapman, M. W.: Morbidity at bone graft donor sites. J. Orthop. Trauma, 3:192–195, 1989.
The morbidity of taking bone grafts was determined on 243 graft sites. The major complication rate was 8.6%, and the minor complication rate was 20.6%. Infection (2.5%), hematoma (3.3%), reoperation (3.8%), pain (2.5%), and drainage (0.8%) were the major problems.

1148. Yu, X. J.: (Classification and treatment of fractures of the tibial plateau.) Chung Hua Wai Ko Tsa Chih, 28:718–722, 1990.
The author classified plateau fractures by displacement. The minimally displaced were of less than 5 mm displacement or 2 mm depression. The results of treatment were good. The moderately displaced group was less than 10 mm and was treated by bolt or wire often by "poking" and fixation. The last group had comminution and a subcondylar fracture. The 30 patients, variously treated, led them to suggest perfect reduction, rigid fixation, and early motion.

1149. Yuan-Zhang, M., Chun-Bo, Z., Ke-Fu, Q., and Yen-Ching, Y.: Traitement des fractures du plateau tibial par manoeuvres et fixation par embrochage percutanées. Acta Orthop. Belg., 49:553–563, 1983.
The authors described manipulative reduction and percutaneous fixation of plateau fractures. They also used a Steinmann pin to reduce local compression fractures. Of the 45 patients reported, 32 were followed more than 1 year with two thirds achieving good to excellent results.

1150. Zachariae, L.: Z. Org. Ges. Chir., 130:399, 1952.

1151. Zachariae, L.: Compression fractures of the lateral condyle. Nord. Med., 49:131–133, 1953.

1152. Zanasi, R., Fioretta, G., and Rotolo, F.: (Guidelines for treating tibial plateau fractures.) Chir. Organi Mov., 68:169–184, 1982–1983.
The authors treated 137 plateau fractures by Zanoli's method, which involves elevation and grafting with internal fixation as needed.

1153. Zandek, M.: Uber knockenfrakturen und pseudarthrosen. Med. Klin. Berl., 20:1104–1106, 1924.

1154. Zander, P.: Ein fall von genu valgum durch fraktur am oberen tibiaende. Mschr. Unfallheilk., 16:235–237, 1909.
This case report involves a 61 year old with a lateral plateau fracture that healed with flexion contracture and valgus at 8 months.

1155. Zanoli, R.: Le fratture del ginocchio. Chir. Organi Mov., 10:463–485, 1926.

1156. Zanoli, R.: Fratture del ginocchio. Chir. Organi Mov., 1928.

1157. Zanuso, G., and Della Grazia: Sulla utilizzazione della vite di Putti nella frattura del piatto tibiale. Ospedale Maggiore, 42–3:118, 1954.

1158. Zecher, S. B., Danziger, M. B., Segal, D., et al: Treatment of high-energy proximal tibial fractures using the Monticelli-Spinelli external fixator: A preliminary report. Am. J. Orthop., 25:49–54, 1996.
Twenty-one high-energy proximal tibial fractures were managed by the Monticelli-Spinelli external fixator. Good and excellent reductions were noted in 15 of 21 cases. Seven pin tract infections and one embolus occurred. Six patients had unsatisfactory results.

1159. Zenker, H., and Springer, H.: Das posttraumatische kniegelenk (Bandverletzung und tibiakopfbruch). Lebensversicherungsmedizin Heft, 9:202–203, 1982.

1160. Zeno, L.: Fractures des tuberosites tibiales. Cir. Ortop. Traum. Habana, 5:224–231, 1937.

1161. Zeno, L.: Fractura de los condilos tibiales. Anal. de Cir., 3:107–115, 1937.

1162. Zeno, L.: Fractures des tuberosites tibiales. Rev. Ortop. Traumatol., 7:32–41, 1937.

1163. Zeno, L.: Z. Org. Ges. Chir., 86:140, 1938.

1164. Zielke: Sur le traitement des fractures des condyles du tibia. Dtsch. Med. Wochenschr., 55:531, 1929.

1165. Zifko, B., and Vlasich, E.: Behandlung der schienbeinkopfbruche und ihre ergebnisse. Arch. Ortop. Unfall. Chir., 66:297–309, 1969.
The authors followed 177 of 310 treated plateau fractures for 4 to 7 years. Good functional results were noted after closed treatment. The author only advocated open treatment in a limited number of cases.

1166. Zimmer, S.: Bermerkung zu der arbeit von E. Lexer: Die richtigstellung der scheinbeingelenkflache durch hebung mit knochenteilen. Zentralbl. Chir., 59:1021, 1932.
This brief discussion involves Lexer's technique for open reduction.

APPENDIX

THE AUTHOR'S TIBIAL PLATEAU FRACTURE SERIES

After becoming interested in tibial plateau fractures during his residency in 1950, the author reviewed all relevant case records dating from 1940 at Los Angeles General Hospital. Every effort was made to induce these patients whose records were available to return for a late follow-up evaluation. The author examined and had x-rays made on those who returned. After completion of the author's residency, additional fractures and follow-ups were gathered from West Los Angeles Veterans' Hospital, UCLA Medical Center, and private practice.

The 1533 collected cases are not consecutive and the patients were not cared for on a protocol basis. These patients were treated by many different orthopedic surgeons with a variety of backgrounds and philosophies. The series reflects treatment performed at the time by a considerable number of surgeons. Although the series has limited value, it tells much about the behavior of fractures and their various treatments. The follow-up studies give valuable information that would be much improved if 100% of patients had been followed instead of 30%.

THE AUTHOR'S 1533 TIBIAL PLATEAU FRACTURES

SOURCE	DATES	NO. OF FRACTURES
Los Angeles County Hospital	1940–1954	683
Los Angeles Veterans' Hospital	1954–1995	311
UCLA Medical Center	1955–1995	332
Private Practice	1953–1995	207
TOTAL		1533

YEARS OF STUDY	FRACTURES	FOLLOW-UP EXAMINATIONS
1940–1949	581	186
1950–1959	166	70
1960–1969	113	78
1970–1979	263	110
1980–1989	274	111
1990–1995	125	11

TREATMENT BY:	NO. OF PATIENTS
The author	256
Other orthopedists	517
Resident with attending	717
Outside case consultations	35

DEMOGRAPHICS	
Age	Mean of 48 years (4–97)
Sex	960 Male; 571 female
Knee	672 Right; 784 left; 35 both
Plateau	1001 Lateral; 219 medial; 307 both

MECHANISM OF INJURY	%
Automobile-pedestrian	42
Automobile-automobile	42
Slip and twist	12
Fall from a height	16
Motorcycle	10
Bicycle	1
Athletics	3
Direct blow	1
Miscellaneous	3

TYPES OF FRACTURE		NO.
Minimally displaced		316
Local compression		415
Split compression		284
Total depression		205
Total subtype	(96)	
Entire subtype	(109)	
Split		48
Rim		73
Compression	(30)	
Avulsion	(43)	
Bicondylar		188
Bicondylar	(166)	
Four part	(22)	

ANTEROPOSTERIOR FRACTURE LOCATION	%
Anterior	2
Anterior to middle	10
Middle	65
Posterior to middle	19
Posterior margin	4

FINDINGS ON ORIGINAL X-RAY SUGGESTING LIGAMENT INJURY (In patients with ligament injuries)	NO.
No findings (only the plateau injury)	54
Wide medial cartilage space	81
Medial widening and femoral avulsion	4
Medial widening and tibial avulsion	1
Medial femoral avulsion	7
Medial tibial avulsion	19
Lateral widening	47
Lateral widening and fibular avulsion	13
Lateral widening and femoral avulsion	11
Lateral avulsion	38

FINDINGS ON STRESS X-RAYS	MEDIAL NO.	LATERAL NO.
No cartilage space opening	117	127
1–2 mm opening	60	49
3–4 mm opening	7	2
5–6 mm opening	19	7
>7 mm	19	6

TIBIAL SPINE AND INTERCONDYLAR EMINENCE FRACTURES (Associated with plateau)	NO.
Anterior spine	126
Posterior spine	18
Both spines	40
Type I	27
Type II	24
Type III	0

SURGICAL APPROACHES USED	BEFORE 1975 (NO.)	SINCE 1975 (NO.)
Medial parapatellar	20	22
Lateral parapatellar	80	54
Inframeniscal	28	125
Inframeniscal with LCL cut	18	8
Medial without arthrotomy	2	7
Lateral without arthrotomy	2	6
Both sides opened	3	21
Midline	1	43
Mercedes Y	0	3
Arthroscopic	0	33

LCL = Lateral collateral ligament.

MENISCAL PATHOLOGY	NO.
Torn and displaced	157
Bucket handle	13
Surgically detached	107

MENISCAL MANAGEMENT	NO.
Not altered	855
Removed for visualization	21
Removed for tear	81
Partial removal	8
Resutured torn meniscus	82
Surgically detached and repaired	107

BONE GRAFT SOURCES	NO.
Local bone	42
Iliac autologous	130
Tibial cortical	23
Fibular head	3
Bank cancellous	30
Bank cortical	4

INTERNAL FIXATION	BEFORE 1975 (%)	SINCE 1975 (%)
Screws	25	38
Bolts	46	12
Plate and bolts	9	2
Buttress plate	2	36
Medial and lateral plates	1	5
Pins or wires	10	2
Bone graft only	7	4
Methyl methacrylate	0	<1
Other	0	1

LIGAMENT REPAIRS (263 Patients With Ligament Injury)	TORN	REPAIRED PRIMARILY (No.)
Medial collateral ligament	130	25
Lateral collateral	112	14
Cruciate ligament	106	18

LOSS OF FRACTURE POSITION	BEFORE 1975 (%)	SINCE 1975 (%)
No loss of position	81	76
1–2 mm	8	9
3–4 mm	7	9
5–6 mm	3	4
7–8 mm	1	2
>8 mm	<1	0

LATER SURGERY REQUIRED	WITHIN 2 YEARS OF INJURY (NO.)	2 OR MORE YEARS AFTER INJURY (NO.)
Hardware removal	83	13
Meniscus removal	12	2
Manipulation for motion	4	0
Ligament reconstruction	2	3
Single condyle osteotomy	3	0
Subcondylar osteotomy	6	13
Bony reconstruction	7	0
Ligament and bony reconstruction	9	2
Total knee replacement	4	13
Arthrodesis	2	3
Arthroscopic adhesion lysis	7	0
Fracture re-reduction	7	0
Bone graft for nonunion	2	0
Miscellaneous	2	0

FOLLOW-UP DATA 2 YEARS OR MORE AFTER A FRACTURE

PATIENTS FOLLOWED BY	NO. OF PATIENTS
Author	352
Other orthopedist	66
Resident	152
Total	570

DIRECTION OF LATE KNEE DEFORMITY	NO.
Valgus	248
Varus	70

LOCATION OF LATE INSTABILITY	NO.
Medial	264
Lateral	66

LOCATION OF TRAUMATIC ARTHRITIS (Moderate-severe)	NO.
Lateral compartment	39
Medial compartment	9
Both compartments	37

LATER PLATEAU FRACTURES IN THE SAME KNEE (NO. = 10)	
Second plateau fracture in the same knee	10

Pelligrini Stieda's ossification	NO.
Adductor region	24

Index

Note: Page numbers in *italics* refer to illustrations; page numbers followed by t refer to tables.

ISBN 0-7216-7015-6

90038

9 780721 670157

HOHL